Managing Physical Stress with Therapeutic Massage

Jeffrey Forman, Ph.D.

THOMSON

DELMAR LEARNING™

Australia Canada Mexico Singapore Spain United Kingdom United States

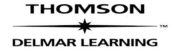

DELMAR LEARNING

Managing Physical Stress with Therapeutic Massage
by Jeffrey Forman, Ph.D.

Vice President, Health Care Business Unit:
William Brottmiller

Director of Learning Solutions:
Matthew Kane

Acquisitions Editor:
Kalen Conerly

Product Manager:
Juliet Steiner

Editorial Assistant:
Molly Belmont

Marketing Director:
Jennifer McAvey

Senior Marketing Manager:
Lynn Henn

Marketing Coordinator:
Andrea Eobstel

Production Director:
Carolyn Miller

Production Manager:
Barbara A. Bullock

Content Project Manager:
Jessica McNavich

Library of Congress Cataloging-in-Publication Data
ISBN 1-4180-1489-3

Notice to the Reader

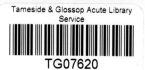
Managing Physical Stress
with Therapeutic Massage

This book is *
the la

About the Author

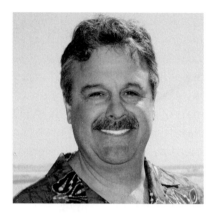

Jeffrey Forman (Ph.D., NCTMB) was born and raised in Boston, Massachusetts. He received his B.S. and M.Ed. from Springfield College in Springfield, Massachusetts. In August of 1976 he traveled west to work as a certified corrective therapist at the Veterans Administration Hospital in Palo Alto, California, where he ran a Physical Restoration Clinic. In April of 1978 he left to become the executive head of the De Anza College Adapted Physical Education Program.

In 1981 he founded his consulting business, Stress Reduction Systems, where he specialized in designing corporate and individual stress reduction programs and his private massage therapy practice. He received his Ph.D. from United States International University in San Diego in 1982. His doctoral research focused on the effects a workday relaxation program has on the stress levels of management personnel. He has been a stress reduction consultant for many multinational corporations and has lectured at many conferences and at colleges and universities in the United States, Denmark, Germany, Greece, Australia, New Zealand, and Japan. In 1987 his book *The Personal Stress Reduction Program* was published by Prentice Hall, Inc.

In 1991 he founded the first massage therapy program at public community colleges in the State of California. In 1992 he received his national certification in therapeutic massage and bodywork. He developed the first massage therapy associate's degree program approved by California's Community College Chancellors' Office and had massage therapy listed as a legitimate vocation in the state community college system. For the past 5 years he has been a member of the planning committee for the AMTA Council of Schools Leadership Conferences. He has also been actively involved in pursuing state regulation of massage therapy in the state of California. His most recent writings and presentations include "How to Run a Successful Massage Clinic," presented at the 2004 AMTA Council of Schools Leadership Conference, and "Status and Trends in California Massage Education," co-authored in 2005. He will serve as chairman of the 2006 and 2007 AMTA leadership conferences. He has been frequently called on by other state colleges for consultations on developing and implementing professional massage therapy training programs. He is a tenured professor and the massage therapy program coordinator at De Anza College in Cupertino, California. He loves to laugh, run, hike in the forest, walk on the beach, fish, cook, garden, travel the world, and enjoy every day to the maximum. He is a teacher, lecturer, author, advocate for the massage therapy profession, and classroom innovator.

Contents

Acknowledgments

Writing this book involved many sets of eyes and the contributions of many individuals, and I'd like to thank all who helped for their time and insight. I'd like to thank my colleague of many years, Rich Schroeder, M.A., coordinator of the Physical Education Division at De Anza College, for his knowledge of fitness, nutrition, and exercise science and for his willingness to read my drafts and give me great feedback. I greatly appreciate the help and feedback provided by another colleague, Kathy Wasowski, P.T., a nationally certified orthopedic specialist, for her extensive feedback on my drafts and her knowledge of pain control, therapeutic exercise, and soft tissue treatment theories and techniques. My appreciation is extended to Eileen Leary, lead research coordinator for the APPLES research project at the Stanford University Sleep Research Center, for her input on the sleep chapter. My thanks go out to Lorilee Turrone, the massage therapy program assistant at De Anza College, for her help organizing this project and her feedback on the chapters. My gratitude is extended to my son, Myles, for all the time he donated to this project posing for sample pictures depicting postural faults, exercises, and massage strokes. I'd like to thank Jessica Joson for helping me stage a preliminary photo shoot and for organizing the photos, and Rachel Boritz, our model. I extend my appreciation to Kalen Conerly, my acquisitions editor at Thomson Delmar Learning, for believing in my vision for this book and working with me from its conception to completion, and Juliet Steiner, my developmental editor, for her dedication, professionalism, skill, and swift feedback. My thanks also go out to Kate Mannix, whom I enjoyed working with throughout the final production process of the book. I'd be remiss if I did not thank my colleague Yanik Chauvin from the council of schools for his tremendous skill and talent as a professional photographer. Finally, I'd like to thank my family and friends for all the support and encouragement they provided me through the past year.

Jeffrey Forman, Ph.D.

Preface

Today's fast-paced world is a fascinating one, in which time seems to fly and stress abounds. We all have our own stresses and strains, and we all have the choice to deal with them proactively or to succumb to them. We can give in to stress and let it destroy our health and psyche, or we can design and implement an action plan to help us evolve physically, spiritually, psychologically, and emotionally to cope successfully with it.

Most of us need to learn ways to slow down, but unfortunately, few individuals truly understand and routinely use the simple strategies that can help them reduce or eliminate their stress. For some, the regular practice of aerobic and postural realignment exercises and eating a well-balanced diet would help them reduce their stress and benefit their minds and bodies by improving blood chemistry, digestion, and bowel function; increasing circulation; lowering blood pressure; improving posture and self image; and decreasing pain. Some need to learn to stop procrastinating, while others need to decide on a meaningful direction for their lives to reduce stress. Many will find stress relief by spending more quality time with their families and friends; others by spending more time sleeping and practicing deep relaxation. Regardless of specific stressors and problems, we must realize that each of us has the power to diminish the negative impact of stress by instituting changes in lifestyles and habits that will help us gain control over our health and happiness. More often than not, however, stress takes control and evolves into an issue where we must seek the help and guidance of health professionals. The incidence of stress-related heath and psychological problems has reached epidemic proportions in this country, and more and more people are turning to massage therapy to help them deal with their stress. In fact, according to a 2005 survey conducted by the American Massage Therapy Association, 26% of consumers who had a massage in the past five years cited relaxation and stress relief as the main reason for getting a massage.

Managing Physical Stress with Therapeutic Massage was developed as a practical guide for helping massage therapists reduce the negative effects of their clients' stress. It is designed as a textbook for college, university, and massage school wellness and physical stress management classes, and as a guide for the practicing therapist. Although this book is written with massage therapy stress reduction treatment programs in mind, it also provides useful information for physical therapists, occupational therapists, athletic trainers, nurses, chiropractors, physical education and adapted physical education specialists, and personal fitness trainers. The tools, tips, and techniques covered in this book are a product of my doctoral research in stress reduction; my years as a college professor of adapted physical education, physical education, and massage therapy; and my years of private practice as a massage therapist and a corporate stress reduction consultant. I wrote this book because stress is an extremely common reason for individuals to seek massage therapy, but there was no book to guide a massage therapist through the step-by-step process of reducing a client's stress by measuring the stress, developing a comprehensive stress reduction plan that involves treatments and client homework, implementing the plan, and then reassessing and evaluating the results.

The goal of this book is to educate massage therapists to help their clients recognize the elements in their lives that need to be changed and then implement those changes—not next month or next New Year's—but now. To reduce stress, clients must stop procrastinating and understand what is causing their stress and how it is affecting them physically, psychologically, socially, and emotionally. A series of simple tests is used to pinpoint the causes of a client's stress; that information is used to develop a personal stress reduction plan. When the plan is implemented the client must then take an active role and do his or her homework assignments on a regular basis to eliminate the factors that are contributing to chronic stress. After the client embarks on the plan, it is constantly reevaluated and revised until a program is found that works. This book can be used as a workbook to educate the client to understand and manage his or her stress. The therapist can also use this book to cope with the stress in his or her own life.

The approach outlined in this book will help both the fledgling and the experienced massage therapist become better at his or her profession. Treatment programs are based on the empirical data ascertained from the assessments, so every treatment is tailored to the individual needs of each client. For more lasting effects and better results after each treatment, clients are given homework assignments. For the readers' convenience, examples of homework assignments for a variety of stress-related problems are listed in the book. Over the course of ensuing treatments the therapist will experiment with different techniques, documenting the effects of each method employed. He or she will use direct manipulative techniques, and if these don't work, he or she will adapt and try gentle indirect approaches. After a series of treatments, he or she will reassess with the original battery of tests to determine if measurable progress was made. Readers will learn how to perform a variety of assessment tests and practice their assessment skills. In addition, the matrix presented in the book is a great reference for a wide assortment of natural stress reduction techniques that they can employ on themselves or as homework suggestions for their clients.

HOW TO USE THIS BOOK

Practicing massage therapists, massage therapy students, and other health care professionals can use the following features of this book to better serve their clients.

In chapters 1 and 2 readers will develop a better understanding of the negative effects that unchecked stress and its incessant sympathetic nervous system arousal have on the human mind and body. They will also learn how to document their client's or patient's stress by completing an in-depth stress analysis that probes the client's physical and psychosocial stress symptoms, diet, postural faults, muscular imbalances, breathing mechanics, and muscle tension. They will experience how to perform a battery of physical assessment tests and how to use that information to develop a client's personal stress profile.

In chapters 3 and 4 readers will improve their understanding of how to use the results of the assessments to design and implement an anti-stress treatment plan for their clients. They will also learn the proper mechanics for breathing, a variety of breathing technique improvement training exercises, how to use focused breathing as a relaxation tool, and massage treatments to help a client breathe easier.

In chapters 5 and 6 readers will comprehend exercise theory and techniques that include normal posture, atypical posture, core strengthening exercises, stretching exercises, and therapeutic exercises that relieve common physical problems, such as forward head, kyphosis, anterior pelvic tilt, and hyperlordosis of the lumbar spine. How to instruct clients to realign their posture and eliminate their habitual bias towards the misalignment that produces their pain and fatigue is also outlined. Controversial and potentially dangerous exercises, fitness training, and aerobic training tips are also outlined in these chapters.

In chapters 7 and 8 the norms for human range of motion are delineated, as are guidelines for performing passive range of motion and the benefits of deep relaxation. Readers will be exposed to a variety of deep relaxation techniques that will help them develop skills to teach their clients how to deeply relax at will and how to incorporate relaxation into massage treatments.

In chapters 9 and 10 readers will develop an improved understanding of the stages experienced in a normal night's sleep, common sleep disorders, natural sleep improvement strategies, and how to perform a massage to help a client sleep more soundly. Readers will also review a variety of pain control strategies, including the use of heat, ice, and massage. Headache relief tips, exercises to reduce eyestrain, and self-massage techniques for the feet, legs, hands, arms, head, face, neck, and chest are also delineated.

In chapters 11 and 12 readers will learn about dietary changes that can help reduce stress, the dangers of fad diets, and information about eating disorders. The reader will also be exposed to strategies for helping clients cope with the psychosocial aspects of their stress. When to refer a client to a professional counselor and practical tips for getting more organized and managing time more efficiently are also outlined. In addition, strategies for reducing decision-making stress, setting appropriate goals, modifying behavior, and working with other professionals in a team approach for reducing a client's stress are also presented.

FEATURES

Unique features of the book include:

- An approachable, easy-to-read writing style.
- Many useful assessment techniques and tips to relieve pain and tension.
- Lots of self-help tips, homework assignments, and exercises for clients.
- Not a lot of theory to bog down the learner.
- An outstanding section on therapeutic exercise.
- Blank copies of forms that can be duplicated and used in treatment programs.

Although there are many self-help books on stress relief that may include massage as a technique an individual can use to manage personal stress, I am not aware of any texts that outline how to develop a comprehensive personal stress reduction program using therapeutic massage skills. Because so many people are suffering from stress, massage therapists who can offer their clients solid guidance on personal stress management will not only add a skill set to their portfolio but will enhance their professional marketability. Massage therapists have a unique opportunity to help people reduce the negative effects of stress on the human body, and this book will greatly help this endeavor.

Jeffrey Forman, Ph.D.

AVENUE FOR FEEDBACK

If you have questions about the book or want information about lectures, workshops, or corporate stress reduction programs, e-mail drjforman@sbcglobal.net or write to:

Stress Reductions Systems
Dr. Jeffrey Forman
P.O. Box 24482
San Jose, CA 95154

Massage Therapy: A Healthy Alternative for Reducing Stress

INTRODUCTION

This book is about healthy ways to relieve **stress.** Of course, you have probably seen a lot of other books on the same topic. What makes this text different is that it is designed as a guide for the health care professional. A personalized, practical, systematic, and easy-to-follow approach is used to help you relieve your client's stress-related physical problems. Stress-induced illnesses are so prevalent in this society that massage therapists, athletic trainers, personal fitness trainers, physical therapists, nurses, and other health care professionals rarely will work a day without seeing clients who suffer from the negative effects of stress. The information presented in this book will help you perform your job more efficiently and effectively and also help you more successfully cope with your own stresses and strains. In addition, this book will be a valuable resource that you can share with your clients so that they can help themselves relieve their stress-related problems.

CONCEPT OF THE BOOK

The idea behind this book is simple. A series of questionnaires and assessment tests reveal the kind and cause of stress the client is experiencing and then pinpoints how it is affecting them physically, psychologically, socially, and emotionally. The results on the Personal Stress Inventory and Stress Log delineate the client's unique Stress Profile. The Stress Profile will be used to tailor massage treatments according to the individual needs of the client. By following the assessments laid out in this book, you will be able to build your client's personal stress reduction program and detail a wide range of exercises and activities that you can use to relieve his or her specific stress-induced problems. By matching the results on the Stress Profile with techniques to relieve them, you build the client's personalized stress reduction program. There is also a chart for matching stresses with coping strategies, which will guide you in building your client's program.

After you design each client's Personal Stress Reduction Program, you must encourage them to implement it for at least 10 weeks; after the 10 weeks you should reassess and check for measurable progress. This program will help clients understand their stress and get to the root of their problems. By eliminating the cause(s) of their stress symptoms they eventually will eliminate their **stressors** and return to balance. Success will require changes, such as adding the routine practice of aerobic and postural realignment exercises; practicing deep relaxation and deep breathing; and making dietary, lifestyle, and behavioral changes to their busy schedule. If they are willing to make the necessary changes, they will succeed. The therapist is a vehicle for change, but the client is ultimately responsible for changing his or her habits and behaviors. This raises the question, "How can massage therapists improve their ability to influence clients to make the changes necessary to improve their health and reduce their stress?"

A strong knowledge base along with professionalism and ethical behavior will help the therapist gain the client's trust and respect. To influence clients to positively transform their lives, the therapist must become a teacher and a persuasive motivator who encourages by example. Therapists must be fit; have good posture; have a professional appearance; take time for routine exercise, deep relaxation, and massage treatments; and essentially practice what they preach. It is much easier for a client to take advice from a therapist who lives his or her life in balance than one who is struggling with his or her own issues. Therapists must give homework and follow up on the assignments to make sure that the client is complying and not procrastinating or avoiding change. Remember that change in itself is stressful. Some people fear change, and many prefer to live in misery rather than enter into an unknown realm. Massage therapists are in the best positions of all alternative health care providers to become stress reduction specialists because they spend more time with clients than other professionals and can tailor treatments specifically to help clients return to homeostasis.

In addition, research has revealed that massage successfully reduces stress. The Touch Research Institutes at the University of Miami School of Medicine has conducted more than 90 studies on the effects of touch therapies on a variety of conditions. The Massage Therapy Foundation has an easily accessible database of massage-related research articles. A sampling of the research pertaining to stress and massage from these two resources has shown that massage therapy may diminish pain from backaches and headaches; relieve the symptoms of fibromyalgia; improve flexibility; decrease smoking cravings and autoimmune problems; enhance immune system function; decrease stress hormone levels, depression, and anxiety; and improve sleep quality and self-image. The table outlined in Appendix 1 categorizes some massage therapy research studies by author and title and the effects on the human body.

Although this is a good start, we need much more research on the effects of different massage treatments on pain, insomnia, anxiety and depression, hormone secretions, and immune function and on how massage stimulates the parasympathetic branch of the sympathetic nervous system to counteract sympathetic nervous system arousal. It is essential that massage therapists learn to administer a battery of assessment techniques and how to accurately document the results so that they can measure and record client progress. They must record baseline data, what techniques were used, and what worked and what did not. They also must learn to reassess after a series of treatments to show clients their progress. Therapists must be able to prove to their clients that their treatments work. Empirical data are essential for more effective treatments and for the advancement of the profession.

STRESS REDUCTION AND RELAXATION TREATMENTS—A NATURAL DIRECTION FOR MASSAGE THERAPISTS

The methods outlined in this book will help you improve your ability to evaluate and treat stress-related physical problems. With so many people suffering from stress-related disorders, relaxation-based treatments can become a large part of your business. A major benefit of performing this type of treatment is that you will not have to work so hard physically because in many instances when working with severe stress problems, less is more. Performing strokes that require less intensity and exertion will help reduce your chance of suffering from repetitive strain injuries and prolong your career. Combining relaxing music or sounds and some heat (unless contraindicated) with conscious relaxation and soothing, calming strokes creates a wonderful healing atmosphere for the highly stressed clients you see. In her book *A Massage Therapist's Guide to Pathology*, Ruth Werner aptly summed up this sentiment when she wrote, "Massage is very much indicated for a person experiencing insomnia. One of the finest gifts massage can offer is a good night's sleep, brought about by the restoration of balance between the sympathetic and parasympathetic nervous systems. For insomniac conditions brought about by pain, massage can serve the dual purpose of soothing the sympathetic reaction, while helping to set the stage for optimum healing of the injury, as long as the pain-causing problem does not contraindicate massage." (Werner 1998:367)

Through massage treatments, therapeutic exercise recommendations, and stress reduction education, massage therapists can help clients realign their posture; recognize and relax excess muscle tension; and improve their ability to breathe properly, sleep more soundly, and relax at will. Many clients need rest, relaxation, sleep, and a caring touch to help them get more in tune with their spirits, minds, and bodies and gain more control over their lives. The stress-reducing massage therapy treatments out-

A Word of Caution!

Please note: If any of your clients have a medical condition, please do not have them perform any of the physical exercises or activities detailed in the book until they have been granted permission by their primary health care provider. Please reinforce: "If it hurts, don't do it," and if they are in doubt, they should ask their doctor, chiropractor, or physical therapist. Also always remember to stay within the specified scope of practice for massage therapists in your state, province, or municipality and avoid making recommendations to clients in the areas of therapeutic exercise, fitness, and nutrition that exceed the limits of your education, training, and right to practice massage therapy.

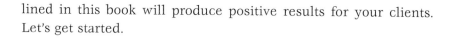

lined in this book will produce positive results for your clients. Let's get started.

WHAT IS STRESS?

Ever since prehistoric beasts chased the first cavemen in search of an easy meal, stress has been with us. Although today's stresses come from different, more modern sources, such as our job, studies, finances, lack of time in the day to accomplish our daily tasks, social responsibilities, family members, the environment, and world events, our bodily reactions are the same. If, like our terrified ancestor, we can sprint to the safety of a cave or otherwise find some outlet for the stress, our bodies quickly return to their normal balanced state. Unrelieved stress, however, keeps us in a state of chronic tension and, just like a hungry beast, eventually will destroy us.

Stress is the body's physical, mental, and chemical reaction to circumstances that frighten, excite, confuse, challenge, surprise, anger, endanger, or irritate. Stressors are events that trigger a stress response and may include physical dangers, political and social issues, work demands and responsibilities, environmental catastrophes, and emotional challenges. The events that cause stress may be good or bad. Good stress **(eustress)** can come from positive situations such as starting a new job or career, getting promoted, writing a book, having a child, or experiencing any situation that you find inspiring or motivating. Bad stress **(distress)** is much more common, coming from such everyday events as unrealistic job deadlines, divorce, money worries, death of a loved one, examinations, neighbors from hell, and even the grind of daily commuting. **Acute stress,** your immediate response to a stressor, is a normal part of life that we must accept. It is normal to have sweaty palms or a racing heart before an exam, a dry mouth before presenting a report, or sleeplessness the night before an important game. However, soon after the event your body should return to its normal balance, or **homeostasis.** Constantly having these physical reactions is an indication of **chronic stress,** which you must find a way to eliminate before your mind and body wear out. Incessant, unchecked **sympathetic nervous system** arousal makes you age more quickly and leads to a wide variety of physical and mental disorders.

Figure 1.1

Stages of the fight-or-flight response

Stage 1: A person is confronted with an emergency situation, danger, or unfavorable conditions that produce the emotions fear, anger, or rage.

Stage 2: The brain instantly interprets the signal, and if it determines the stimulation is a real threat, the brain stimulates the nervous, endocrine, and immune systems to quickly prepare for battle or evacuation. This reaction prepares the body to exert high levels of physical energy during a struggle for survival.

Stage 3: The body remains in this state of alarm or activation, maintaining the threat-induced physiological changes until the danger is over.

Stage 4: The body returns to homeostasis when the threat is eliminated.

WHAT EFFECT DOES STRESS HAVE ON THE BODY?

In the early part of the twentieth century Walter Cannon, a physiologist from Harvard University, was the first to coin the word homeostasis, referring to the body's ability to adapt to a variety of situations to maintain a relative consistency in its internal environment. He conducted a series of animal studies to determine the mechanisms involved in regulating and controlling the various self-righting mechanisms of the body. He was the first to research the body's natural defenses that create an immediate physiological reaction when we experience rage and fear. He postulated that fear is associated with the urge to run or escape and that rage or anger prepares the body to attack and dominate in a life-or-death struggle. The terms **fight or flight** have been commonly associated with his findings. Figure 1.1 outlines the stages of the fight-or-flight response.

Canadian researcher Hans Selye conducted extensive research on the fight-or-flight response, particularly the body's physiological response to chronic stress. Studying rats, Selye (1956) noted that prolonged exposure to stress produced several physiological adaptations. He called the changes induced by prolonged unchecked stress **the general adaptation syndrome.** Figure 1.2 outlines the stages of general adaptation syndrome.

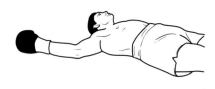

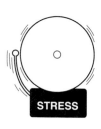

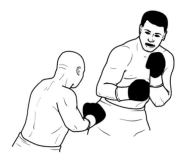

Alarm

Resistance

Exhaustion

Stage 1: Alarm Reaction—As a threat is perceived, the flight-or-fight response is activated and changes occur to the nervous, endocrine, cardio-vascular, integumentary, and immune systems.

Stage 2: Resistance—The body is mobilized to combat the stressor. It tries to revert back to homeostasis, but it never fully returns to normal because the threat is never entirely eliminated. The metabolic rate is increased, and one or more organs, endocrine glands, or bodily systems may be working in excess.

Stage 3: Exhaustion—The body's resources have been depleted and the stressed individual gets sick, an organ or bodily system breaks down, or the body dies because of the excess demands placed on it.

Figure 1.2

General adaptation syndrome

THE PHYSIOLOGY OF STRESS

The rats that Selye (1956) overstressed developed serious physical problems that included an enlargement of the adrenal cortex because of the constant release of the stress hormones aldosterone and cortisol; bleeding ulcers of the stomach and small intestine; a decrease in white blood cell count; and damage to structures of the lymphatic system, including shrinkage of the spleen, thymus, and lymph nodes. When extrapolated to humans, the noted physiological changes resulting from stress can seriously affect a person's ability to fight infections and disease and reduce his or her overall health and the quality of life experienced.

Let's look at the dramatic example (depicted in Figure 1.3) of how humans respond to a threat. You are hiking in the woods when suddenly you come face to face with a hungry mountain lion. The fear that you experience results in an immediate response by the sympathetic branch of the **autonomic nervous system** (ANS), the endocrine and the immune systems. Table 1.1 summarizes the stress-induced physiological changes that occur in the body when the fight-or-flight response is activated.

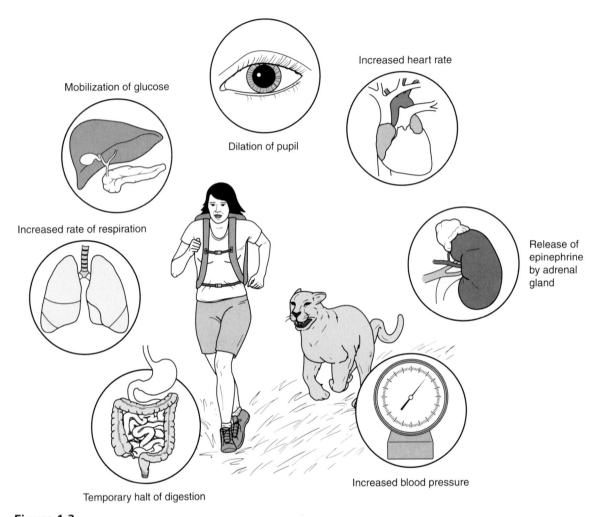

Figure 1.3

The fight-or-flight response

The chain of events that comprises a stress response includes the response of the brain; hypothalamus; and the pituitary, thyroid, and adrenal glands. The association among these structures is outlined in Figure 1.4. When we encounter a stressor, sensory organs take in the information, such as the smell of a fire, the sound of a gunshot, the taste of poison, or the sight of a mountain lion on the trail, and pass the message to the brain. It is important to note that in addition to the physical triggers, psychological and emotional reactions and interpretations of stressors also can activate this

TABLE 1.1

Summary of the Body's Stress-Induced Physiological Changes

Affected Organ or Body Part	Physiological Changes
Pupils of the Eye	Pupils dilate to improve visual sensitivity or acuity.
Heart	Dilation of the coronary arteries occurs. The rate and volume of blood pumped is increased and blood pressure rises.
Cardiovascular System	Vasodilation of the arteries that increases the blood flow to the brain, heart, and major muscle groups of the arms and legs occurs. Blood-clotting mechanisms start up, decreasing clotting time if injured.
Lungs	Breathing becomes faster and deeper because more oxygen is required by the brain and musculature during strenuous activity.
Liver	Fats are mobilized and broken down into sugar. Glycogen, the storage form of glucose, is broken down into glucose for quick energy.
Stomach and Intestines	Digestion is temporarily halted as the blood is shifted to the major muscle groups because digestion is a nonessential activity in an emergency.
Skin	Increased perspiration and decreased surface temperature occur.
Muscles	The muscles tense and tighten. More oxygen and sugar are delivered, which increases muscular strength.
Mouth	The saliva in the mouth dries up.
Spleen	The spleen contracts and releases red blood cells needed to carry oxygen.
Thyroid	Release of thyroid hormone increases the overall metabolic rate.
Adrenal Medulla	Adrenalin is released to reduce muscular fatigue.
Adrenal Cortex	Cortisol is released to help mobilize glucose to satisfy the body's energy demands.
Brain and Nervous System	Blood sugars and fats flow to the brain for energy needed. All senses are heightened.
Immune System	Mobilization of white blood cells is increased in case of an injury.

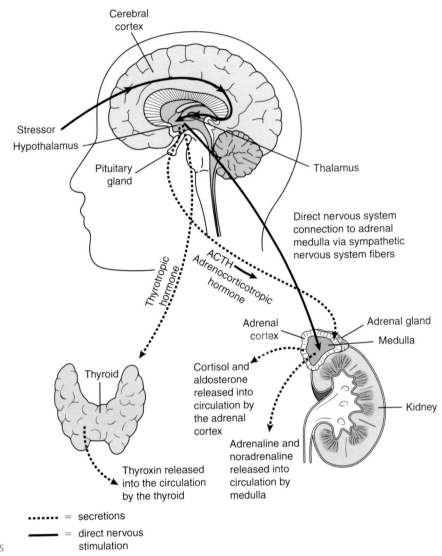

Figure 1.4

The response of the brain, hypothalamus, pituitary, thyroid, and adrenal glands to stress

response. The brain responds to stressors by activating the endocrine and autonomic nervous systems. After a threat is perceived, the brain sends nerve impulses to stimulate the hypothalamus. The hypothalamus in turn activates the sympathetic branch of the autonomic nervous system, initiating the stress response. Impulses travel along sympathetic nerves to the adrenal medulla, which then releases the substances called catecholamines—the hormones epinephrine (adrenaline) and norepinephrine (noradrenaline). This release of epinephrine and norepinephrine dilates the coronary arteries; accelerates the heart rate; increases the force of heart muscle contraction; dilates the arteries that feed the major muscles of the arms and legs that are needed to fight or flee; and constricts the arteries to the muscles that are not necessary in an emergency situation, such as the smooth muscles of the intestine, which reduces digestive activity. These hormones also dilate the pupils and the bronchioles to improve visual acuity and increase ventilation, increase metabolic rate, and release glucose from the liver to provide more oxygen and energy needed to combat stress. This sympathetic nervous system arousal prepares the body to expend energy and supplies the skeletal muscles with the necessary nutrient-rich oxygenated blood to fuel the required energy demands.

The hypothalamus then stimulates the pituitary gland to release ACTH (adrenocorticotropic hormone), which passes through the bloodstream to the adrenal cortex. The adrenal cortex secretes a number of hormones, among them a glucocorticoid, cortisol, and a mineralocorticoid, aldosterone. Cortisol increases the availability of energy to the body by increasing a process that occurs in the liver called gluconeogenesis, which essentially forms glucose out of the available glycogen and amino acids. In addition to mobilizing glucose, cortisol also serves as an anti-inflammatory agent. Aldosterone is an important hormone for regulating the body's blood pressure and electrolyte balance. It acts on the kidneys and the sweat glands to regulate salt and potassium levels and raises the blood pressure to transport the extra nutrients and oxygen needed by our bodies during a stress reaction. Some studies have reported that during chronic stress cortisol and aldosterone have been shown to suppress the immune system by reducing the number of T cells, which locate, identify, and destroy mutant cells.

The thyroid gland also is involved in the body's reaction to stress. In response to a stressor the hypothalamus also stimulates the pituitary gland to release thyrotropic hormone, which stimulates the thyroid gland to secrete the hormone thyroxin. Thyroxin increases the body's overall metabolism or basal metabolic rate, blood pressure, heart rate, and rate of respiration. In addition, thyroxin also mobilizes energy stores, can reduce tiredness and increase feelings of anxiety, and in some cases can lead to insomnia.

The immune system is a network composed of the bone marrow, which supplies the lymph tissue with stem cells used to fabricate lymphoid cells; the thymus, where the stem cells mature into

T lymphocytes; the lymph nodes; spleen; and parts of the associated lymphoid tissue located in the abdomen, where the T cells and B cells occasionally, in the course of their travels throughout the body, inhabit (Seaward, 1994). The link between chronic stress and the immune system comes from the sympathetic nervous system fibers that descend from the brain to the bone marrow, the thymus, the spleen, lymph nodes, and the lymphoid tissues. Long-term activation of the fight-or-flight response, as a result of unchecked sympathetic nervous system engagement, wears out the normal natural immune system ability to produce antibodies and respond to signals of **antigens.** This makes people more susceptible to the negative immunological effects of stress. For primitive humans, the energy expenditure required in escape or fight helped reverse the stress-induced physiological changes and allowed their body to quickly return to homeostasis. In today's world we all too often cannot run from or fight the cause of our stress. Society will not accept us running away and hiding or smacking our bosses with a club each time they yell at us. Everyday stress triggers the same kinds of responses to prepare your body to combat any imposing threat. Unfortunately, many individuals have not incorporated healthy activities that naturally help reverse these physiological changes induced by stress. The problem is that the human body pays a price each time it is overstressed. And the more intense the stress or the longer it lasts, the higher the price.

THOUGHTS AND EMOTIONS MAY CREATE DISTRESS

The stress of daily living and events that occur in the world and in our lives affects our internal state of emotional tension. How we think, interpret, react, and cope with these events in our daily lives can create emotional reactions that can strain our minds and bodies. The mind and the body are inseparable, and emotions associated with anticipation and even imagination can produce a physical stress response. Even if an incident is insignificant, unimportant, and inconsequential in the whole scheme of things, if the mind blows it out of proportion it can negatively affect the body. For example, intimate relationships bring up situations where loyalty, jealousy, and competition create irrational emotional responses. Just talking to someone of the opposite sex can

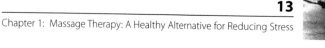

spur some significant others into fits of anger, rage, fear, and depression that create real physical stress. In actuality nothing happened, but because of the mental overreaction a full-blown stress response may raise their blood pressure, redden their face, make them nauseous, interfere with their sleep, or make them behave in ways that they may later regret.

THE RIGHT AMOUNT OF STRESS

It must be emphasized that not all stress is bad. A certain amount is necessary for life and actually acts as a catalyst for achievement. The optimal amount of stress actually can improve physical performance, focus, and concentration. In fact, we would never accomplish much without deadlines. If you start on a project when it is assigned and gradually whittle away at it, the deadline is a positive, exhilarating influence that spurs you on to greater achievement. Procrastination or an unworkable timeline results in distress that can damage a person's physical and mental health. The goal is to strive to balance your life so that you have the right amount of stress. In fact, too much or too little stress can have a similar negative impact on the human condition. The Stress Load Symptoms Chart in Figure 1.5 compares an individual with the right amount of stress with those with the stress underloads and overloads that may lead to physical and mental breakdowns.

THE PRICE WE PAY FOR STRESS

The excessive wear and tear from a stress imbalance may produce physical and psychological disorders, premature aging, and even early death. In fact, an estimated 80 percent of all illnesses that plague modern society are either precipitated or aggravated by stress (Girdano, Dusek, & Everly, 2005). Herbert Benson, MD, of Harvard Medical School believes that between 60 percent to 90 percent of visits to physicians are prompted by stress-related conditions (Benson, 2001). In 1998 in the *Journal of Clinical Psychiatry* it was reported that in 90 percent of the visits to primary care physicians there were no organic complaints (Katon and Walker, 1998). It is also estimated that job-related stress and strain costs American industry $300 billion annually as a result of absenteeism, reduced productivity, workers' compensation claims,

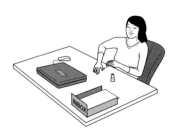 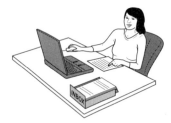 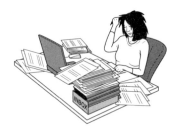

Too Little Stress	**The Right Amount of Stress**	**Too Much Stress**
Dull thinking	Clear thinking and clear perception	Cloudy thinking
Irritability	Calmness under duress	Irritability
Decreased motivation	Highly motivated	Motivated but overloaded
Lethargic performance	Efficient and effective job performance	Reduced quality of work
Apathy	Positive attitude	Not enough time in the day
Lack of direction and challenge	Task oriented	Apathy
Negativity	High energy and expectations	Reduced judgment and recall
More accidents	Effective decision-making and problem solving	More accidents
Changing appetite	Excellent memory recall	Changing appetite
Erratic interrupted sleep	High creativity	Sleep-onset insomnia
Increased absenteeism	Normal sleep patterns	Increased absenteeism
More alcohol and drug abuse	Work is a positive challenge	More alcohol and drug abuse
Strained relationships	Naturally exhilarated	Chronic fatigue
Anxiety		Social withdrawal
Procrastination		Strained relationships
		Decreased creativity

Figure 1.5

Stress Load Symptoms Chart *(Adapted from Goldberg [1978:40])*

insurance and medical fees, and training new employees because of job turnover. It was reported in the 2001 issue of *Health and Stress*, the newsletter of the American Institute of Stress, that "Surveys show that 75 to 90 percent of all visits to primary care physicians are for stress related complaints or conditions. As indicated, job stress is far and away the leading source of stress for American adults. Health care expenditures are nearly 50% greater for workers who report high stress levels and the $300 billion dollar estimate for job stress costs may now have to be revised upward." (*Health and Stress*, Number 3, 2001)

The national stress problem is growing because the number of families with both parents working has increased markedly over the past 30 years. With both parents working there is less time to perform household tasks and to have quality time with each other, with children, and for themselves. Compounding the situation, Americans are spending more time at work. In addition, corporations do not spend enough on preventive health care. In fact, only 3 cents of every dollar spent on health care in the United States is for prevention, yet the average return for every dollar invested in illness-preventing programs is $5.00 (*Business & Health Bulletin*, January, 2000). Stress is an international problem and is being documented throughout the world. The World Health Organization reported on 1997 statistics that indicated that work-related diseases and injuries cost 4 percent of the world's gross product (World Health Organization, 1999). A 2004 study by psychologists Suzanne Segerstrom, PhD, of the University of Kentucky and Gregory Miller, PhD, of the University of British Columbia reviewed 293 independent studies reported in peer-reviewed scientific journals between 1960 and 2001. Their major findings were that stress alters immunity; short-term stress actually amps up the immune system, preparing the body to fight injury or infection. They also found that long-term stress (chronic stress) causes much wear and tear and eventually will break down one of the body's systems, and that older and already sick individuals are more prone to suffer from stress-related problems (Segerstrom and Miller, 2004).

Throughout the literature, stress has been linked to heart disease, high blood pressure, strokes, and immune system disorders. A specific (but by no means exhaustive) list of diseases that may be stress induced are outlined in Table 1.2.

Stress-related problems are so rampant because many people do not know safe, healthy, and successful ways of coping with modern stresses. Too often, people under stress try to artificially escape it through alcohol; self-medication with illegal drugs; or prescription muscle relaxants, tranquilizers, and sleeping pills. These escapes merely suppress stress symptoms and lead to other serious problems, such as addiction, liver damage, impotence, fatigue, nausea, drowsiness, gastric irritation and bleeding, mental confusion, and psychoses.

TABLE 1.2

Diseases with Potential Links to Stress

Condition Name	Description and Relationship to Stress
Allergies	A defense of the body against foreign substances. Long-term stress depletes supplies of cortisol, which limits the body's ability to quell antigen-produced inflammation.
Amenorrhea	Stress can cause the absence or abnormal stoppage of the menstrual cycle.
Asthma (extrinsic, intrinsic, and mixed)	Bouts of difficulty breathing, shortness of breath, and wheezing as a result of excess mucus secretion or spasm or swelling of the bronchi. Emotional stress and allergens have been direct contributors to this disorder.
Arteriosclerosis (hardening of the arteries)	Occurs as plaque buildup in the walls of the arteries, making them grow thicker and less elastic. Exacerbated by stress, poor diet, high blood pressure, smoking, and lack of proper exercise.
Atherosclerosis	Lipids floating in the blood start to adhere to the lining of major arteries as a result of stress, lack of exercise, poor diet, high blood pressure, and smoking.
Cancer (breast, prostate, and lung cancer)	Body cells mutate and multiply uncontrollably. Long-term stress reduces the body's T-cell production, which impairs the ability to locate, identify, and destroy mutant cells.
Chronic Fatigue Syndrome	Incapacitating fatigue that may be accompanied by aches, pains, insomnia, fever, and swollen lymph nodes. The immune system is overworked as it continues fighting a nonexistent infection long after the original infection has been destroyed.
Coronary Artery Disease	Physiological changes induced by stress such as increased heart rate, blood pressure, and cholesterol can lead to blockage of a coronary artery and death to areas of the heart muscle.
Drug and Alcohol Abuse	Addiction and alcoholism are unhealthy and all too frequently used as attempts to escape from stress.
Eating Disorders (anorexia nervosa, bulimia, binge eating)	Low self-esteem, a poor self-image, and stress can lead a person to self-starvation and purging to maintain weight or to bouts of overeating. Depression, anxiety, anger, and loneliness are common companions to these disorders.
Heart Attack (myocardial infarction)	Damage to the heart muscle that results from the blockage of a coronary artery. Stress is a big contributor to heart attacks.

(continued)

TABLE 1.2—continued

Diseases with Potential Links to Stress

Condition Name	Description and Relationship to Stress
Hypertension (high blood pressure)	Excess pressure of the blood against the walls of the arteries that emotional stress, a poor diet, and lack of exercise can contribute to.
Hives (urticaria)	An allergy or emotional stress can create small, red, hot, itchy spots on the skin that may come and go.
Immune System Disorders	The immune system changes as a result of chronic stress and can make a person more susceptible to chronic fatigue, the common cold, and the flu.
Irritable Bowel Syndrome (spastic colon, irritable colon, and mucus colitis)	A condition of the digestive tract that varies among individuals. Symptoms may include cramps, constipation, gas, diarrhea, and bloating. Stressful events can flare up this condition.
Migraine Headaches	Emotional stress, tension. and dietary factors can cause these debilitating vascular headaches. After an initial vasoconstriction the arteries of the head dilate and the blood vessels become engorged with blood, producing throbbing pain.
Myofascial Pain	Head, neck, shoulder, and back pain in the muscles and fascia can be the product of habitually poor posture, injury or accidents, or stress-induced excess muscle tension.
Neuroses	Stress can increase anxiety, tension, and nervous irritability and contribute to neurotic conditions.
Raynaud's Syndrome (phenomenon and disease)	Spasm and constriction of the small arteries of the hands and fingers; feet and toes; and sometimes the nose, ears, lips, and tongue. Emotional stress, anxiety and tension, or another disease can cause episodes of this disorder.
Temporomandibular Joint (TMJ) Dysfunction	Popping and pain in front of the ear where the mandible meets the temporal bone. Emotional stress can contribute to jaw clenching, teeth grinding, tight musculature, and pain when chewing.
Tension Headaches	Headaches that are caused by poor posture and excess muscle tension in the musculature of the head, neck, and suboccipital region.
Trichotillon	A rare, compulsive, hair-pulling disorder. Some feel that stress, anxiety, and depression can contribute to this rare disorder.

SUMMARY

Now that we have a better understanding of what stress is, what causes it, and its effects on the human mind and body, the next step is to learn how to measure and document it. Before moving on to the next chapter, some key points to remember are as follows:

- Use the results of assessments and questionnaires in this book to develop your client's unique stress profile.

- Use the client's stress profile to tailor his or her stress reduction treatment program.

- Implement the client's individualized program for 10 weeks and then reassess.

- A strong knowledge base, along with professionalism and ethical behavior, will help the therapist gain the client's trust and respect.

- More research is needed to determine the effects of massage treatments on the measurable manifestations of stress.

- Stress is part of life, and it's most beneficial to learn and use natural techniques to cope with it and help the mind and body return to balance.

- The fight-or-flight response is a primitive mechanism, still active in modern humans, which instantly mobilizes the body's defenses to repel or avoid a threat.

- The brain, hypothalamus, pituitary, adrenal cortex, adrenal medulla, thyroid glands, and the immune system are all part of the body's complex reaction to stress.

- The hormones epinephrine and norepinephrine, released by the adrenal medulla; cortisol and aldosterone, released by the adrenal cortex; and thyroxin, released by the thyroid, all contribute to the dramatic physiological changes that occur as the body tries to cope with stress.

- As much as 80 percent of all disease has been attributed to stress-related origins.

- Unchecked stress can lead to a wide variety of physical, psychological, and emotional problems.

- Stress-related illness and absenteeism costs the world economy billions of dollars each year.

Assessment Techniques for Measuring Stress

To successfully combat clients' stress, massage therapists must learn how to measure and document its effects on the clients' body and how to help them recognize the controllable factors in their lives that are contributing to it. Before treatments begin it is essential to objectively measure the client's stress level and the effect it is having so that you can determine the effectiveness of your treatment programs. Baseline data can then be compared with post-treatment program results to determine the relative effectiveness of the massage and stress reduction techniques used. Every client is unique, and this information is vital to the development of beneficial personalized stress reduction treatment programs. This chapter will outline how to administer a battery of assessment tests to measure the stress response of clients and to isolate the changeable elements in their lives that may be contributing to it. Aside from many of the posture and flexibility assessment techniques used in this chapter, the results are not compared with norms; rather, clients are compared with themselves. After a series of treatments, over a minimum period of 10 weeks, the client is retested. Ten weeks of treatments and personal stress reduction program implementation is enough time for the client to institute lifestyle changes and achieve significantly measurable progress in a variety of areas.

Ideally, 2 hours should be scheduled for the first session with a new client. You need that much time to administer the collection of tests outlined in this chapter, review the results with the client, perform the initial treatment, and give them a homework assignment. However, if your client is pressed for time, you can shorten the initial visit by assigning some parts of the Personal Stress Inventory (PSI) as homework. Also, there are other useful quick assessment tools presented in Chapter 5 that might fit their schedule better. The therapist can also pull bits and pieces from the battery of assessment tools presented to design his or her own streamlined version of the PSI.

These tests are necessary to establish the cause of your clients' distress. The ensuing assessments will disclose where and how stress is affecting them physically, psychologically, behaviorally, and emotionally. This compilation of tests will help you evaluate their posture, muscular imbalances, muscle tension, flexibility, diet and exercise habits, sleep quality, weekly schedule, relaxation practice, breathing mechanics, and overall lifestyle in an attempt to pinpoint and isolate specific causes of their stress. To successfully reduce stress, clients must take an in-depth look at their physical health, psychological health, and overall lifestyle. Recording this information will bring them face to face with their problems and help you measure their progress. It's vital that they are honest and complete when doing the assignments. These evaluations will uncover their physical stress symptoms, psychosocial stress, the time of the day they are most stressed, and other factors and habits that contribute to their stress level.

If the client does not have 2 hours for the full first examination and treatment, an option is to have them complete the PSI Section 1 at home. To save time, you can also get empirical data from the quick body scan outlined in Chapter 5. You can adapt the evaluation and treatment to the client's schedule and needs, but it is great experience to become familiar with the entire group of tests included in this chapter. Many clients love this evaluation because it gives them information on how their bodies are out of balance and what factors are contributing to their distress. This improves their understanding of what they need to do and the changes they need to make to relieve their problems. Clients also love when the post-test results demonstrate that their stress reduction program is helping them achieve improvements.

Before we begin taking physical measurements, it is important for the massage therapist to know which of their eyes is dominant. The results that you ascertain will be more accurate and consistent if you take your readings with the same eye.

DOMINANT EYE TEST

Hold your extended arms out in front of you with your shoulders flexed to 90 degrees. With your hands, shape a small circle about the size of a golf ball and look through this circle at an identifiable object across the room from you. Figure 2.1 demonstrates the proper hand position for this test. Without moving your hands or your head, first close one eye and then the other. The eye that the object is in focus with is your dominant eye; you should always focus with that eye when performing physical tests and measurements.

Please note that the posture and flexibility analyses used in this book are intended to help you reveal your client's postural faults and muscular imbalances so that you can accurately document where a treatment program starts and can chart their progress over the course of a treatment program. They are not intended for the purpose of diagnosis, which is beyond the scope of practice of massage therapists.

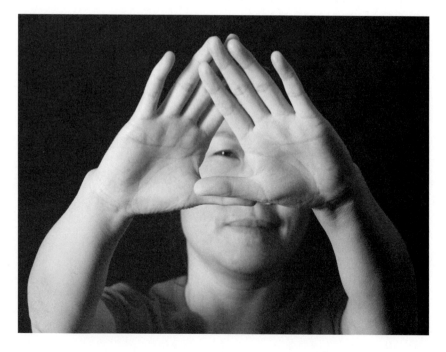

Figure 2.1

Hand position for dominant eye test

ADMINISTERING THE PERSONAL STRESS INVENTORY

The PSI is designed to help you gather the information necessary to formulate your client's personal stress profile, which you then use to develop a personal stress reduction program. Section 1 of the PSI studies clients' physical and psychosocial state of being. It summarizes their history of stress-related disorders; stress symptoms; medications taken; nutritional habits; stimulants ingested; and sleep, exercise, and relaxation habits. Section 1 also identifies the situations that cause or add to their stress, such as work, school, friends, family, money, decision-making, lack of achievement, lack of control over their lives, and lack of motivation. Section 2 checks their posture, flexibility, muscle imbalances, lung capacity, breathing mechanics, and where they carry their pain and tension. Have your client dress for this appointment in loose, comfortable clothing or in a swimsuit. Now make a copy of the blank PSI located in Appendix 2, and let's begin.

Personal Stress Inventory, Section 1, Part A: Physical Symptoms of Stress

Instruct the client to use the following scale to answer the questions and circle those that apply.

1 = Never	2 = Rarely	3 = Sometimes
4 = Often	5 = Always	

To what extent do you experience the following?

    1 2 3 4 5   Sweaty palms

    1 2 3 4 5   Cold hands and feet

    1 2 3 4 5   Tension headaches

    1 2 3 4 5   Migraine headaches

    1 2 3 4 5   Teeth grinding

    1 2 3 4 5   Neck pains

1 2 3 4 5   Uncontrollable muscle spasms

1 2 3 4 5   Pains in the shoulder, upper back, or both

1 2 3 4 5   Low back pain

1 2 3 4 5   Pain down the back of your leg(s)

1 2 3 4 5   Shortness of breath

1 2 3 4 5   Susceptibility to minor illness

1 2 3 4 5   Poor-quality sleep

1 2 3 4 5   Hair, eyelash, or beard pulling

1 2 3 4 5   Nail biting

1 2 3 4 5   Frequent trips to the toilet

1 2 3 4 5   Gastrointestinal pain or discomfort

1 2 3 4 5   Diarrhea

1 2 3 4 5   Constipation

1 2 3 4 5   Nausea

1 2 3 4 5   Chronic fatigue

1 2 3 4 5   Binge eating

1 2 3 4 5   Do not eat because you fear becoming fat

1 2 3 4 5   Bulimia

1 2 3 4 5   General malaise

1 2 3 4 5   Cold sores, hives

1 2 3 4 5   Restless legs or feet (toe or finger shaking)

1 2 3 4 5   Repetitive joint cracking (neck, knuckles, etc.)

Personal Stress Inventory, Section 1, Part B: Psychosocial Symptoms of Stress

Continue using the same scale:

1 = Never	2 = Rarely	3 = Sometimes
4 = Often	5 = Always	

How frequently do you experience the following? Circle the answers that apply.

1 2 3 4 5   Not enough time in the day

1 2 3 4 5   Trouble concentrating (difficulty thinking clearly)

1 2 3 4 5   Anxiety from causes that you cannot pinpoint

1 2 3 4 5   Irritability

1 2 3 4 5   Strained relationships

1 2 3 4 5   Easily aroused to hostility or anger

1 2 3 4 5   Job dissatisfaction or prolonged unemployment

1 2 3 4 5   Depression

1 2 3 4 5   Taking work home with you

1 2 3 4 5   Thinking about work even when relaxing

1 2 3 4 5   Being a workaholic

1 2 3 4 5   Trouble turning off your mind at night

1 2 3 4 5   Decision-making anxiety

1 2 3 4 5   Stressful dreams

1 2 3 4 5   Nonstop rushing around

1 2 3 4 5   Low motivation

1 2 3 4 5   Pessimism

1 2 3 4 5   Worrying

1 2 3 4 5   Lack of control over your life

1 2 3 4 5   A short-fused temper

1 2 3 4 5   An unhappy home environment

1 2 3 4 5   Isolation or loneliness

1 2 3 4 5   Procrastination

1 2 3 4 5   Panic attacks

1 2 3 4 5   So impatient that you finish others' sentences

1 2 3 4 5   Functioning subnormally or missing work because of drug or alcohol abuse

Personal Stress Inventory, Section 1, Part C: Diet, Exercise, Deep Relaxation, and Lifestyle Evaluation

Circle the diet that best describes your eating habits on a typical day.

a. Lots of fruit and vegetables (salads), whole grains, and legumes; less than 30% of all food consumed comes from fat; at least two glasses of dairy products (unless allergic) each day; low cholesterol; little sugar; more fish, turkey, and chicken than red meat.
b. Lots of fast food, junk food, soda, and grease.
c. Meat and potatoes.
d. Vegetarian.
e. A combination of _____ and _____.

How many cups of stimulants do you drink each day (include coffee, tea, hot chocolate, and soda)? _____

List the name and dose of any medications you are currently taking (including appetite suppressants and vitamin pills):

_____

_____

How frequently do you practice a form of deep relaxation (such as meditation) each week?

Never _____ Days a week _____ Duration _____

How frequently do you participate in vigorous, nonstop aerobic activities that elevate your heart rate to your target range?

Never _____ Days a week _____ Duration _____

How often do you perform postural realignment or stretching exercises?

Never _____ Days a week _____ Duration _____

How frequently do you lift weights, perform calisthenics, or participate in any other activities that tone your muscles?

Never _____ Days a week _____ Duration _____

What time of the day do you feel most stressed? What happens at these times (i.e., commute in traffic, children fighting at the dinner table, the daily meeting with the boss)? Use more paper if necessary.

_____

_____

The following factors are common contributors to stress. Put them in the order that you think they contribute to your stress level. Put a 1 next to the element that causes the most stress, then

a 2 next to your second biggest stressor, and so on down the list.

_____ Job or lack of a job

_____ Studies

_____ Family members

_____ Social relationships

_____ Sexual issues

_____ Financial issues

_____ Health

_____ Living situation

_____ Environmental pollution

_____ The world situation

_____ Other _____

List three lifestyle or behavioral changes that you think may

improve the quality of your life. _____

_____

_____

_____

_____

List some ideas for coping with, or eliminating, your stressors.

Include even the most bizarre alternatives that you can imagine.

Don't inhibit your creativity. _____

_____

_____

Personal Stress Inventory, Section 2, Part A: Posture Evaluation

You will need some masking or athletic tape and a cloth measuring tape to complete this part of the PSI. Peel off two 18-inch pieces of tape and place them on the floor in the shape of a plus sign (+) with one piece bisecting the other at a right angle. For the standing evaluations, instruct your clients to stand with the tips of their toes on one line and their feet equidistant apart from the center (bisecting) line. To get a true evaluation, they must not be allowed to stand at attention. Instruct them to stand in their relaxed habitual posture, and then compare what you see with the pictures in the PSI. On the copy of the PSI, record which picture most closely resembles the client's posture. Additional methods of evaluating posture will be discussed in the Chapter 5.

Forward Head

Normal Posture   Mild   Moderate   Severe

Comments _____

Kyphosis

Normal Posture   Mild   Moderate   Severe

Comments _____

Forward Head

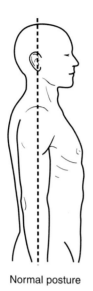 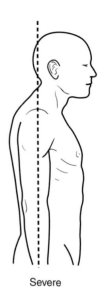

Normal posture   Mild   Severe

Figure 2.2

Forward head

Kyphosis

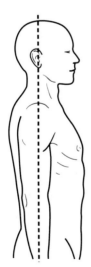 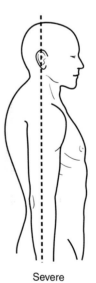

Normal posture   Mild   Severe

Figure 2.3

Kyphosis

Elevated Shoulder

R or L   Normal   Mild   Moderate   Severe

Comments _____

_____

Head Tilt

R or L   Normal   Mild   Moderate   Severe

Comments _____

_____

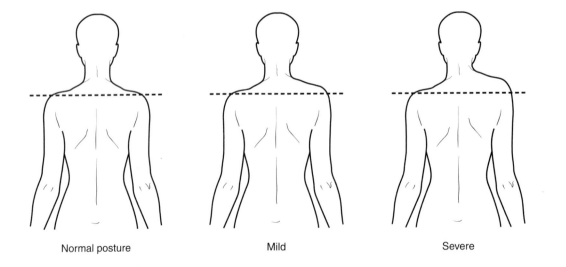

Elevated Shoulder

Normal posture   Mild   Severe

Figure 2.4

Elevated shoulders

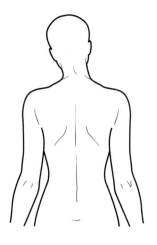

Figure 2.5

Head tilt

Elevated Hip

R or L   Normal   Mild   Moderate   Severe

Comments _____

_____

_____

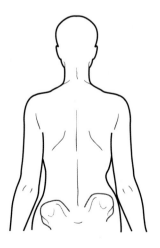

Figure 2.6

Elevated hip

C or S Curve of the Spine

For this test just compare one side of the body to the other. The

C and S curves are named on the side of the convexity. The S

curves are named left thoracic right lumbar and right thoracic

left lumbar. Check all clients for rib cage rotation, and record

the side that they rotate to.

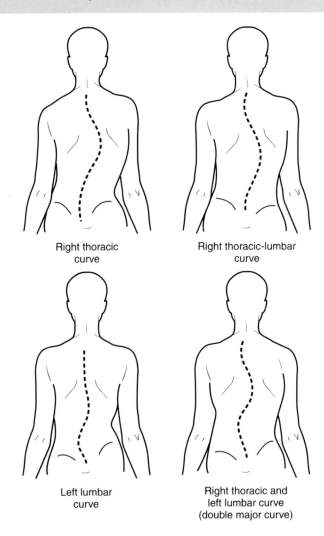

Right thoracic
curve

Right thoracic-lumbar
curve

Left lumbar
curve

Right thoracic and
left lumbar curve
(double major curve)

Figure 2.7

C or S curve of the
spine

Normal	C right	C left	LTRL	RTLL

Rib Cage Rotation L R

Comments _____

Hyperlordosis (Exaggerated Lumbar Curve and Anterior Pelvic Tilt)

Normal Posture	Mild	Moderate	Severe

Comments _____

Hyperlordosis

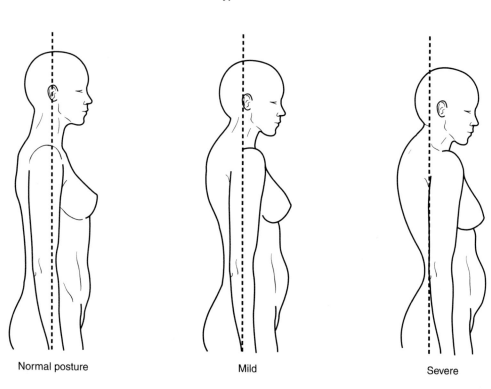

Normal posture   Mild   Severe

Figure 2.8

Hyperlordosis

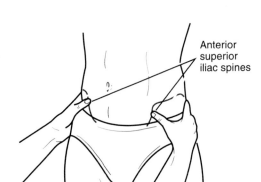

Anterior
superior
iliac spines

Figure 2.9

ASIS rotation

ASIS Rotation

Normal   Right low _____ inches   Left low _____ inches

Comments _____

Leg Length

To measure for imbalances in leg length in the supine position, first flex the hips and knees, bringing the heels to the gluteals. Place your thumbs just below the client's medial malleoli and lower both legs, extending them fully; then give a gentle pull. Use your dominant eye to check how well the malleoli line up by comparing the location of your thumbs, or you can measure the difference between the bottoms of the heels. If they line up equally, mark normal; if there is a difference, note the side that is short and then measure how many inches short it is.

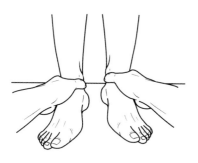 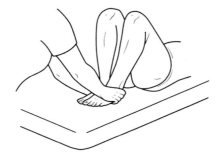

Figure 2.10

Leg length

Equal length _____   Left short _____ inches

Right short _____ inches

Comments _____

Personal Stress Inventory, Section 2, Part B: Flexibility Evaluation

Excess tightness in muscles can contribute to poor posture, pain, fatigue, and joint and skeletal problems. Evaluate the following muscle groups and check their lengths compared to the pictures. Have the client try to assume the positions indicated without warming up first. Instruct them not to strain or cause any pain or injury. Record the appropriate positions they can comfortably attain.

Hip Flexors

R Normal Length	Mild	Moderate	Severe
L Normal Length	Mild	Moderate	Severe

Comments _____

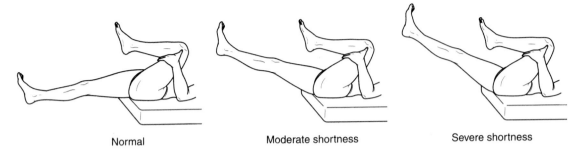

Normal   Moderate shortness   Severe shortness

Figure 2.11

Hip flexors

Quadriceps

R Normal Length   Mild   Moderate   Severe

L Normal Length   Mild   Moderate   Severe

Comments _____

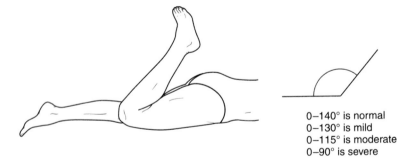

0–140° is normal
0–130° is mild
0–115° is moderate
0–90° is severe

Figure 2.12

Quadriceps

Low Back

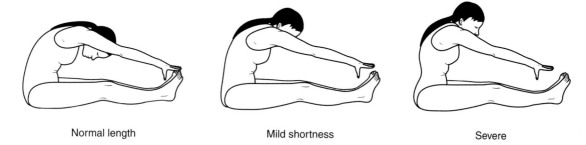

Normal length   Mild shortness   Severe

Figure 2.13

Low back muscles

Low Back Muscles

Normal Length   Mild   Moderate   Severe

Comments _____

Hamstrings

R Normal Length   Mild   Moderate   Severe

L Normal Length   Mild   Moderate   Severe

Comments _____

Hamstring

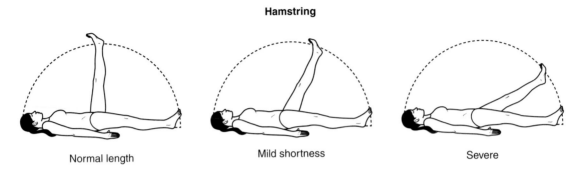

Normal length   Mild shortness   Severe

Figure 2.14

Hamstrings

Hip Lateral Rotators

Measure the distance from the bottom of the patella perpendicular to the table. Compare sides.

R _____ inches   L _____ inches

Comments _____

Hip Adductors

R Normal Length	Mild	Moderate	Severe
L Normal Length	Mild	Moderate	Severe

Comments _____

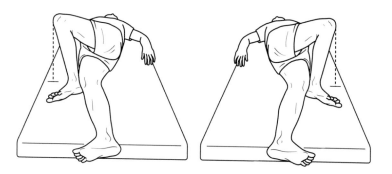

Figure 2.15

Hip lateral rotators: compare the sides. Measure the knee's distance from the table

Hip Adductors

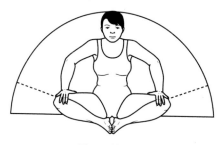

Normal length

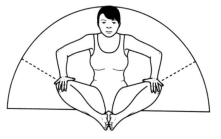

Mild shortness

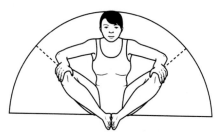

Severe

Figure 2.16

Hip adductors

Tensor Fasciae Latae and Iliotibial Tract

Position the client sidelying with his or her backside close to the edge of the table. Have the client gently flex the bottom hip and knee for stability. Stand behind the client, place your top hand on the iliac crest, and press down firmly to prevent lateral flexion of the pelvis. Have the client flex both the top hip and knee to 90 degrees. Next support the top knee with your hand and forearm and bring the hip back into extension and complete abduction. Next lower the extended hip into as much adduction as the client's range of motion allows. While testing, prevent the pelvis from laterally flexing and do not let the hip being tested flex or internally rotate. Normal for this test is when the thigh drops into adduction slightly below the horizontal or about 10 degrees. For more specific data measure the distance from the bottom of the knee perpendicular to the table.

R Normal   Inches from table _____

L Normal   Inches from table _____

Comments _____

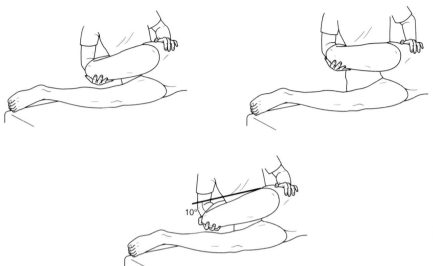

Figure 2.17

Tensor fasciae latae and iliotibial tract

Gastrocnemius

Place the hands on the wall, extend one knee completely, and slide the foot flat on the ground back as far as possible. The foot should be kept straight ahead, and the heel should not rise up. Measure the distance from the toes to the wall. Compare sides.

R _____ inches

L _____ inches

Comments _____

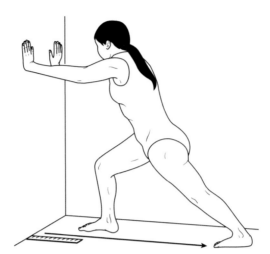

Figure 2.18

Gastrocnemius

Soleus

Place the hands and the sole of one foot on a wall, raising the toes as high as they can comfortably go. Flex the knee and bring the patella toward the wall; then measure the distance from the patella to the wall.

R _____ inches

L _____ inches

Comments _____

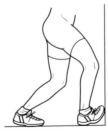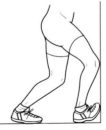

Figure 2.19

Soleus

Longitudinal Arch, Calcaneal Tendon Angle, and Toe Deviations

Observe the client's feet while he or she is standing barefoot.

Look for a flat or extra high arch, deviations of the calcaneal tendon angle, hammer toes, and big toe deviations.

R Longitudinal arch: Normal _____ Flat _____ High _____

L Longitudinal arch: Normal _____ Flat _____ High _____

R Calcaneus tendon angle: Straight   Medial deviation

L Calcaneus tendon angle: Straight   Medial deviation

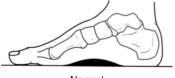

Normal

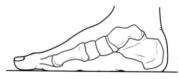

Flattened

Figure 2.20

Longitudinal arch

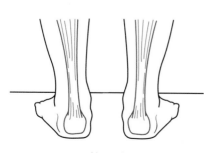

Normal

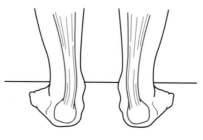

Pronated

Figure 2.21

Calcaneus tendon angle

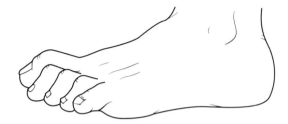

Figure 2.22

Hammer toes

R Toes: Normal deviation observed

L Toes: Normal deviation observed

R Big toe: Normal   Lateral deviation observed

L Big toe: Normal   Lateral deviation observed

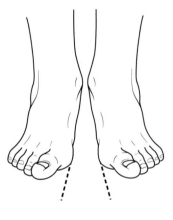

Figure 2.23

Big toe deviation

Neutral Position for Shoulder Rotation and Shoulder External Rotation:

R Normal	Mild	Moderate	Severe
L Normal	Mild	Moderate	Severe

Comments _____

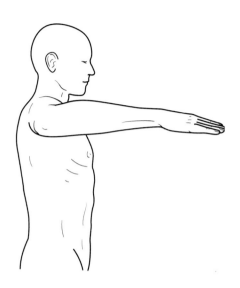

Figure 2.24

Neutral position for shoulder rotation

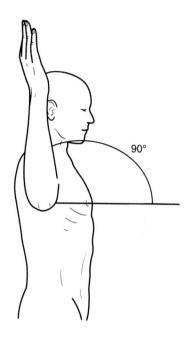

90°

Figure 2.25

Normal shoulder external rotation

Shoulder Internal Rotation:

R Normal	Mild	Moderate	Severe
L Normal	Mild	Moderate	Severe

Comments _____

Shoulder Flexion

R Normal	Mild	Moderate	Severe
L Normal	Mild	Moderate	Severe

Comments _____

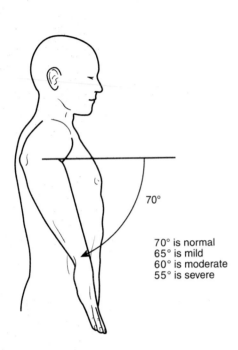

70°

70° is normal
65° is mild
60° is moderate
55° is severe

Figure 2.26

Normal shoulder internal rotation

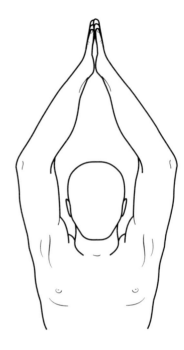

Normal shoulder flexion

Figure 2.27

Shoulder flexion: 180 degrees normal

Shoulder Extension			
R Normal	Mild	Moderate	Severe
L Normal	Mild	Moderate	Severe
Comments _____			

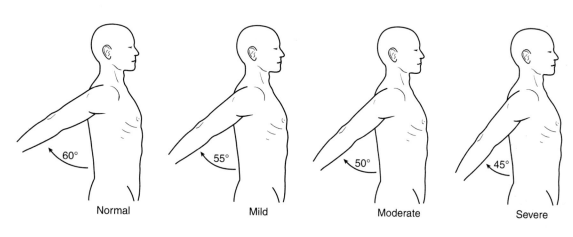

Normal	Mild	Moderate	Severe
60°	55°	50°	45°

Figure 2.28

Shoulder extension

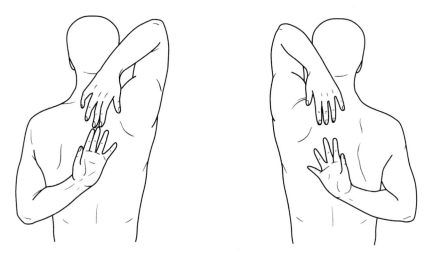

Normal   Mild restriction

Figure 2.29

Over and under

Over and Under

R over   Normal (Fingers touch) _____ inches between fingers

L over   Normal (Fingers touch) _____ inches between fingers

Comments _____

Personal Stress Inventory, Section 2, Part C: Muscle Tension Evaluation

Now let's evaluate and map areas of tension and pain in your client's body. Draw a dot on the points that are hypertonic. Draw an X on those that are painful; use wavy lines (∼) for points that the client reports radiate pain. Press all over the client's body from the top of the head to the bottom of the feet.

Personal Stress Inventory, Section 2, Part D: Breathing Evaluation

The way a person breathes can contribute to his or her level of stress. You will be evaluating five breathing factors that include the following: the length of inhalation, length of exhalation, shoulder elevation, action of the diaphragm, and overall control. Have clients sit in a chair and relax. Use your clock or stopwatch to measure the time it takes for them to fully inhale and exhale. Instruct them to take long, slow, deep, complete breaths in through the nose, breathing as slowly as possible. Then instruct them to release the breath, exhaling through their nose as slowly as possible. Record the time it takes for them to inhale and exhale. Perform two trials, and record them both.

Trial 1

Inhalation _____

Exhalation _____

Trial 2

Inhalation _____

Exhalation _____

Now perform the following tests. Place your hands on their upper trapezius muscles and have them continue to take long slow breaths in and out.

1. Do the client's shoulders move when they breathe? YES   NO

Next place your hands on the client's diaphragm just below the xiphoid process and check the action of the diaphragm. (If the person practices the principles of Pilates, place your hands on the sides of the rib cage in the same region.)

2. When the client begins to take air in, does the action of the diaphragm push your hands out away from the client's body? YES   NO

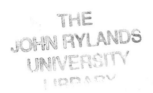

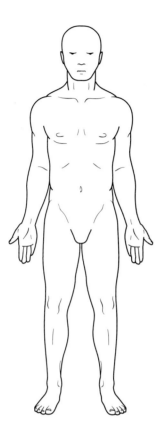

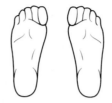

Figure 2.31

Sole of the foot

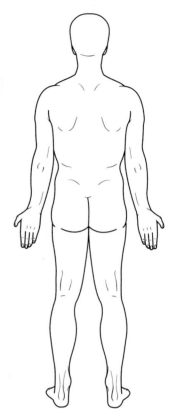

Figure 2.30

Front view of the body

Figure 2.32

Back view of the body

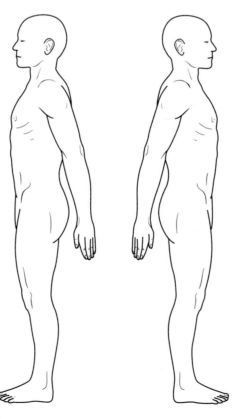

Figure 2.33

Side view of the body

3. Next ask the client if it feels to him or her that the inhalation travels from the bottom to the top of the chest. YES　　NO
4. Ask the client if his or her breathing feels deep, relaxed, and coordinated. YES　　NO

This completes the PSI. The next chapter will explain what the results mean and how to develop a personal stress reduction program from the information gathered from the tests.

STRESS LOG

The PSI questions and assessment tests should begin to get your client thinking about how stress presents itself in day-to-day life. Often, clients are excited after taking the PSI because it gives them new insights into their habitual way of being. Make good use of their excitement by giving them the following 1-week homework assignment designed to increase their awareness of the causes of their stress and pain even further.

Ask clients to chart their behavior and reactions to stress over one typical week. Instruct them to slip a small notebook or mini voice recorder into their pocket, backpack, or briefcase and carry it with them for a whole week. At the end of each day they should record their results on the Stress Log summary form located in Appendix 3.

Whenever they experience a stress reaction they should record the time of day, what caused it, and how they physically and mentally reacted to it. (Please tell them not to perform this activity while driving.) It is essential that they really tune into their body's messages to accurately pinpoint their physical manifestations of stress. Also have them note if they did anything to reverse the stress (how they coped with it) and if their actions were successful. If they are under stress, they will soon see a pattern developing of its causes and successful coping strategies. Furthermore, a week's worth of stress laid out in black and white should open their eyes to what may be an astonishing number of daily stresses, both large and small. Figure 2.34 provides an example of Stress Log entries. Have each client bring the completed log to their next appointment, which you should now schedule for the following week.

Sample 1-Week Stress Log Entry

Figure 2.34 provides an excerpt from a sample 1-week stress long entry.

Date or day	Time of day	Stressor	Physical reaction	Psychological reaction	Coping techniques
Monday	7:30 AM	Woke up late Rushing around	Stiff neck Pounding heart Sweating	Fear, guilt and anxiety that I will be late for work again. Angry with myself. My client will be waiting.	Drank coffee and cranked up the stereo. Drove fast
Monday	8:15 AM	Speeding ticket	Headache, shortness of breath, shoulder pain	Nervous Embarrassed, worried about the cost	Took a deep breath

Figure 2.34

Sample stress log

SUMMARY

Some important points to remember are as follows:

- Assessment tests are needed to help pinpoint and document the cause of your clients' distress.

- Baseline data will be compared to the post-test results after 10 weeks of treatments and implementation of their personal stress reduction program

- To successfully reduce stress clients must evaluate their overall lifestyle and then be willing to make the changes that are indicated.

- Always use your dominant eye when recording data on physical measurements.

- Evaluating the client's posture, muscle imbalances, muscle tension, flexibility, diet and exercise habits, sleep quality, weekly schedule, deep relaxation practice, breathing mechanics, and lung capacity and lifestyle will provide you with the data needed to develop his or her personal stress reduction program.

- Assign the client some stress reduction homework after each treatment.

Developing an Anti-Stress Plan

This chapter will present how to develop personalized, effective stress reduction treatment programs for your clients. The first step in designing an anti-stress plan is to get as much information about the client as possible. The tests in Chapter 2 were administered to record baseline data on the condition of the client before the start of treatment. These tests reveal a great deal of subjective information and extensive objective data, which, in essence, develop a time-sensitive snapshot of the client's physical, psychological, emotional, and social stress responses; body balance; and problems he or she is experiencing. The next task is to process the pertinent information and design a treatment program that will help return the client to homeostasis. In other words, the client is at point A and he or she needs to get to point B. The question is: How does the therapist get him or her there? The rest of this book presents a wide variety of practical techniques to help in this endeavor. The basic steps involved in developing, implementing, recording, and measuring the success of a treatment program are detailed in Figure 3.1, with discussion following.

The initial session with a client seeking stress reduction treatments should begin with a concise medical and health history that provides the therapist with essential data, such as contact information, history of medical problems, allergies to oil or lotion, depth of pressure preferred, areas to avoid, contraindications, music preference, and the client's goals and expectations for the treatments. The information garnered from the initial client interview should also include when the problems began; the location, frequency, intensity, and duration of the problems; and activities of daily living that exacerbate and relieve symptoms. It's a good idea for the therapist to reevaluate and restructure his or her

**How to Design and Implement Effective Stress
Reduction Treatment Programs**

1. Administer a medical and health history form to get essential background and subjective information on the client.

2. Perform assessment tests, Personal Stress Inventory (PSI), and Stress Log for stress-specific subjective information and baseline objective data acquisition.

3. Use the Stress Profile Summary Chart to synthesize the PSI, Stress Log, and health history form data and develop the client's stress profile.

4. Record essential data on chart records using SOAP (*S*ubjective, *O*bjective, *A*ssessment, *P*lan) format.

5. Design a stress reduction program based on the individual needs of the client.

6. Implement the plan.

7. Thoroughly document treatments and client self-help assignments.

8. Through trial and continuous revision, try different strokes and techniques to help the client reduce or eliminate his or her negative stress responses.

9. Reinforce all positive behavioral changes made by the client.

10. Retest after 10 weeks of treatments and program implementation to document measurable progress.

Figure 3.1

How to design and implement effective stress reduction treatment programs

current intake form so that the questions are not redundant with those asked on the Personal Stress Inventory (PSI). Refer to Appendix 4 for a sample client health history/intake form. The next step is to try to get more specific stress-related subjective data and objective information for use in developing the client's unique **stress profile.** Appendix 5 provides a sample pretreatment status form that can be used before each massage treatment session.

The data from the PSI and Stress Log are combined with the information ascertained from the intake form and the pretreatment status form to help develop each client's stress profile. This information should be condensed in the Stress Profile Summary Chart found in Appendix 6. The summary chart helps the therapist conveniently examine all the factors contributing to a client's distress, which helps in the design of an anti-stress plan. The summary also offers a handy comparison of the client's posture, flexibility, painful points, and breathing mechanics before treatment with the client's situation after a series of treatments.

The stress profile includes all the 4 and 5 responses to the questions in Section 1, Parts A and B that indicate that the client is often or always experiencing the selected physical, psychological, emotional, or social stress symptoms. The stress profile will also include pertinent information about the client's diet, exercise habits, and deep relaxation practice garnered from Section 1, Part C. In addition, the stress profile documents objective visual and palpable findings from Section 2, such as all deviations from the norm in regard to the client's posture, flexibility, muscle tension, and breathing mechanics. Other observations, such as atypical gait patterns, tender points, trigger points, and any other pertinent information, also are included in the client's profile. Any patterns of stressors and stress-related problems uncovered in the Stress Log should also be recorded. After the client's stress is documented and summarized the therapist will use the data and his or her critical thinking skills to forge the client's personal stress reduction treatment program.

When completed, the stress profile is shared with clients because it will help them understand the toll that stress is taking on their life. It will also help clients realize that a variety of factors contribute to their stress and that changes in their lifestyle, behaviors, exercise, and eating habits may be needed to reverse its course. It is hoped that clients will grasp the concept that every problem area disclosed must be dealt with by the therapist and themselves over the course of the treatment program. It is essential that the clients acknowledge and accept the fact that to succeed at reducing or eliminating their stress they cannot just lay there and receive relaxing massage treatments—they must play an active role.

INTERPRETING THE PERSONAL STRESS INVENTORY AND STRESS LOG RESULTS

Let's take a look at what the PSI results indicate. Section 1, Part A records the client's physical stress symptoms, and Part B provides information on the client's psychosocial and emotional stress symptoms. For Section 1, Parts A and B, 1 and 2 (never and rarely) responses indicate that the client is coping successfully. Even a 3 response is normal because it is normal to sometimes experience these manifestations of stress. However, all 4 and 5 (often and always) responses are danger signals that indicate chronic stress problems that must be dealt with. On the summary chart, list each of the client's 4 and 5 responses on Section 1, Parts A and B.

Section 1, Part C evaluates the client's diet, exercise, and deep relaxation practice habits and lifestyle factors that may be contributing to their stress. The types of food eaten, amount of calories consumed, and amount of stimulants ingested and medications taken can have a tremendous impact on the health, self-concept, and stress level of a client. The practical dietary changes to reduce stress outlined in Chapter 11 should be shared with the client when indicated, unless prohibited by your scope of practice. In addition, clients should check the side effects of any medications that they are taking and then compare it with their symptoms in Section 1, Parts A and B. The therapist should never recommend that the client stop taking a prescribed medication; however, it is a good idea for everyone to compare their stress symptoms to determine possible side effects of a drug. If a correlation is found, then the client should consider speaking to his or her doctor to see if there are alternative medications that may be better for them.

Section 1, Part C investigates clients' deep relaxation or meditation practice, aerobic training, frequency of postural realignment exercise practice, and muscle strengthening and toning activities performed each week. The author recommends that clients perform deep relaxation or meditation for 20 minutes at least 3 times a week and aerobic exercises that elevate their heart rate to the target range for 20 to 50 minutes at least 3 times a week. If postural abnormalities and muscular imbalances are uncovered in the PSI, then it is recommended that clients perform brief bouts of the stretching, strengthening, and postural realignment exercises recommended in Chapter 5 for their particular problems throughout each day. In addition, if the clients' muscles are hypotonic and they need to burn more calories each day, then they should possibly add three bouts of weight lifting or calisthenics to their weekly schedule. If clients fail to fulfill the minimum requirements of areas in Part C, record it on the Stress Profile Summary Chart.

This section also pinpoints the time of day that the client is most stressed and what factors are contributing to it. Record the client's top three rank-ordered stressors, his or her response to three lifestyle or behavioral changes that would help him or her, and his or her ideas for coping with or eliminating their stress. Chapter 12 offers suggestions to help clients cope with behavioral issues uncovered by the tests. Record all pertinent information from Section 1, Part C on the summary chart.

Section 2, Part A gives an in-depth look at the client's posture. A normal response is great and does not go on the summary chart because the client does not need to work on that area. However, all the areas of the body where the client demonstrates a mild, moderate, or severe deviation or an imbalance in inches should be noted on the summary chart. Section 2, Part B puts the client through a flexibility analysis to determine any muscular imbalances that can be contributing to atypical posture, pain, and discomfort and should be added to a treatment program. Record the imbalances on the summary chart.

In Section 2, Part C the therapist uses his or her palpation skills to feel and examine the client's body, searching for the painful **hypertonic** areas that must be treated. Record each area of the body that is painful when pressed with gentle to moderate pressure and then have the client rate its severity on a 1–10 scale. Also note those points that radiate pain when pressed and where the pain radiates.

Part D checks the client's lung capacity and breathing mechanics. The following pattern is considered normal on this test: The inhalation lasts at least 6 seconds, and the exhalation lasts at least 2 seconds longer than the inhalation, or at least 8 seconds. The shoulders do not move during inhalation or exhalation. The breath in begins when the diaphragm flattens and either the abdomen pushes forward or the lower rib cage widens in the lateral direction. The lower, middle, and upper ribs separate as the inhaled air progresses by filling the bottom; middle; and, finally, the upper lobes of the lungs. The client's breathing should feel deep, relaxed, and coordinated. Record the client's results on the summary chart.

USING THE DATA TO CREATE A STRESS REDUCTION PLAN

Now that the client's stress profile has been developed, it's time to use the information to develop a personal stress reduction program. Before beginning, however, the therapist should research medical diagnoses that he or she is unfamiliar with in a **pathology** book or a medical dictionary to determine if he or she is qualified to work on this client. If the therapist does not understand a condition or medical problem, he or she should ask a mentor or the client's primary care physician if massage is indicated. When in doubt, refer out.

When satisfied that to the best of your knowledge you will do no harm to this client, simply match each of the client's problems with the specific massage and stress reduction techniques provided in the rest of this book to create the client's personal stress management plan. Remember that all treatment sessions should be recorded on chart records using the SOAP (*Subjective, Objective, Assessment, Plan*) format. Appendix 7 offers a brief review of SOAP note charting. Appendix 8 offers a sample of a blank SOAP note form and an example of a completed SOAP note form.

The anti-stress plan should address pain control first because pain can seriously detract from the quality of a person's life and may significantly influence many other stress symptoms. Eliminating pain may require the use of ice or heat, trigger point work, postural realignment and kinesthetic awareness training, muscle tension reduction, deep relaxation, proper breathing, aerobic exercise, stretching and strengthening of imbalanced musculature, positional release, gross or specific myofascial release, self-massage, or something as simple as buying a new mattress or neck pillow or removing a wallet from a back pocket when driving. In addition to massage, it may be necessary to include other elements in a stress management program, such as breathing training; aerobic exercise; core strengthening; flexibility training; dietary changes, such as less caffeine, eating more roughage, and balancing intake with expenditure; postural realignment; deep relaxation; sleep improvement; pain control; and time management skills. The therapist must remember that all of the parts make up the whole person and an effective stress reduction plan is a comprehensive plan that encompasses every aspect of a client's life. Clients must realize from the start that no wonder drug can eliminate their stress and no person can do it for them. The therapist lays out a plan for the client, which requires a series of treatments over a 10-week period. Each treatment may use different strokes and techniques and require the client to perform different exercises or other homework. The client and therapist are a team working together with a common goal. The therapist must adapt treatments as the client's condition changes. Clients must be ready to make changes in their habits and lifestyle and accept the ultimate responsibility for their health and for reducing their stress. To be successful, it is necessary that clients make the indicated changes in their behavior and lifestyle, take responsibility for their actions, and improve their self-discipline. They must be encouraged to actively work at changing the elements of their lives contributing to their negative stress, or the painful consequences will happen just as sure as the sun sets each day.

After each massage session the therapist must assign homework or self-help tips for the client to practice between treatments. Try to limit instructions to only three new activities each week because any more may create more stress and confusion for the client. Each exercise will help the client build a strong foundation for coping with stress. All activities instructed must be practiced for the entire program. The following homework examples may be inappropriate for your client and are offered as examples only. At the end of the first treatment instruct each client in exercises to help them reduce their forward head, round shoulders, and tight hip flexor muscles; provide them some basic dietary tips, such as eliminating caffeine or eating more vegetables; and show them how to safely use heat or ice to reduce their pain at home. During the next treatment, follow up by asking them how their homework went. Tell them to keep practicing those activities and then instruct them in diaphragmatic breathing exercises, kinesthetic awareness training, and deep-relaxation instruction to add to their repertoire. At the third week, discuss the benefits of walking and show the client some self-massage techniques. For the fourth week's homework, have the client develop a weekly schedule on paper that shows when they have scheduled time to practice their healthy activities (stretching, self-massage, walking, or deep relaxation) and when they are taking time for themselves and their family. Creating and implementing this type of weekly stress reduction schedule is highly recommended homework for all stress reduction clients. For the fifth week's homework, have the client set three realistic and attainable short-term and long-term goals and discuss strategies of how they plan to achieve them.

The therapist must tailor the stress reduction program and homework assignments to the specific needs of the client. The client must implement the plan, and the therapist should reinforce when clients positively change any of their behaviors that contribute to their stress. The massage therapist must guide the client on the path to health and balance in his or her life through education, encouragement, and treatments to relax and rebalance them. The client must stick to the plan, and he or she will enjoy the benefits of a healthier, less stressful life.

SUMMARY

Before we move on to the next chapter to start learning specific techniques to help your clients overcome stress, let's review the following key concepts:

- Use the Stress Profile Summary Chart to condense the pertinent data from the client's PSI, Stress Log, and medical/health history form.

- Design a stress reduction treatment plan according to your client's particular needs.

- Document all treatments using the SOAP charting format.

- Ensure that clients take an active role in their stress reduction programs.

- Give the client simple homework assignments after each treatment and follow up at the next session.

- As the client's condition changes, ensure treatment sessions evolve accordingly.

- Reinforce positive behavioral changes made by the client.

Breathing for Relaxation

The first component to consider adding to your client's stress reduction treatment and training program is proper breathing techniques. In the book *Science of Breath,* Swami Rama reinforced the importance of proper breathing when he stated, "If there is a correspondence between personality type and pattern of breathing, then the yogi states categorically that by changing the pattern of breathing we can transform the personality, for when the mind is disturbed, the breath is disturbed and becomes shallow, rapid and uneven. By consciously making the breath deep, even, and regular, we will experience a notable release of tension and an increased sense of relaxation and tranquility" (Rama, 2005:84). Breathing is the key to relaxation. If clients can learn to control their breathing, then they can relax any time and place that they desire. This chapter will review the anatomy involved in the breathing process, the mechanics of breathing, common breathing faults, and breathing exercises to improve coordination and tempo. In addition, the relationship between breathing and posture, how to use focused breathing as a relaxation tool, and massage techniques to help your client breathe easier will be outlined.

BREATHING IS LIFE AND THE KEY TO RELAXATION

Breathing is essential for life. From the moment we are born until we die every cell in our body requires a constant supply of oxygen and the removal of excess carbon dioxide, the byproduct of cellular metabolism. Unfortunately, many people lack control over their breathing, and they breathe incorrectly because of skeletal abnormalities, emotional distress, obesity, or simply bad habits. Generally, we breathe without thinking about technique or how it affects our lives, but breathing can have a profound impact on our health. Breathing is both a voluntary and involuntary process that can be consciously modified through training.

Guiding our clients to focus on their breathing, slow it down, use proper mechanics, and eliminate unnecessary muscular activity can have an extreme impact on relieving the physical manifestations of stress. For optimal health, it's essential that clients learn to balance and control their breathing because imbalances can lead to a variety of physical problems, such as pains in the neck, shoulders, back, and chest; insomnia; poor circulation; hypertension; headaches; anxiety; and panic attacks. Everyone can benefit from the routine practice of breathing exercises.

Depending on a person's level of activity and respiratory system health, humans breathe 12–20 times a minute, which translates to 17,280–28,800 times each day. When a person is calm, his or her breathing is slow, deep, smooth, and relaxed. The breathing style demonstrated by many highly stressed individuals resembles panting or gasping for air. The stressed-out individual's breathing is quick and shallow and uses mostly the middle and upper rib cage and the upper lobes of the lungs. This method of breathing is very inefficient because the rib cage alone does not expand enough to fulfill all the body's needs for oxygen and the removal of carbon dioxide. Combining this inefficient breathing with forward head and round shoulders will further restrict expansion of the ribs and may recruit contraction of accessory breathing muscles, which can lead to muscle tension and pain. This sort of breathing may alter the body's normal blood gas levels, which can lead to agitation, dizziness, anxiety, fatigue, and cloudy thinking.

THE ANATOMY OF RESPIRATION

In the book *Muscles: Testing and Function*, the authors list the primary muscles of respiration as the diaphragm, the intercostals, and the abdominals (Kendal, McCreary, and Provance, 2005). The diaphragm initiates **inspiration** and **expiration;** portions of the external and internal intercostals assist with inspiration, and some branches assist with expiration. The lower abdominals, particularly those with slight or no trunk flexion function, are the chief muscles called on to force air out when oxygen demands are increased. The accessory muscles are the scalenes, sternocleidomastoid

(SCM), serratus anterior, pectoralis major and minor, upper trapezius, latissimus dorsi thoracic erector spinae, iliocostalis lumborum, quadratus lumborum, serratus posterior superior and inferior, levatores costarum, transverses thoracis, and the subclavius (Kendal, McCreary, and Provance, 2005). Recruitment of these accessory muscles as a result of pulmonary disease, obesity, poor posture, lack of fitness, and improper breathing mechanics can lead to pain and discomfort from the head to the pelvis. Massage treatments for clients who breathe improperly should check for hypertonicities in each of these muscles and stretch or relax them as indicated. Let's help our clients eliminate this preventable pain, fear, and anxiety through our massage treatments and by instructing them to breathe using proper mechanics.

THE MECHANICS OF PROPER BREATHING

Proper breathing is a smooth, coordinated progression of movements that starts in the dome- or parachute-shaped diaphragm muscle, the principal muscle of respiration. The diaphragm is located at the base of the rib cage, where it separates the thoracic and abdominal cavities. The diaphragm has numerous bony attachments. The anterior attachments include the posterior aspect of the xiphoid process of the sternum and the seventh through twelfth ribs and the costal cartilage of those ribs. The posterior attachments include the twelfth ribs and upper lumbar vertebrae. During inhalation, the diaphragm flattens, allowing more room for the lower lobes of the lungs to expand downward in the chest cavity. This increase in thoracic volume created when the diaphragm flattens decreases the air pressure in the lungs. The higher-pressure atmospheric air readily flows in, filling the lungs to equalize the pressure. Simultaneously, the abdominal area just above the belly button pushes out and the lower ribs spread laterally. The inhalation then progresses from the bottom to the middle of the chest as the middle part of the rib cage expands. Finally, the inhalation ends when the upper ribs elevate and separate, allowing the top of the lungs to expand and fill. The shoulders should remain stationary throughout the entire breathing cycle. Figure 4.1 outlines the action of the diaphragm and ribs during inhalation and exhalation.

During a normal exhalation, the diaphragm relaxes and resumes its normal dome shape, reducing the volume and increasing the pressure in the thoracic cavity, which passively forces air out.

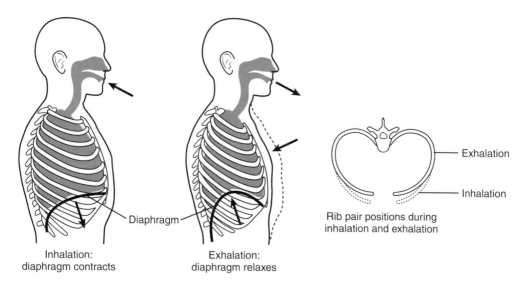

Inhalation:
diaphragm contracts

Exhalation:
diaphragm relaxes

Diaphragm

Exhalation

Inhalation

Rib pair positions during
inhalation and exhalation

Figure 4.1

Action of the diaphragm and ribs during inhalation and exhalation (adapted from Sebel, 1985)

The relaxation and elastic recoil of the lungs, abdominals, and rib muscles also passively force air out. The abdominals (rectus abdominis, external and internal obliques, and the transverse abdominis), the quadratus lumborum, and the latissimus dorsi can be called on to assist with forced exhalation during periods of exertion. These muscles can also be voluntarily contracted to help an individual experiencing the respiratory panic induced by an asthmatic attack make more room for air in the lungs and relieve distress.

COMMON BREATHING FAULTS

Many clients fall into one of the following patterns of improper breathing. Increasing clients' awareness of their specific breathing faults and empowering them with proper breathing technique will allow them to adjust their breathing pattern to prevent pain and tension.

Shallow, Rapid Breathing

Shallow and rapid breathing, which uses only the upper and middle chest, can lead to pains in the upper chest musculature, an inadequate supply of oxygen, and a decrease in the body's normal carbon dioxide level. This type of breathing is less efficient and requires the heart and lungs to work harder and the body to burn more energy than slow, deep, diaphragmatic breathing. In extreme cases, this type of breathing can lead to hyperventilation, black-outs, and a change in the body's normal pH. Help the client learn to breathe more diaphragmatically, relax tight muscles, and slow down and take more complete full breaths.

Elevating the Clavicles and Shoulders

Unless you are running or performing another demanding aerobic activity, shoulder action is not needed to breathe properly. Elevating the shoulders and clavicles during respiration can lead to headaches and pains in the neck, shoulders, and upper back. We need to help clients eliminate all unnecessary muscular activity. Massage treatments should help clients eliminate unnecessary contraction of their scalenes, SCM, levator scapulae, and upper trapezius while breathing.

Inhalation Longer Than Exhalation

Inhalations that are longer than exhalations can lead to overinflated lungs and breathing distress on mild exertion. Training a client to exhale for 2 seconds longer than they inhale will slow their breathing and help relieve this problem.

Poor Posture and Skeletal Deformities Can Impair Breathing

Kyphosis and severe **scoliosis** may prevent the chest cavity from fully expanding, which inhibits the client's ability to take complete breaths. Severe forward head can also alter an individual's breathing mechanics. Massage treatments should help clients improve their **kinesthetic awareness** of their posture and rebalance their musculature. Therapists should also stretch out clients' shortened rib cage muscles and instruct them to breathe properly while in proper postural alignment. Seated work on the edge of the table with the clients' feet on a footrest will best accomplish this task.

Paradoxical Breathing

Paradoxical breathing occurs when a client expands his or her chest while simultaneously contracting his or her abdominals. This can occur when a client is startled, is surprised, or is merely attempting to look good. Have you ever been watching a thrilling movie at the theater and heard the whole audience gasp when the villain jumps out of the dark and attacks the hero? Have you ever seen an ex-athlete on the beach lifting his chest up and sucking in his protruding abdomen when a pretty girl passes by? These are examples of paradoxical breathing. In paradoxical breathing, the diaphragm is essentially pulling back up into the chest cavity, forcing air out of the lungs and shrinking the size of the chest cavity (Rama, 2005). This is an inefficient way to breathe. Clients must be instructed to let their diaphragm flatten and allow the lower abdomen to push out when they begin to take air in so that they can use their entire chest capacity.

Sleep Apnea

Sleep apnea occurs when a sleeping person's airway temporarily shuts down and he or she stops breathing for up to 60 seconds at a time. Snoring and constant fatigue are associated with this disorder. This topic will be addressed in more detail in Chapter 9.

BREATHING TIPS

Whenever possible, inhale through the nose because the nose adjusts the temperature and adds moisture to the air inhaled. Also, the mucus and hair in the nasal membranes filter out dust and microbes so that clean air passes to the lungs. In addition, by using your nostrils to meter your breath, like the air vents on an airplane, you will gain greater control over your respiration.

If your nose is frequently blocked, use a saline nose solution to help clear it. A great product is the NeilMed sinus rinse, which is a modern way of doing an Indian practice called **neti** or nasal wash. Never use over-the-counter nasal spray products because, although they may temporarily provide relief, the mucus membranes will soon rebound and swell up and the nasal passages will block up more than they were originally.

Water exercises are great for people with breathing difficulties. The hydrostatic pressure of the water compresses the chest and ribs and helps a person get a more complete exhalation. The resistance of the water also improves circulation and helps strengthen the diaphragm and the muscles that assist inspiration. You don't even have to swim because you can get great results from walking in the water or deep water running.

DEEP BREATHING EXERCISES

The following exercises will help improve your clients' breathing mechanics, tempo, and control. Work with your clients to help them master these techniques. Have the client practice them as homework between treatments while listening to soft music and silently repeating the following passive suggestions:

My neck and chest muscles feel totally relaxed.

My shoulders and arms feel warm and heavy.

I feel limp and loose, relaxed and comfortable.

My body feels limp like a rag doll.

I feel quiet and warm.

My mind and body are completely relaxed.

 EXERCISE 1

Breathe in for 4 seconds (or longer) through the nose, and then exhale for 6 seconds (or longer) through the nose. Repeat three times. As clients progress have them increase the time of their inhalation and exhalation. Always remember to exhale longer than inhaling.

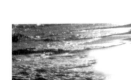 **EXERCISE 2**

Inhale 4 seconds through the nose and exhale 6 seconds through the mouth, either through pursed lips or by making a hissing, buzzing, or humming sound. Repeat three times. To progress, increase the times.

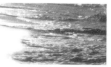

EXERCISE 3

Inhale 4 seconds through the nose, hold the breath for 4 seconds, and then exhale as slowly as you can for at least 6 seconds. This pause in breathing helps the client relax his or her mind and body. Progressively increase the length of time of the inhalation and the exhalation.

EXERCISE 4

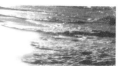

If your nose is clogged, use a sinus rinse before performing this alternate nostril breathing exercise. To begin, exhale completely and then take a slow, full inhalation through your nose. When your inhalation is complete, close off the right nostril with the tip of your right thumb and then slowly exhale through the left nostril. This is followed by an inhalation through the left nostril. When your exhalation is complete, press the left nostril with the right index finger, remove your right thumb from the right nostril, and exhale through the right nostril while blocking the left nostril. Repeat three times for each nostril. To progress, relax your mind and focus all of your awareness on your breathing.

EXERCISE 5

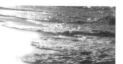

With the client's chin tucked down and the head brought back into proper postural alignment, instruct the client to inhale for 4 seconds through the nose while you grasp your client's upper arms and raise his or her shoulders up and back. Then instruct the client to exhale for 6 seconds while he or she lets the shoulders sink slowly down. This helps the client learn to relax tight levator scapulae and upper trapezius muscles. It also helps stretch out the chest musculature. This can be performed standing, kneeling, or sitting.

EXERCISE 6

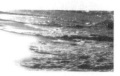

While standing in the anatomical position, have clients take a long, slow, complete inhalation while slowly abducting their shoulders and raising their arms above their head. Their inhalation should last until their hands touch above their heads. Then they should exhale and slowly lower their arms, metering their exhalation so it lasts until their arms return to the anatomical position.

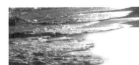

EXERCISE 7

This exercise is performed with the client seated on the edge of the table with his or her feet on a footstool, or the client can be sitting in a chair. The massage therapist is kneeling on the table behind the client or standing behind the client in a chair. Have clients clasp their hands and place them with the palms on the back of their heads. The therapist places his or her hip gently in the client's back and then reaches over the client and grasps his or her upper arms. The therapist then gently raises the client's arms first in a superior direction and then back in a posterior direction. Instruct the client to relax, breathe diaphragmatically, and gently squeeze his or her scapulae together. If the client is comfortable, hold this stretch for 20 seconds and release. This will open up the chest, which will help the client take more complete breaths.

EXERCISE 8

For clients who have difficulty activating their diaphragms, have them lie on their backs on your table and place a book, a light ankle weight, or one of their hands on their diaphragm. Instruct them to elevate the object when they inhale and let it fall naturally when they exhale.

BREATHING AS A RELAXATION TOOL

Mastering focused breathing is a giant step toward learning how to successfully cope with stress and tension. Focused breathing unlocks an innate natural relaxation mechanism that exactly reverses the damaging physiological changes to the body caused by prolonged, unchecked stress. Focused breathing, in particular, helps calm the mind and body, reduces muscle tension and blood pressure, and counteracts dangerous chemical and hormonal changes brought on by stress.

The following breathing exercises develop the proper technique of slow, steady, smooth, relaxed, controlled breathing. To instruct the client in these breathing exercises, the room must be quiet and warm. Use bolsters and pillows to make the client comfortable on your table. Soft music and indirect lighting are also helpful.

FOCUSED BREATHING EXERCISES

Once the client is comfortable with deep breathing, you can progress to the focused breathing techniques. These advanced breathing techniques induce deep relaxation by having the client concentrate on the breathing process itself. The total concentration in these exercises helps them to relax and relieve their stresses because it forces them to stop thinking about their problems. Constantly dwelling on negative thoughts and worries, even when supposedly relaxing, is a major plague of the highly stressed. If your client has these kinds of destructive thought patterns, focused breathing techniques will help them break them and deeply relax at will. Record these instructions or read them out loud to the client with soft, relaxing background music. Speak slowly and evenly.

Focused Breathing Session 1

Instruct clients to passively allow themselves to relax when they listen to the following focused breathing instructions. Relaxation is a passive skill that requires no effort; they should not try forcing themselves to relax. To begin, say the following to your client:

> Take a long, slow, deep, relaxing, complete breath in through the nose, and when you are ready exhale as slowly and fully as you possibly can through your nose. Place all of your conscious awareness on your breathing, turn off all unnecessary thoughts, tune out all distracting noises, and silence your internal voice. Continue to breathe slowly, smoothly, and quietly. In your mind, picture fresh, clean, oxygen-rich air flowing through your nose and passing through your throat and chest until it reaches your lungs. Picture and feel your lungs expanding to their maximum and then emptying totally, like large pink balloons filling completely and then collapsing totally when empty. When you inhale, feel your belly button push out and your lower ribs separate. Feel your breath filling the bottom, the middle, and finally the top of your lungs, as your rib cage gently expands. When you exhale, feel all the muscles in your body from the top of your head to the tips of your toes totally relax. Let all of

your breath passively flow out of your lungs. Feel loose and limp, warm and heavy, and deeply, deeply relaxed. Now, think of nothing but the movement of air within yourself. Remember that each breath is nourishing your entire body with fresh oxygen-rich blood and each exhalation is cleansing your body. If your thoughts stray from your breathing, bring them back and focus your entire awareness on your breathing. (Pause for 10–15 seconds.)

Continue to concentrate on your breathing while passively relaxing all the muscles of your scalp, forehead, face, and jaw. (Pause for 10–15 seconds.)

Slow your breathing and feel this wave of relaxation spreading down to the muscles of the front of your neck, the sides of your neck, and the back of your neck and shoulders where so much tension accrues. Let each exhalation melt your muscles even more as this wonderful feeling of relaxation spreads down to all the muscles of your chest and abdomen. Your breathing is slow and full and very efficient. You feel calm and peaceful. Focus all of your awareness on your breathing until you hear my voice again.

At this point, let the music play for 5–10 minutes without speaking, and then say to your client:

When I count to 3, you will open your eyes and feel much better than you did before. Your heart rate is slower, your blood pressure is reduced, your eye muscles are relaxed, and your ability to use oxygen is improved. When you open your eyes you will feel totally relaxed and refreshed. One, two, three; eyes open.

Focused Breathing Session 2

Instruct the client to passively relax as you read them the following focused breathing script.

To begin, take a long, slow, deep complete breath through your nose, filling your lungs to capacity. Hold the breath briefly and when you are ready, exhale through your nose as slowly and fully as you possibly can. Repeat this breathing three times. Continue this relaxed breathing and focus all of your awareness on it. Now count your breaths from 1 to 10. When you reach 10, count back down to 1. If you lose count, don't worry; simply return to the number 1 and start again. Focus all of your thoughts on your breathing, and relax.

Now focus your concentration on a point an inch below your navel. Feel it rise with each inhalation and fall with each exhalation. Feel gravity pulling your body down. Let all the weight of your body go, giving in to the force of gravity. Your arms and hands feel warm, heavy, and deeply relaxed. Your legs and feet feel warm, heavy, and deeply relaxed. Feel your entire body totally relax more and more with each breath and each rise and fall of this point on your abdomen. Silently pause for 5 minutes.

Now let your thoughts drift to your perfect place of relaxation. It could be a mountain, the ocean, the desert, the forest, or wherever you are most relaxed and peaceful; let your thoughts flow freely there. Silently pause for 2 minutes.

When I count to 3, you'll open your eyes and feel much better than before. When you open your eyes, you will still be totally relaxed but awake and alert so that you can enjoy this wonderful feeling of total relaxation for the rest of the day. One, two, three; eyes open.

MASSAGE TREATMENTS TO HELP A CLIENT BREATHE EASIER

Here are some basic tips for helping your client breath easier by combining breathing instruction and the application of massage strokes. An in-depth stress-reducing massage sequence of strokes and timing will be addressed later in the book, after all the elements that comprise a stress reduction massage treatment are covered.

In the Personal Stress Inventory you have recorded each client's length of inhalation and exhalation, the action of their diaphragm, whether they are using the lower lobes of their lungs, their overall coordination and control, whether they are tensing accessory muscles, and how many breaths they take per minute. Fourteen breaths per minute is considered the normal rate of respiration for adults (Sebel et al., 1985). The first goals of a stress reduction treatment program are to slow down clients' rate of respiration and to improve their breathing mechanics so that they are breathing more diaphragmatically and efficiently without unnecessary muscular activity.

Have clients relax and focus their awareness on their breathing while you are working. Have them slow their rate of respiration, and instruct them to always practice proper breathing mechanics. Pay close attention to the clients' breathing at all times, and, if possible, try to coordinate your breathing with theirs. This will help you tune in to their body more, which will help you know when to instruct them to breathe or to slow down their breathing. The clients should breathe and relax when you are pressing uncomfortable points; holding the breath is not allowed because this will inhibit the flow of oxygen and the removal of waste. Instruct them to breathe through these points and to use the warmth of your hand as biofeedback to pinpoint these hypertonic areas so they can consciously help them melt away.

Every muscle fiber in the body needs oxygen, nutrients, and the removal of waste products; therefore, begin your treatment with circulation-improving strokes and progress to some light friction. Deep pressure is not needed for this type of treatment. Start the client prone, unless the client does not like having his or her face in the face cradle, in which case start him or her sidelying. After about 20 minutes prone, progress to the supine position and finish with a few minutes of seated work for breathing instruction and postural realignment.

In the course of the massage, address all of the primary and accessory muscles of respiration, remembering to spend more time working on all the palpable muscles that attach and have influence on the sternum, clavicle, ribs, and scapulae. In the prone or sidelying positions, remember to seek out and try to disperse all areas of hypertonicity along the base of the skull, the SCM, the upper trapezius, levator scapula, serratus anterior and serratus posterior, the thoracic erector spinae, and latissimus dorsi.

In the supine position assess the diaphragm, intercostals, abdominals, scalenes, SCM, subclavius, and pectoralis major and minor. You should also massage where the ribs meet the sternum and the tips of the ribs and perform the anterior thoracic and diaphragm releases. Perform gentle gliding strokes and gentle friction in between all the ribs both prone and supine. Figures 4.2 through 4.8 illustrate some techniques for working on the intercostals, the rib

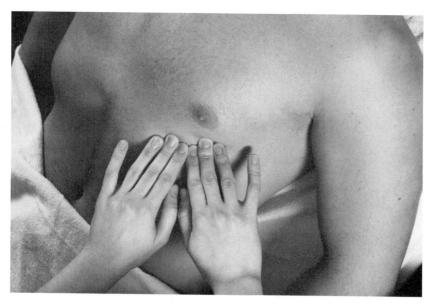

Figure 4.2

Massage to the intercostals

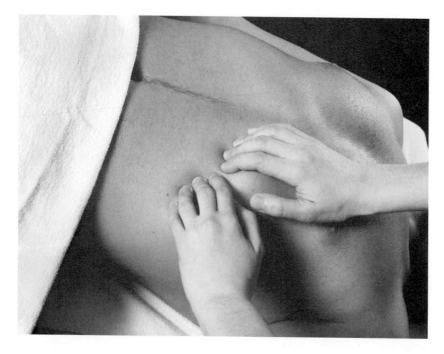

Figure 4.3

Massage to the rib tips

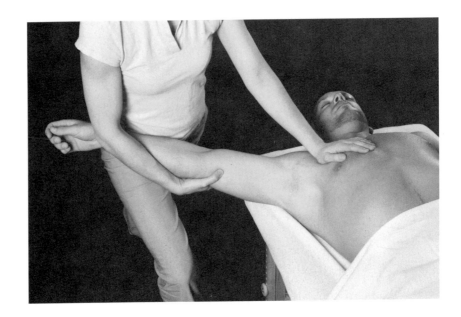

Figure 4.4

Massage to pectoralis major

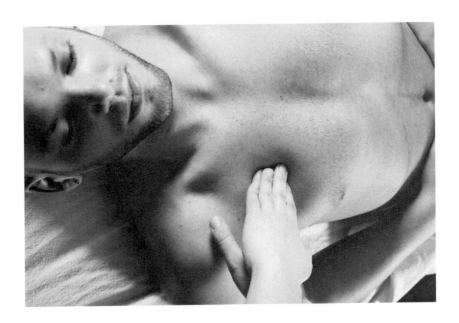

Figure 4.5

Massage to pectoralis minor

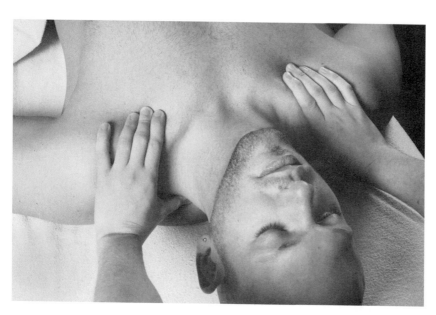

Figure 4.6

Massage inferior to the clavicle

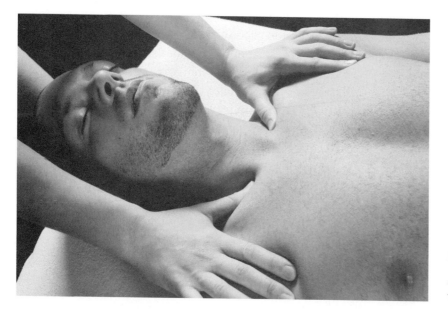

Figure 4.7

Massage just behind the clavicle

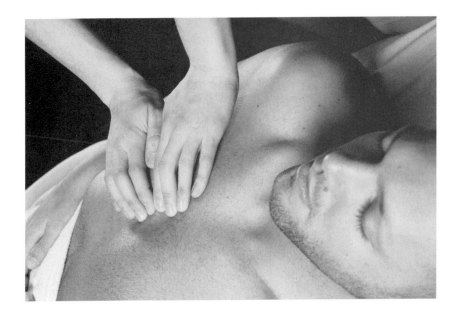

Figure 4.8

Massage along the sternum

tips, the pectoralis major and minor, and inferior to and just behind the clavicle and by the sternum. The therapist can also use gravity, pillows, and bolsters to help stretch out and relax tight musculature.

Gliding strokes, gentle friction, and positional release techniques are effective in releasing tension in the scalenes and SCM. Figures 4.9 and 4.10 illustrate positional release techniques for these muscles.

The anterior thoracic release is performed in the supine position. One hand is placed under the client, on the upper thoracic vertebra, over the spine with the metacarpal phalangeal joints, placed under the spinous processes of the vertebrae. The top hand is placed at the junction of the sternum and clavicle. While holding this spot, project warmth and caring from your hand and instruct the client to slow his or her breathing, relax the muscles, and let all the tension float away. Figure 4.11 demonstrates the hand positions for the thoracic release.

The diaphragm release is also performed in the supine position. Place one hand under the client by the junction of the lower thoracic and upper lumbar vertebrae over the spine with the metacarpal phalangeal joint placed under the spinous processes of the vertebrae. Place the other hand just below the xiphoid process. While holding this spot, project warmth and caring from your hand and instruct the client to slow his or her breathing, relax the

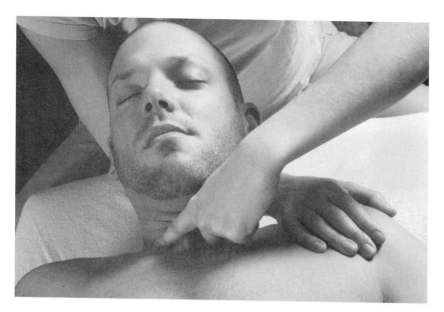

Figure 4.9

Positional release techniques for the scalenes

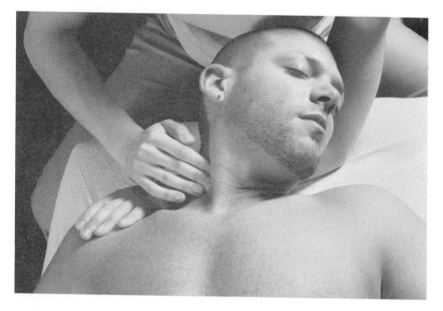

Figure 4.10

Positional release techniques for the sternocleidomastoid (SCM)

muscles, and let thoughts grow peaceful. When performing this release, it is essential that you tune in to the client's breathing. Let your hand rise with each inhalation, and when exhaling apply gentle pressure toward the client's back. Figures 4.12 and 4.13 demonstrate the hand positions for the diaphragm release.

When you have finished addressing all of the client's needs in the supine position, the next step is to work on the client seated.

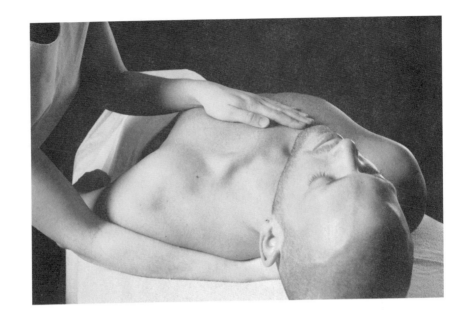

Figure 4.11

Thoracic release, top
and bottom hand
position

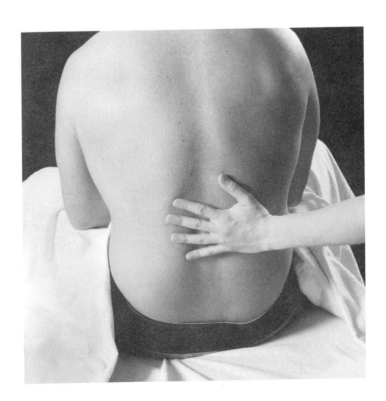

Figure 4.12

Diaphragm release,
bottom hand position

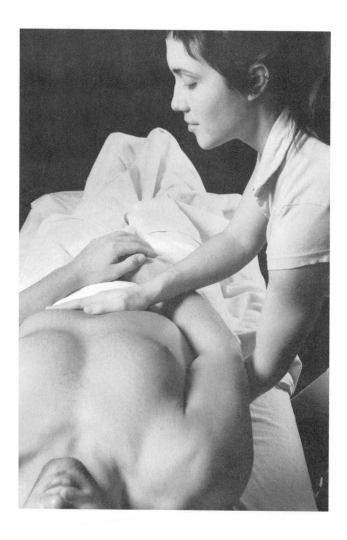

Figure 4.13

Diaphragm release, top hand position

The seated position is used to conclude this treatment because it gives you a chance to check and correct the client's posture and breathing mechanics. The client is placed on the side edge of the table with his or her feet on a footrest; don't just let the legs dangle because this may tighten up the hip flexor muscles that you have just relaxed. Make sure that your client is wearing a bathing suit or is properly draped so that he or she can relax during this portion of the treatment. You can simply use a clothespin to hold the sheet in place so the client can relax more. The proper position for seated work is demonstrated in Figure 4.14.

The next step is to have clients lower their chin toward their chest and bring their head and shoulders gently back so that the

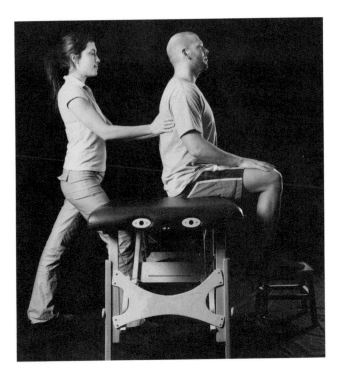

Figure 4.14

Seated work

lobe of the ears lines up with the acromion processes of the scapulae. We will discuss postural realignment and kinesthetic awareness training in more detail in the following chapter. Try to encourage clients to keep their chins down and not let their eyes point up because this will contribute to tight suboccipital muscles. This is a good time to use breathing exercise 5 to relax the levator scapulae and upper trapezius muscles and breathing exercise 7 to stretch out tight pectoralis major muscles.

The next step is to check the client's breathing. Instruct the client to once again bring his or her head and shoulders back into balance. You place your fingertips on each of the client's upper trapezius and then instruct the client to place one hand on his or her diaphragm. Have the client take some deep full breaths and reinforce that, on inhalation, the hand will push out and, on exhalation, it will fall back. You are feeling for shoulder movement when the client is breathing. Have the client relax any unnecessary muscular activity and shoulder movement. Then when you have him or her breathing diaphragmatically with no shoulder motion, instruct the client to simultaneously rebalance the head and neck to find a spot where there is no tension and pain. This is "the position" to try to assume whenever he or she is experiencing neck pain and tension during the day.

Before your client leaves, assign homework and book his or her next appointment. Have the client build a new weekly schedule that incorporates focused breathing practice 3 days a week for 15–20 minutes. Encourage the client to assume "the position" and practice a few breathing exercises every day or whenever he or she feels the stresses and strains of life building up. After the client leaves and the treatment is still fresh in your mind, it will reduce your stress to immediately complete the SOAP (Subjective, Objective, Assessment, Plan) note chart.

SUMMARY

Now that you have started your clients on the path to better breathing, the next components to consider adding to their stress reduction programs are improving their kinesthetic awareness, rebalancing their musculature, and improving their posture. Before we proceed, let's review the following key concepts:

- Breathing control is the key to relaxation.

- Improper breathing mechanics can lead to pain, insomnia, poor circulation, hypertension, headaches, anxiety, and panic attacks.

- During a normal inhalation the diaphragm flattens and the abdominal area just above the umbilicus pushes out as the lower ribs spread laterally and the lower lobes of the lungs fill first. The mid part of the rib cage expands as the breath spreads to the middle of the chest; then the upper ribs elevate and separate as the top part of the lungs expand and fill.

- During a normal exhalation the diaphragm relaxes and resumes its normal dome shape, passively forcing air out. The relaxation and elastic recoil of the lungs, abdominals, and rib cage also passively force air out.

- The abdominals, quadratus lumborum, and the latissimus dorsi can be voluntarily contracted to assist with exhalation. This is particularly useful information for individuals experiencing respiratory distress because of overinflated lungs. They can contract these muscles to force air out and make room for a deep breath.

- Common breathing faults include shallow and rapid breathing using only upper and middle chest, elevating the shoulders and clavicles, inhaling longer than exhaling, paradoxical breathing, and sleep apnea.

- When the Personal Stress Inventory indicates, the client should practice breathing exercises to increase his or her lung capacity and improve overall breath control.

- Exercising in the water improves the circulation and helps strengthen the muscles of respiration.

- Breathing exercises can be combined with active and passive stretching activities.

- Focused breathing combines diaphragmatic breathing with deep relaxation. It should be practiced 3 days a week for 15–20 minutes.

- For clients who have breathing difficulties, address all the primary and secondary muscles of respiration in the course of massage treatments.

- When clients feel the stresses and strains of life building up, they should use "the position" to realign their head, neck, and shoulder posture, combined with a few deep diaphragmatic breaths to help them relax.

- Diaphragmatic breathing can help clients relax any time and any place that they feel stressed.

Improve Posture to Reduce Stress

The next vital component to consider adding to your client's personal stress reduction plan is postural rebalancing. **Posture,** or body alignment, refers to the overall balance of the body and its parts. When the body is in balance, the gravitational stresses and strain on the joints and the soft tissues are minimal, less energy is expended, and movement is more efficient. Maintaining good posture while standing, sitting, and moving protects the body from injuries caused by the impact of gravity. Habitually poor posture, lack of proper exercise, sports injuries, accidents, congenital structural deformities (such as unequal leg length or scoliosis), and a poor kinesthetic sense of what proper carriage feels like can all alter the body's normal balance. Pain, spasm, headaches, dizziness, decreased flexibility, and wear and tear on the joints and bones can all result from the effects of gravity on an asymmetrical body. If your client demonstrates atypical posture and muscular imbalances in Section 2 of the Personal Stress Inventory, then postural realignment exercises are an important addition to his or her personal stress reduction plan. This chapter discusses normal posture, additional assessment tools, commonly seen muscular imbalances, and postural deviations; it also includes the therapeutic exercises to help correct these imbalances.

NORMAL POSTURE

Normal posture refers to the ideal alignment of the body along its axis and throughout all of the joints in the body. Unfortunately, most human bodies do not resemble this norm; in fact, this standard is demonstrated infrequently. To improve our understanding of the balance between skeletal and soft tissues in ideal posture we must first look at some alternative techniques for evaluating it. Figures 5.1 and 5.2 detail an anterior, posterior, and side view of an individual standing in ideal body alignment.

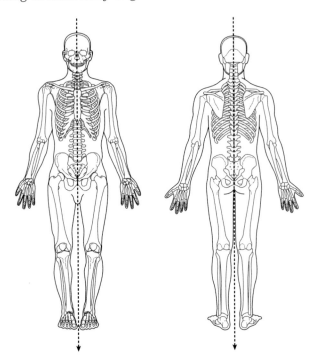

Figure 5.1

Anterior and posterior view of ideal alignment

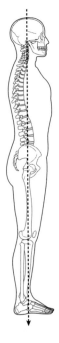

Figure 5.2

Side view of ideal alignment

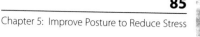

Measuring Deviations from Normal Posture

In the Personal Stress Inventory you were instructed to compare the client's relaxed posture to the pictures in the book. This is a quick way of performing a simple posture analysis and acquiring objective data on clients. Another method of evaluating posture is with a **plumb line** (gravity line) and a posture grid. A string with a weight attached or a professional plumb bob is used to give a stationary point or fixed point of reference on which to base the evaluation. The client's posture is assessed from the front, back, and each side of the body to determine any asymmetries in alignment. The plumb line is always lined up at the feet and is not moved during the analysis because a consistent gravity line provides the most accurate results.

When taking a lateral or coronal view of a plumb line to assess the client's alignment in the sagittal plane, have the weight positioned just in front of the lateral malleolus. This lateral view provides information on the anterior/posterior balance of the body as well as any atypical rotational curves. A body in perfect alignment will have the gravity line run just anterior to the lateral malleolus, posterior to the patella through the knee joint, through the center of the greater trochanter of the femur, through the bodies of the lumbar vertebrae, through the tip of the shoulder (the acromion process of the scapula), and up through the ear (external auditory meatus) to the top of the skull (at the area of the coronal suture). Furthermore, the eyes should be level, the knees should be extended straight (not flexed or hyper-extended), and the pelvis should be in a neutral position when the body is in ideal alignment.

In the anterior/posterior direction, the human body normally has three curves: a cervical lordosis, a thoracic kyphosis, and a lumbar lordosis. A neutral pelvis means that the anterior superior iliac spines (ASIS) are lined up in the same vertical plane as the symphysis pubis and that both ASIS are located on the same horizontal plane (Kendal, McCreary, and Provance, 2005). In many individuals the ASIS and the posterior superior iliac spines (PSIS) line up on a fairly horizontal plane, but because this is not true for everyone, particularly women, this measurement is unreliable. When a gravity line from the ASIS falls anterior to the pubic symphysis, the condition is known as an anterior pelvic tilt. The exaggerated lumbar curve that occurs when the pelvis is tilted anteriorly is a condition known as hyperlordosis. When an individual has hyperlordosis, the hips are flexed, the lumbar spine is hyperextended, and the normal mild lordotic curve is increased. Measuring the angles of vertebral curves is beyond the scope of massage therapy; however, the numbers are included here for information purposes.

Although the numbers may vary for age and sex, in the general population a person considered to have ideal posture will have a cervical region lordosis of 30–35 degrees, a thoracic kyphosis of 40 degrees, and a lumbar lordosis of 40–45 degrees. Figure 5.3 demonstrates how these angles are measured (Neumann, 2002:276). In the lateral view, abnormal rib cage and trunk rotation can also be observed and noted.

Posterior pelvic tilt occurs when on a vertical plane the pubic symphysis is rotated anterior to the ASIS. This posture, known as flat back, is demonstrated by the reduction of the normal lumbar lordosis. In a person with flat back the hips may be extended and the lumbar spine may be flattened. Sway back is another posture associated with posterior pelvic tilt and absence of the normal lumbar lordosis. A person with sway back generally has an exaggerated long thoracic curve and no lumbar curve that brings the upper trunk back into a kyphotic position. The body attempts to compensate for the round

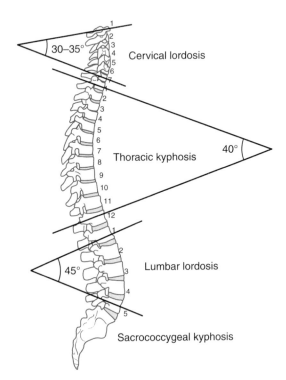

Figure 5.3

Measuring spinal angles

upper back by moving the head forward and hyperextending the hips and knees (Kendal, McCreary, and Provance, 2005).

Continuing up the body, the relationship of the acromion process to the vertical gravity line provides additional information about whether a client has kyphosis or round shoulders. The relationship of the ear lobe to this same vertical line can quickly reveal forward head positioning.

When taking a mid-sagittal view of the client's frontal plane the body is positioned so that the plumb line falls equidistant to the heels and then travels up between the legs and through the middle of the pelvis, the vertebral column, and skull. This view of the front side of the client gives us information on the lateral or side-to-side balance of the body. Normally, the ASIS of both hips are in the same horizontal plane. Lateral pelvic tilt occurs when one ASIS is rotated downward and the opposite hip is higher. A client with ideal lateral posture will have his or her feet straight ahead and not inverted or everted, the patellae will be straight ahead with the knees not knocked or bowed, the ASIS will be on the same horizontal plane, the clavicles and shoulders will be level, and the head will not be tilted.

A sagittal view of the client's dorsum is used to observe the calcaneal (Achilles) tendon angle, PSIS and hip level balance, straightness of the spine, rib cage rotation, shoulder and scapulae positioning, and head tilt. A client with ideal lateral posture viewed from their posterior would demonstrate calcaneus tendons that run in a straight line from the calcaneus to the mid calf, level posterior superior iliac spines and hips, no lateral deviations of their vertebral column or rotation of their rib cage, scapulae that lie flat against their back with no part protruding, level relaxed shoulders, and a level head. Lateral curves of the vertebral column are known as scoliosis. Scoliosis is named according to the convexity. Frequently, the rib cage rotates along with the vertebrae, a factor that may cause pain and inhibit normal breathing mechanics. Different forms of scoliosis are demonstrated and named in Figure 5.4.

A functional scoliosis, resulting from soft-tissue imbalances, will disappear when a client bends forward into trunk flexion. This type of scoliosis responds well to therapeutic exercises and posture training. A structural scoliosis will not disappear when bending forward and is the result of skeletal changes. Although surgery most often is needed to correct structural deformities of the skeleton,

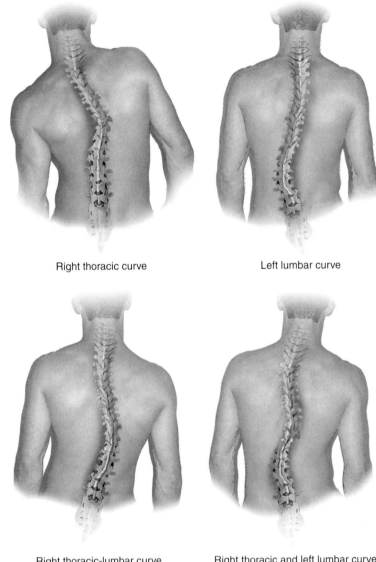

Right thoracic curve

Left lumbar curve

Right thoracic-lumbar curve

Right thoracic and left lumbar curve
(double major curve)

Figure 5.4

Different forms of
scoliosis

exercise and posture training can help relieve the symptoms and prevent the problem from getting worse.

Another way to record posture and flexibility data that is gaining in popularity is to take pretreatment digital photographs of the client and then use a photo draw program to draw in horizontal and vertical lines to assess body balance. These photos can be used to determine deviation from the ideal, to develop programs, and to demonstrate progress to clients when compared to post-treatment photos. This is also an excellent technique to use on a client who does not have the time for the full battery of tests that the Personal Stress Inventory requires. In addition to the aforementioned static tests for posture and body balance, it is important to observe your client's posture when he or she walks and sits because individuals can vary greatly in their alignment during these different activities.

DYNAMIC POSTURE

Observing a client's dynamic posture and body balance while walking provides valuable information on how efficiently clients carry themselves when moving. Walking is the intentional loss and gain of balance during forward progression. Humans use a bipedal reciprocal form of gait, which means that the opposite arm and leg swing forward simultaneously. Walking gait is divided into a series of phases called the swing phase, heel strike, foot flat, mid-stance, heel rise, and toe off.

The swing phase refers to the period of time from toe off to heel strike when one leg is off the ground. If the pelvis drops more than 5 degrees on the unsupported side during the swing phase, it is an indication that the opposite gluteus medius muscle is weak. This exaggerated drop of the pelvis on the unsupported side during unilateral weight bearing is known as a **Trendelenburg sign.**

The heel strike occurs just after the swing phase when the heel makes contact with the ground. After heel strike, the weight shifts to the lateral border of the foot and then to the ball of the foot during foot flat, midstance, and heel rise. Toe off is the final propulsive phase of gait.

Casually observe your client walk as he or she enters your office. Note the position of the feet, knees, pelvis, hips, arms, shoulders, neck, and head. Look for symmetry, smoothness, foot drop with peroneal flip, hip hiking, knee hyperextension, walking up on the toes, limps, and unusual muscular activity.

QUICK BODY SCAN

Another assessment technique for the therapist to experiment with is the 10-minute, toe-to-head, quick body scan. The therapist can gain a great deal of information by performing a visual inspection of the client during the initial meeting. Look at the client's face, checking for forehead and jaw tension, eye position, and neck muscle hyper-tonicities and imbalances. Check to see if the client's breathing is relaxed or if he or she is using inappropriate muscular activity. Then watch the client walk barefoot, looking at the smoothness of gait and how all the joints in the body line up. Finish by checking the client's relaxed standing posture from the front, back, and both sides. Use the following guidelines when performing a quick body scan.

10-Minute Quick Body Scan

1. Have the client walk barefoot and look at the quality and smoothness of movement. Start from the feet and scan up. How does the client's body balance compare to norms?
2. Check the client's arches and feet. Are the arches flat, normal, or high? Are the feet neutral, inverted, or everted? Are the toes out, in, or straight ahead?
3. Are the client's calcaneus tendons straight or medially deviated?
4. Are the patellae straight ahead or rotated medially or laterally? Are the legs (knees) knocked, bowed or straight, flexed or hyperextended?
5. Are the client's ASIS equal or is one rotated and one higher?
6. Is the client's pelvis neutral or tilted anteriorly or posteriorly?
7. Are the client's clavicles and shoulder positions equal?
8. Are the client's scapulae level and symmetrical?
9. Is the tip of the client's shoulders (acromion process) in the vertical gravity line?
10. Is the client's head in balance over the neck and shoulders?
11. Are the client's eyes straight ahead, or are they tilted up?

Now that you have reviewed different ways to assess posture, the next step is to recognize the factors that contribute to it. Understanding the commonly seen skeletal changes and patterns of muscular imbalances that frequently contribute to physical problems will make for more effective treatments.

MUSCLE IMBALANCES

Many postural faults are caused by muscular imbalances—that is, one group of muscles is stronger than its opposing group, which pulls the body out of balance. The concept called tensegrity has been adapted from structural engineering and applied to the human body to describe the essential balance between the bones, muscles, and connective tissues needed for humans to counteract gravity and be functional. The muscles and the **fascia** are the guy wires that support and hold up our framework, much like the steel cables supporting a suspension bridge. Just as a suspension bridge will collapse when its steel cables are overtaxed, our muscles and fascia will break down when the force of gravity is applied to a misaligned skeleton. When the normal balance of the skeleton is altered, pain and tension are produced. From our feet up to our heads, all of our body segments must align. An imbalance in one part of the body affects the bones, muscles, ligaments, and fascia in the rest of the body. The body will compensate for a deviation by seeking an adapted point of balance. These adaptations must be corrected, or physical problems will occur. Using the tensegrity principle, Figure 5.5 depicts a model of a structure in balance and one under stress. Fortunately, the soft tissues are pliable and plastic-like and therefore can be remolded and reshaped through exercise and massage to rebalance the body.

If the muscles and fascia are not rebalanced through exercise, the skeletal system may be permanently altered, causing pain and deformity. Imbalances caused by the soft tissue are called functional, and those that involve the bones are called structural. Structural problems are much harder to resolve than functional problems. Many times the only way to resolve structural problems is through surgery, whereas functional problems respond well to corrective exercises. Poor posture is very common. Many clients unconsciously develop

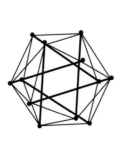

A structure in balance

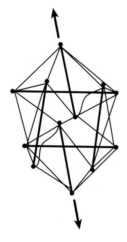

A structure under stress

Figure 5.5

Tensegrity models

bad postural habits because their body alignment is out of the realm of their conscious awareness. Clients need feedback about their postural imbalances to become aware of the problem. They need to be shown the difference between their habitual deviated postural alignment and their realigned, corrected posture. Feedback will allow the client to learn to recognize what proper posture feels like and how to self-correct whenever they feel themselves deviating.

Kinesthesia is a term that refers to conscious proprioception or the internal feeling or sense of how one's body and parts are aligned while standing, sitting, and moving. If we can rebalance our clients' body alignment and reeducate their kinesthetic sense so that they can feel what proper posture feels like, our treatments will have a more lasting impact. It is essential that clients recognize when they are falling back into deviated posture patterns and make a conscious effort at assuming the corrected position.

COMMON POSTURE FAULTS AND MUSCLE IMBALANCES

There is a wide variety of opinion on the muscle imbalances that contribute to the postural faults that will be discussed. The information presented is a synthesis of Janda (1988), Dalton (1998), and Kendal, McCreary, and Provance (2005). Every body is different, so the actual imbalances your client may demonstrate could be slightly different.

Upper and Lower Crossed Syndromes

Vladimir Janda coined the term **"crossed syndromes"** to describe frequently seen combinations of tight and weak muscles that alter the body's normal balance. Tight muscles on the front of the body combine with tight muscles on the posterior to overpower their weak antagonists and alter the normal balance of joints. For example, tight or short pectoralis major and minor combine with tight levator scapulae and upper trapezius muscles to overpower the weak deep neck flexors and lower scapulae stabilizers. When lines are drawn between the tight and weak muscles, they form a cross (Janda, 1988). These body-crossing imbalances occur in the cervical, thoracic, and lumbar region of the body. Figure 5.6 illustrates this concept.

Upper crossed syndrome can contribute to forward head, increased thoracic kyphosis, internal rotation of the humerus,

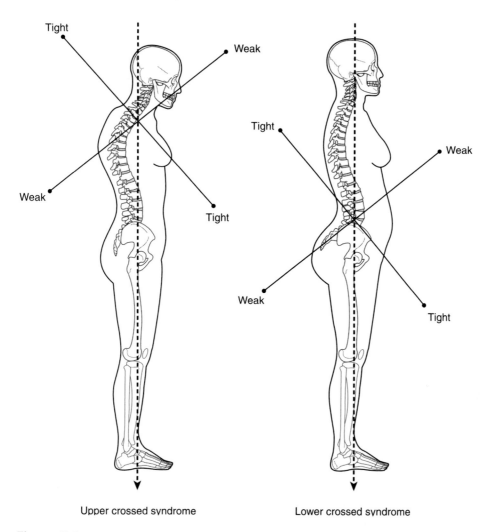

Tight

Weak

Weak

Tight

Tight

Weak

Weak

Tight

Upper crossed syndrome

Lower crossed syndrome

Figure 5.6

Upper and lower crossed syndromes

headaches, rotator cuff impingements, thoracic outlet syndrome, and shoulder instability. Individuals with upper crossed syndrome demonstrate tight upper trapezius, levator scapulae, sternocleidomastoid, scalenes, suboccipitals, and pectoralis major and minor. Their weak muscles are the lower and middle trapezius, rhomboids, serratus anterior, infraspinatus, teres minor, hyoids, and the longus capitis and colli.

Lower crossed syndrome can lead to anterior pelvic tilt, hyperlordosis, hip flexion, knee pain, hamstring pain, and low back pain.

Figure 5.7

Summary of the muscular imbalances in upper and lower crossed syndromes and their associated problems

Upper Crossed Syndrome

Too tight	*Too weak*
Upper Trapezius	Lower and Middle Trapezius
Levator Scapulae	Rhomboids
Sternocleidomastoid	Serratus Anterior
Scalenes	Infraspinatus
Suboccipitals	Teres Minor
Pectoralis Major and Minor	Hyoids
	Longus Capitis and Colli

Associated Problems

Forward Head   Headaches   Shoulder Instability
Increased Thoracic Kyphosis   Rotator Cuff Impingements
Internal Rotation of the   Thoracic Outlet Syndrome
  Humerus

Lower Crossed Syndrome

Too tight	*Too weak*
Iliopsoas	Abdominals
Rectus Femoris	Gluteals
Lumbar Extensors	Vastus Medialis
Hamstrings	Vastus Lateralis
Tensor Fasciae Latae	
Hip Adductors	
Piriformis	
Quadratus Lumborum	

Associated Problems

Anterior Pelvic Tilt   Hyperlordosis   Hip Flexion
Knee Pain   Hamstring Pain   Low Back Pain

Clients with lower crossed syndrome may demonstrate tight iliopsoas, rectus femoris, hamstrings, lumbar extensors, tensor fasciae latae, hip adductors, piriformis, and quadratus lumborum. Their weak muscles may include the abdominals, gluteals, vastus medialis, and vastus lateralis. Figure 5.7 summarizes the muscle imbalances in upper and lower crossed syndrome and their associated problems. Before we discuss exercises to relieve these problems we will discuss postural faults in regard to specific body areas.

Forward Head

> Tight muscles: Sternocleidomastoid, scalenes, suboccipitals, frequently the pectorals, upper trapezius, and levator scapulae are also short.

> Weak muscles: Lower cervical and upper thoracic erector spinae, hyoids, longus capitis, and colli.

See Figure 5.8.

Kyphosis

Tight muscles: Pectoralis major and minor, upper trapezius, and levator scapulae. Also the anterior deltoid, intercostals, and upper abdominals are frequently too tight.

Weak muscles: Lower and middle trapezius, rhomboids, serratus anterior, thoracic erector spinae, infraspinatus, and teres minor.

See Figure 5.9.

Hyperlordosis

Tight muscles: Iliopsoas, rectus femoris, hamstrings, lumbar extensors, tensor fascia latae, hip adductors, piriformis, quadratus lumborum.

Weak muscles: Abdominals, gluteals, vastus medialis and lateralis.

See Figure 5.10.

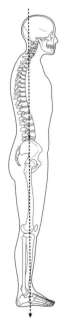

Figure 5.8

Forward head

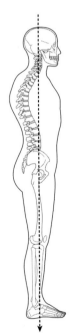

Figure 5.9

Kyphosis

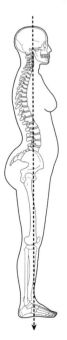

Figure 5.10

Hyperlordosis

Flat Back

Tight muscles: Anterior abdominals, hip extensors, and possibly the hamstrings.

Weak muscles: Iliopsoas and the low back erector spinae.

See Figure 5.11.

Sway Back

Tight muscles: Upper rectus abdominus, upper internal oblique abdominals, gluteals, and hamstrings. At times the intercostals are also tight.

Weak muscles: Iliopsoas, lower abdominals (particularly the external oblique), the upper thoracic extensors, and the deep neck flexors.

See Figure 5.12.

Massage therapists performing stress reduction treatments can greatly assist a client's return to balance by applying massage strokes appropriately, suggesting stretching and strengthening activities,

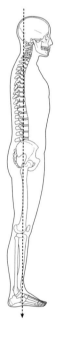
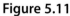

Figure 5.11

Flat back

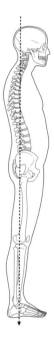

Figure 5.12

Sway back

and improving the client's kinesthetic awareness. By stretching out muscles that are too tight and by strengthening muscles that are too weak, the massage therapist is acting like a structural engineer for the body, shoring the structure to prevent collapse. It is important to note that the **scope of practice** of massage therapy must be adhered to in the area of therapeutic exercise. Some massage therapy programs do not require training in this field, and some states prohibit a massage therapist from recommending exercises. If you have not been properly trained in the application of therapeutic exercises and postural realignment or your state or province, or local jurisdiction prohibits you from making these sort of recommendations to your clients, refer them to a physical therapist, adapted physical education specialist, or a chiropractor when the need arises. If your massage therapy training does not cover therapeutic exercises and postural realignment in its curricula, then it behooves you to take a class in it as part of your continuing education.

MASSAGE AND POSTURAL REEDUCATION

The massage therapist should not do this type of work with a client who has an acute problem (the first 48–72 hours after an accident or injury) and with individuals who have recently had surgery. Whenever you have doubts or questions, refer your clients to a physical therapist, osteopath, chiropractor, or their primary care physician. Talking with a mentor may be useful with specific cases or techniques. Any chronic problems that do not resolve with massage should be referred out to the appropriate professionals. After a client is released from physical therapy or his or her primary care provider approves massage therapy treatments and mild physical conditioning, the techniques outlined in this chapter can be extremely helpful. Remember to err on the side of caution. Always start clients out slowly and gradually build up their strength and endurance.

Massage therapists are in a great position to be posture reeducators. The tests in this book have helped you evaluate your clients' bodies and record their postural faults and muscular imbalances. To rebalance a client's posture, you have to help him or her stretch out tight muscle groups, strengthen weak ones, and then improve awareness or perception of what proper posture feels like. You have to select the appropriate exercises for his or her particular problems. As part of a treatment program, teach the client the appropriate activities for their condition for them to do as homework. Observe them performing

TABLE 5.1

A Quick Guide for Posture Improvement

- Summarize your client's postural faults and muscular imbalances.

- Select the strengthening and stretching exercises appropriate for your client's particular problems from those described in the rest of the chapter.

- Teach your client how to properly perform the designated exercises.

- Observe and correct improper form.

- Modify or adapt exercises and programs according to your client's limitations and progress.

- Have your client add the total body strengthening and stretching exercise program to his or her weekly schedule three days a week.

- Reinforce the need for quick postural realignment and stretching breaks periodically throughout the day.

- Have your client make a conscious effort to be more aware of his or her posture, to correct it when it deviates and to try to keep it correct. This is especially important when sitting, driving, or working in front of a computer for long periods of time.

- Instruct your client that when he or she feels pain in the neck, shoulders, back, or has a headache to check his or her posture, correct it, and to breathe diaphragmatically. As he or she exhales, encourage him or her to relax all the tight muscles.

the activity, and make sure that they are using proper form. If an exercise or activity causes pain and discomfort, modify or eliminate it from the client's program. Have the client add this strengthening and stretching exercise program to his or her weekly schedule 3 days a week. Also encourage clients to take posture realignment and stretching breaks throughout each workday or whenever they feel neck and or shoulder tension, a tension headache, or back pain. Encourage them to remember whenever they feel stressed during the day "the position," outlined in Chapter 4, in which their head is lined up over their neck and shoulders and there is no neck tension, their shoulders are back and relaxed, and they are breathing diaphragmatically. Table 5.1 summarizes the steps on how to incorporate posture training into your stress reduction treatment programs.

Instruct your clients to follow the following rules while performing their homework exercise program. To avoid pain and injury it is vital that they warm up before stretching and cool down and stretch after performing strengthening activities.

General Rules for Performing Therapeutic Exercise

Warmup: Actively moving the major joints through a gentle range of motion 10–20 times will raise the core temperature of the body and prepare the muscles and fascia for action. Of course, massage will also warm up the muscles and fascia. Never stretch without first warming up the area being stretched.

Stretch: Use flexibility techniques to stretch out the tight musculature.

Strengthen: Use strength-building techniques for the client's weak musculature.

Stretch again: Always cool down and stretch after aerobic and strength-development exercises.

TRAINING OPTIONS

The following exercises may be used for musculoskeletal rebalancing during treatments and some taught to clients for use in their personal stress reduction home programs. Using massage strokes combined with active client muscle contraction and movement; active assistive, passive, and manual resistance exercises; and positional release as part of massage treatments will be discussed in subsequent chapters. According to the needs of your client, select from the following training options.

1. The client slowly assumes a stretching posture and gently lets his or her muscles lengthen and relax for 20–90 seconds. The client can also modify the angle of stretch throughout the course of the activity. This option is great for relaxation and for stretching out tight musculature because it helps reeducate the muscle spindles that the lengthened position is the proper position to be in.
2. Gently stretch a muscle for 20 seconds. Then after relaxing for a few seconds refine the angle of the stretch and stretch it again for 20 seconds. Repeat this procedure as many as 4 times.
3. The client moves through an exercise 10–20 times (repetitions), or for a specified time, for 1–3 sets. This helps build strength, tone, flexibility, and endurance. As the client increases his or

her strength and endurance, weights can be used to progressively increase the difficulty.

4. The client contracts one muscle group to stretch its antagonist. When an agonist contracts, it shuts off or reflexively inhibits the contraction of the opposing muscles. This is called reciprocal inhibition. For example, with the leg fully extended bring the toes toward the nose by contracting the tibialis anterior muscle. Actively contracting the tibialis anterior, the agonist for dorsiflexion, will reflexively inhibit the antagonistic muscle, the gastrocnemius, and help stretch out the calf.

5. The client moves actively through the range of motion and then the therapist, or the client, uses manual force to anchor a muscle while he or she stretches in the direction opposite to the tightness. This will help release myofascial restrictions.

6. Clients actively move through the range of motion, and when they reach the end of their range, the therapist applies a few pounds of force in the desired direction for 2 seconds; this is called assisted force. After the 2 seconds of pressure the client returns to the starting position. This can be done in sets of 10, and different angles can be used to effectively stretch the different directions that the muscle fibers run. This system of stretching is known as active isolated stretching or the Mattes method (Mattes, 2000).

7. Applying slight resistance to a movement can relax tight muscles and in many instances improve limited range of motion. The client actively moves a tight joint through its range of motion, and when he or she reaches a sticking point, the therapist manually resists the client's movement for 6 seconds. After a brief pause the client actively attempts to move further through the range. This technique, which can be repeated 3 or 4 times, is called resisted force or muscle energy technique.

8. Contract-relax-antagonist-contract (CRAC) can be used to improve flexibility only after the client has been adequately warmed up. Clients are asked to move a joint actively through their range of motion as far as they comfortably can. When they reach the end of their range of motion they contract the muscle group that they are trying to stretch for 6 seconds against resistance provided by the therapist, an immovable object, or their own hands. Tell the client to just meet your resistance and not to try to overpower you. The contraction and resistance phase is followed by a brief post-isometric contraction 2-second relax-

ation pause, which is then followed by the contraction of the muscle group antagonistic to the one you are trying to stretch. For example, when trying to stretch the hamstrings, position the client supine and instruct him or her to slowly raise the fully extended leg into hip flexion as far as it can comfortably go. Then have the client resist your pressure, contracting the hamstrings for 6 seconds. After the resistance instruct the client to relax for 2 seconds, which is followed by the contraction of the quadriceps to actively move them into increased hip flexion.

SAFE POSTURAL REALIGNMENT, FLEXIBILITY, AND STRENGTHENING EXERCISES

The following exercises are an excellent resource to share with your clients when they need to rebalance their musculature.

Exercises to Safely Improve Neck Flexibility

The following neck exercises will reduce muscle tension and restrictions in movement.

Neck Flexion

Standing, bring the chin back horizontally, then flex the neck and lower the head to the chest to stretch the suboccipital and cervical extensors muscles. A variation is to rotate the neck 45 degrees before flexing. This can also be performed supine. Have the client lie supine, rotate his or her neck 45 degrees, and then actively flex the neck while tucking the chin toward the chest. At the end of the range the therapist assists the stretch with a few pounds of pressure to stretch out the levator scapulae. See Figures 5.13 and 5.14.

Neck Lateral Flexion 1

Relax the shoulders, let them drop toward the ground, and then tilt an ear to the shoulder. Reverse and repeat. See Figure 5.15.

Neck Lateral Flexion 2

While clasping on to a chair or edge of the massage table with one hand, reach over the head with the other hand to gently assist with lateral flexion. See Figure 5.16.

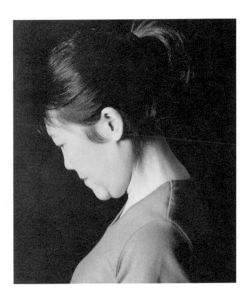

Figure 5.13

Neck flexion

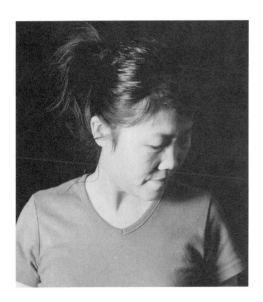

Figure 5.14

Neck flexion with rotation

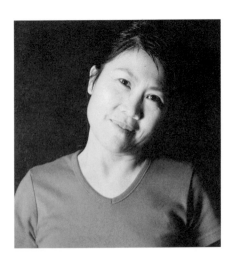

Figure 5.15

Neck lateral flexion 1

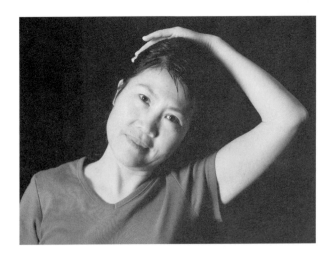

Figure 5.16

Neck lateral flexion 2

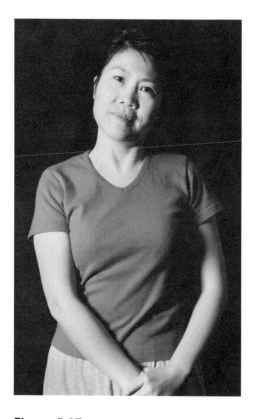

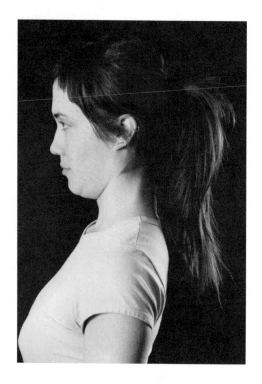

Figure 5.17

Neck lateral flexion 3

Figure 5.18

Chin down, head back

Neck Lateral Flexion 3

Grasp the wrist and pull it down and across the body while laterally flexing the neck to the opposite side of the arm being held. See Figure 5.17.

Exercises to Reduce Forward Head

Use the following exercises to help reduce forward head posture.

Chin Down, Head Back

Tilt the head forward, chin to the chest, and then bring the head back to the vertical gravity line. Position the eyes straight ahead. See Figure 5.18.

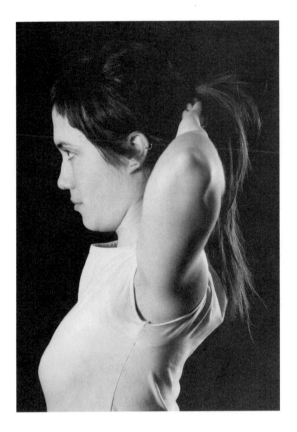

Figure 5.19

Chin down, head back
with resistance

Chin Down, Head Back with Resistance

Bring the head back, keeping the eyes and chin level while placing
the hands behind the head and applying manual resistance. See
Figure 5.19.

Mirror Exercise

Have the client look in the mirror while you help them adjust their
posture in the reverse direction of their deviations. Adjust their eyes
straight ahead to relax their suboccipital muscles. Try to help them
find a spot where they have no neck tension. See Figure 5.20.

Back Against the Wall

Place the back against the wall and flatten the lower back, bring the
shoulders back, and finally bring the head back while keeping the
chin down, eyes level. See Figure 5.21.

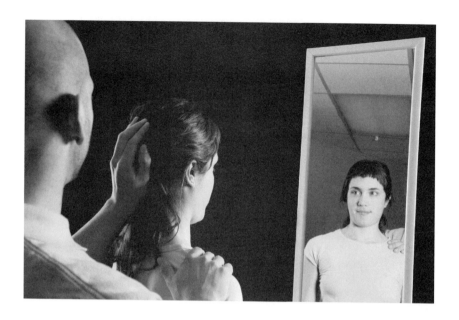

Figure 5.20

Mirror exercise

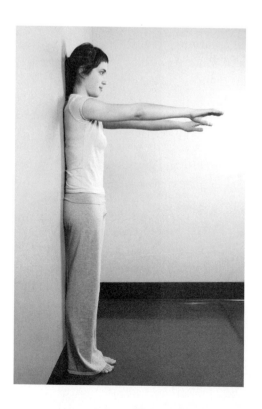

Figure 5.21

Back against the wall

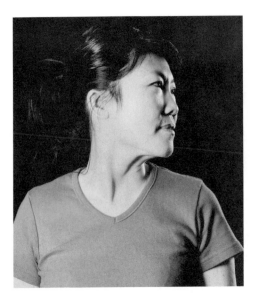

Figure 5.22

Neck rotation 1

Neck Rotation 1

Rotate the head to the side while keeping the eyes and chin level. See Figure 5.22.

Neck Rotation 2

Actively turn the head into neck rotation and at the end of the range assist it further with 2 pounds of force (training option 6) or resist rotation (training option 7). See Figures 5.23 and 5.24.

Neck Rotation 3

Rotate the neck and then lift the chin slightly while anchoring and pressing the pectoral area just beneath the opposite clavicle in an inferior and lateral direction. See Figure 5.25.

Neck Rotation with a Shoulder Press

Place the left thumb and index finger around the outside edge of the client's left ear and place the right hand on the client's right shoulder with the heel of the hand on the client's upper trapezius and the fingers beneath the front edge of the clavicle. Rotate the client's head to the left as far as comfortable and then press the right shoulder in an inferior and lateral direction. If the right shoulder is internally rotated it should also be pressed into the table. See Figure 5.26.

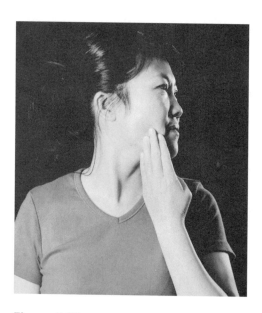

Figure 5.23

Neck rotation 2

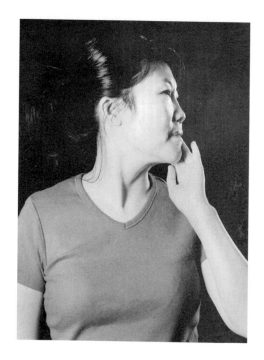

Figure 5.24

Neck rotation 2 with
resistance

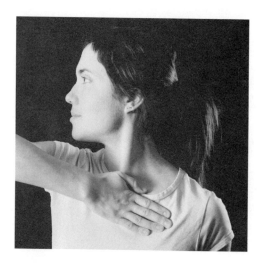

Figure 5.25

Neck rotation 3

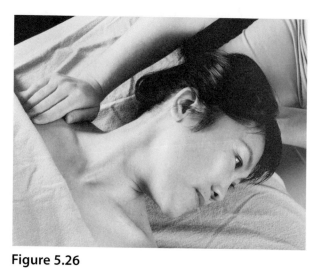

Figure 5.26

Neck rotation with
shoulder press

Exercises to Reduce Kyphosis and Round Shoulders

The following exercises can help reduce functional kyphosis and bring the shoulders back into a more balanced alignment.

Chest Stretches

Standing, cross the arms in front of the chest (shoulder horizontal adduction) and then bring the elbows back while squeezing the scapulae together in the rear (shoulder horizontal abduction). This first stage of this exercise stretches out the rhomboids and the middle and lower trapezius, whereas the second stage strengthens the first three and stretches the pectoralis major. See Figures 5.27 and 5.28.

Hand Clap

Standing, clap the hands in front of the chest and behind the back or above the head and behind the back. This is a great warmup activity.

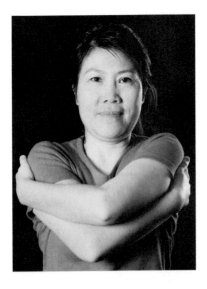

Figure 5.27

Shoulder horizontal adduction

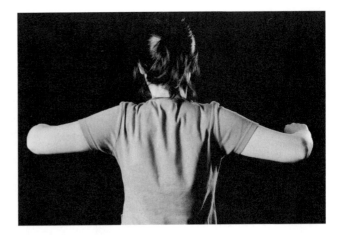

Figure 5.28

Shoulder horizontal abduction

Scapulae Squeeze

Standing, have clients clasp their hands together behind their back interlacing their fingers. If they have difficulties clasping their hands, have them hold on to their opposite forearm, the ends of a towel, a belt, a cane, or a piece of PVC pipe. Next have them pinch their gluteus maximus together so that they straighten up. Finally, have the client squeeze their scapulae together and raise their arms up in the rear in a superior direction. The therapist can also raise the clients' arms, but make sure that you communicate and work slowly and within their pain tolerance. This exercise tones the gluteals, stretches out the pectoralis major and anterior deltoid, and strengthens the middle and lower trapezius and rhomboids. See Figure 5.29a and b.

Up and Under Triceps Stretch

Standing, raise the right arm over the right shoulder and point the fingers down the back and then place the left arm behind the back with the fingers pointing up the back. Clients should try to touch

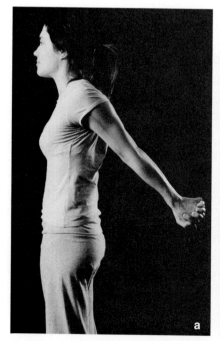
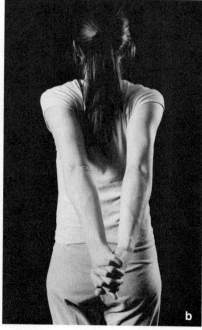

Figure 5.29

Scapula squeeze.
a: Lateral view;
b: Posterior view

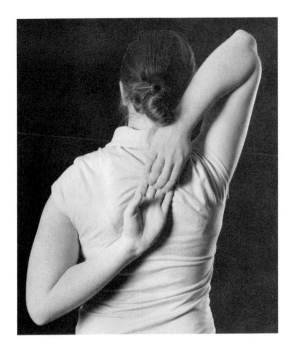

Figure 5.30

Up and under triceps stretch

their fingers together, but if they can't, they can use a towel or a cloth strap to try to walk their fingers together. This stretches out the triceps, teres major, and the latissimus dorsi. See Figure 5.30.

Doorway Chest Stretch for Pectoral Muscles

Place the hands on a door frame and stride through the open door, stretching out the chest musculature. Try this stretch while placing the hands high (45 degrees above horizontal), medium (horizontal), and low (45 degrees below horizontal). This stretches out the pectoralis major and minor and anterior deltoid. See Figure 5.31.

Hands Behind Head 1

Seated or standing, have clients interlace their fingers behind their heads, bring their chin down, move their head back, and then squeeze their scapulae together in the rear. This stretches out the chest and strengthens the scapula adductors. See Figure 5.32.

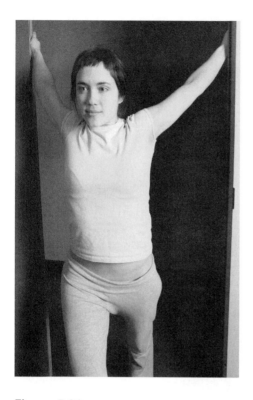

Figure 5.31

Doorway stretch

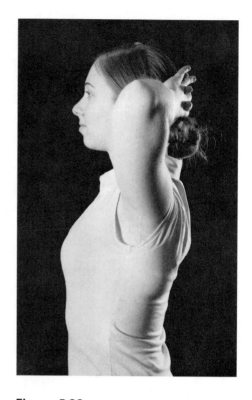

Figure 5.32

Hands behind head 1

Hands Behind Head 2

Start in the same position as the previous exercise; however, the client is passive for this stretch. The therapist kneels on the table behind the client or stands behind their chair and gently stabilizes the client's back with their hip. The therapist then reaches over the client's forearms and grasps his or her upper arms and raises them up in a superior direction. When the vertical range is maximized, the force is then directed in a posterior direction to stretch out the chest musculature. Pay attention to the end feel on the stretch so as to not overpower the client. See Figure 5.33.

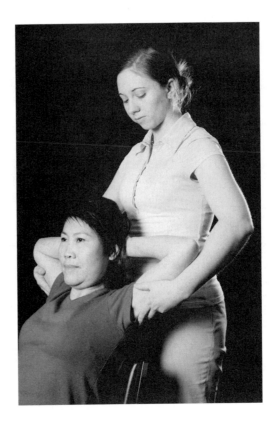

Figure 5.33

Hands behind head 2

Wall Arm Raise

Stand with the back to the wall and flatten the low back. Next move the shoulders and neck back toward the wall. Place the arms horizontal to the ground, back against the wall, and keep the arms against the wall. Have the client slide his or her arms up as far as possible. The eventual goal is perpendicular to the ground. See Figure 5.34.

Single Arm Chest Stretch

Standing, with the right arm horizontal to the ground, place the right hand on the wall and rotate the torso counterclockwise. Try different angles with the arm to get the stretch that the client most needs in the pectoral region. See Figure 5.35.

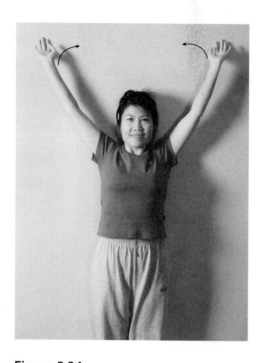

Figure 5.34

Wall arm raise

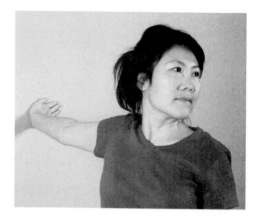

Figure 5.35

Single arm chest stretch

Prone Horizontal Abduction

Have the client lie prone with his or her arms out to the sides of the body. Have the clients raise arms up, squeezing the scapulae together. Start just lifting against gravity and progress to a dumbbell in each hand. Once again use different angles to strengthen and tone the scapular adductors and stabilizers. See Figure 5.36.

Supine Chest and Shoulder Stretch 1

Have the client scoot to the edge of the table and horizontally abduct his or her shoulder off the table at different angles (high, medium, and low) and above the head into shoulder flexion. Let gravity do the work. See Figure 5.37.

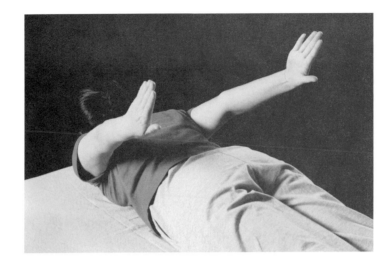

Figure 5.36

Prone horizontal
abduction

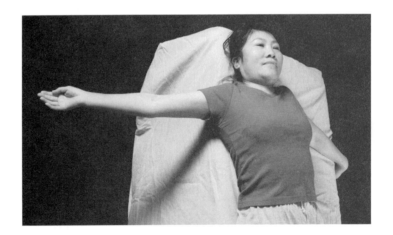

Figure 5.37

Supine chest and
shoulder stretch 1

Supine Chest and Shoulder Stretch 2

Another option is to have the client scoot to the edge of the table and horizontally adduct the shoulder. The therapist then places his or her knuckles on the lateral aspect of the client's pectoralis major and grasps the client's forearm. The therapist compresses the fibers of the pectoralis major, with the force directed toward the sternum or the clavicle, while lowering the client's arm in different angles to stretch the different angled fibers of the muscle. Another option is for the client to actively abduct the shoulder while the therapist

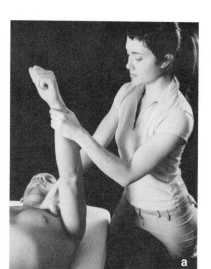 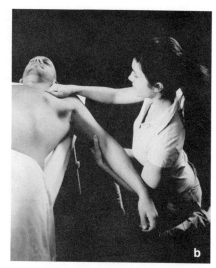

Figure 5.38

Supine chest and shoulder stretch 2. **a:** Starting position; **b:** Ending position

strips the muscle from the distal toward the proximal attachment of the muscle. See Figure 5.38a and b.

Shoulder Exercises

The following exercises will help the client maintain normal shoulder mobility.

Shoulder Circles

Standing with palms up, do small, medium, and large circles of the shoulder joint to warm it up before stretching. See Figure 5.39.

Shoulders Rolls

Standing or seated, instruct clients to take a deep breath and raise their shoulders up, then squeeze their scapulae together as they bring their shoulders back, and then exhale as they lower the shoulders down. The therapist can also grasp the client's upper arms and passively move the client through this activity. See Figure 5.40.

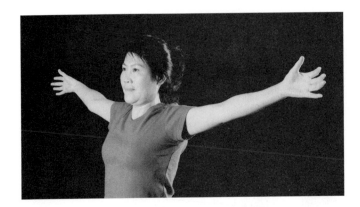

Figure 5.39

Shoulder circles

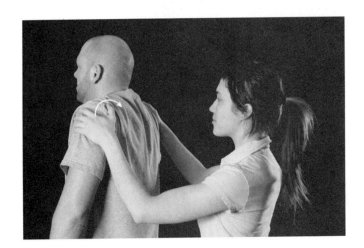

Figure 5.40

Passive shoulder rolls

Shoulder Horizontal Adduction

Standing, horizontally adduct the left shoulder and use the right forearm or hand behind the left elbow to assist with the stretch. Stretch three different angles: high, middle, and low. See Figure 5.41.

"ITWMV"

"ITWMV" is a series of shoulder exercises that are performed standing. From the anatomic position the client first brings his or her extended arms through the sagittal plane into shoulder flexion, forming an "I" shape. The client should bring the chin down and head back and then move the upper arms back next to the ears. The

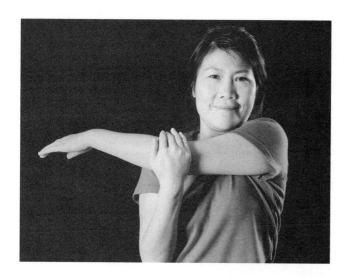

Figure 5.41

Shoulder horizontal adduction

goal is 180 degrees of shoulder flexion. Next, lower the arms and have the client horizontally abduct his or her shoulders with elbows extended to make a "T" shape. It is important for the client to squeeze his or her scapulae together when bringing the arms back. After the "T" the client can lower the arms slightly as he or she flexes the elbows, points fingers to the ceiling, and then squeezes the scapulae together in the rear to make a "W" shape. To make the "M" shape follow the same procedure as the "W" except point the finger tips to the ground. The "V" shape is performed by bringing the shoulders back halfway between the "I" and the "T." Figure 5.42 demonstrates the "W."

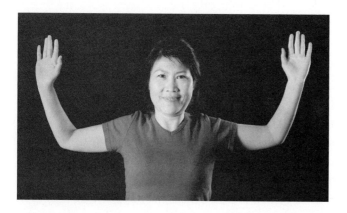

Figure 5.42

The "W" stretch

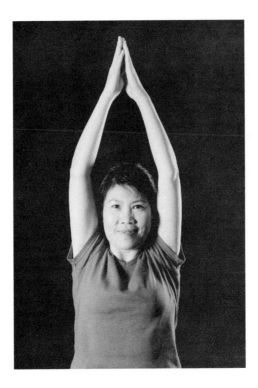

Figure 5.43

Overhead arm raise 1

Overhead Arm Raise 1

Standing, take a long, slow, deep breath as you abduct the shoulders in the coronal plane. Meter the breath so the inhalation lasts until the hands touch above the head. It's important to keep the palms up so the greater tubercle of the humerus doesn't impinge on the acromion process of the scapula during this movement. After the hands touch overhead, exhale and slowly lower the arms, metering the breath so that the exhalation lasts until the hands touch by the sides. See Figure 5.43.

Overhead Arm Raise 2

Standing, clasp the hands in front of the body and then extend the elbows and turn the palms down to stretch the forearm, wrist, and finger flexors. Next have the client raise the arms up into shoulder flexion, in the sagittal plane, as he or she takes a long, slow, deep breath in. When shoulder flexion is reached have the client push the palms to the ceiling as if someone is pulling his or her hands and arms with a rope. After the peak of this stretch have the client

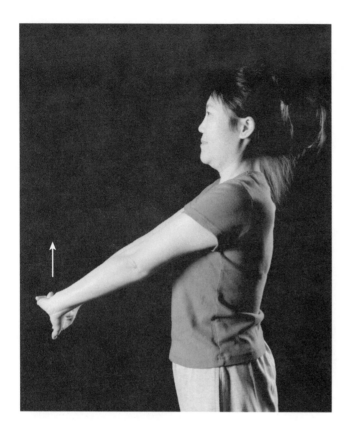

Figure 5.44

Overhead arm raise 2

release the hands and let the arms descend in the coronal plane as he or she slowly exhales, metering each breath until the hands touch by the sides. See Figure 5.44.

Single Arm Raise

Have the client raise one arm overhead, fully extend the wrist of the elevated hand, and then lift his or her head to look at that hand for 5 seconds before switching. The down hand should be swung softly behind the back. See Figure 5.45.

Shoulder External and Internal Rotation

Standing or seated, start in the neutral position with the shoulder abducted to 90 degrees and the elbow flexed to 90 degrees, with the forearm and hand parallel to the ground. For external rotation rotate the hand up to the ceiling, and for internal rotation rotate the hand

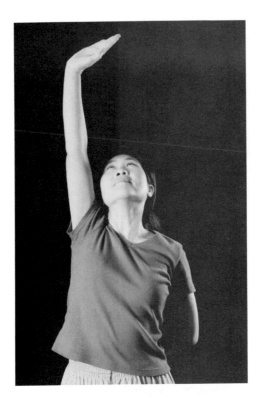

Figure 5.45

Single arm raise

toward the floor. This stretch can also be performed in a doorway, stepping through the door with the forearm and hand on the wall or doorjamb to help increase the stretch. For individuals who experience undue discomfort from this position it can also be performed with the upper arm next to the rib cage on the side of the chest. External rotation is away from the midline, and internal rotation is toward the midline. See Figures 5.46, 5.47, and 5.48.

Hang from a Bar

Find an elementary school with an outside playground; grasp onto a horizontal bar above the head and hang to stretch out the chest, shoulder girdle, vertebral column, lumbosacral junction, and sacroiliac joint. If the client is very tight, have him or her choose the lowest bar to stretch from and have the client bend his or her knees to control the stretch. Feel the soft tissues lengthen, relax, and rebalance. See Figure 5.49.

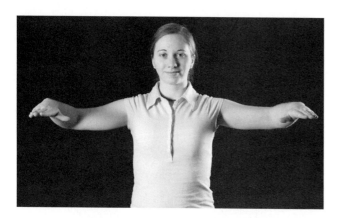

Figure 5.46

Shoulder rotation, neutral position

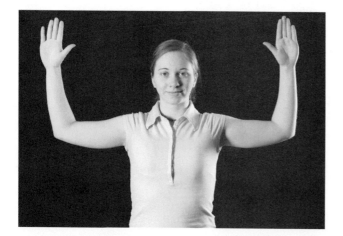

Figure 5.47

Shoulder external rotation

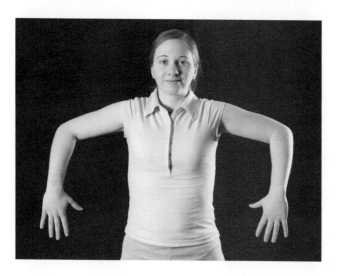

Figure 5.48

Shoulder internal rotation

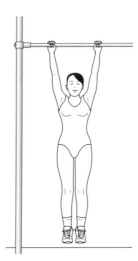

Figure 5.49

Hang from a bar

Rotator Cuff Exercises

To perform rotator cuff toning exercises with therapeutic rubber bands or tubing, tie the tubing to a fixed object about hip high to ensure safety.

Supraspinatus

When working the right supraspinatus have the left shoulder face the band's point of attachment. Reach across the body to grab the band securely in the right hand and proceed to abduct the shoulder 10–15 degrees away from the right side of the body. Work slowly and smoothly.

Infraspinatus and Teres Minor

When working the right infraspinatus and teres minor have the left shoulder face the band's point of attachment. Reach across the body and grasp the band securely in the right hand, and have the right upper arm on the side of the body next to the rib cage and the elbow flexed to 90 degrees. Keeping the upper arm next to the side at all times externally or laterally rotate the shoulder.

Subscapularis

When working the right subscapularis have the right shoulder facing the band's point of attachment. Start with the right shoulder externally rotated, the right upper arm on the side of the body next to the rib cage, and the elbow flexed to 90 degrees. Grasp the band securely and move it across the torso in front of the body into shoulder internal rotation. Always keep the upper arm against the side.

Forearm and Finger Stretching Exercises

These forearm and finger stretching exercises are useful for relieving tension in the wrist and forearm muscles.

Forearm Flexor Stretch 1

Clasp the hands in front of the chest, extend the elbows, and rotate the hands so the palms face away from the body. This stretches the forearm, wrist, and finger flexors. See Figure 5.50.

Forearm Flexor Stretch 2

Extend the right elbow and wrist and then use the left hand to apply force to the metacarpals of the right hand and stretch out the flexors. See Figure 5.51.

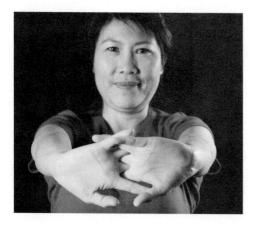

Figure 5.50

Forearm flexor stretch 1

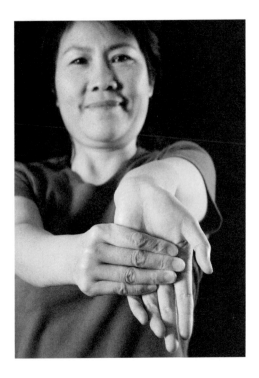

Figure 5.51

Forearm flexor stretch 2

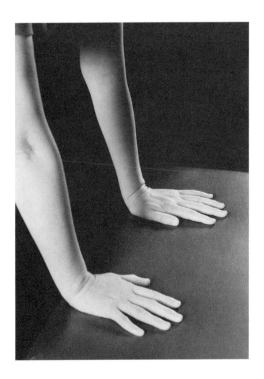

Figure 5.52

Forearm flexor stretch 3

Forearm Flexor Stretch 3

Place both hands palms down on a table and extend the wrist to stretch the flexors. Start with the fingers at 12 o'clock; after stretching there experiment with different angles for a more effective stretch. See Figure 5.52.

Forearm Extensor Stretch

In front of the chest raise the left arm to 90 degrees of shoulder flexion, with the elbow extended and the wrist flexed. Use the right hand to apply gentle force to the metacarpals of the left hand and, if desired, to the fingers to stretch the finger extensors. See Figure 5.53.

Spiders Doing Pushups on a Mirror

Touch the fingertips together and then move the palms together and apart. See Figure 5.54a and b.

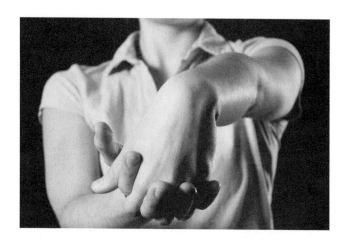

Figure 5.53

Forearm extensor
stretch

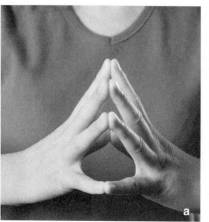
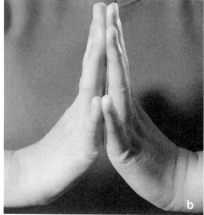

Figure 5.54

Spiders doing pushups
on a mirror. **a:** Starting
position; **b:** Ending
position

Finger Opposition

Touch the thumb to each fingertip. Start by touching the little
finger, and progress by moving to the index finger and then back.

Finger Extension

Start with the fists gently closed with the elbows flexed in front of
the chest; then extend elbows. Follow with complete extension of
the fingers.

Thumb Circles

Move the thumbs in circles in each direction. Some can also move
fingers in circles too.

Exercises to Stretch the Hip Flexors

Stretching the hip flexors is an essential component for preventing and relieving back pain.

Hip Flexor Stretch 1

Lie on the back and bring the left knee to the chest, grabbing under the knee to avoid hyperflexion of the knee; keep the right leg with the knee extended flat on the table. The hip flexor of the straight leg is the one being stretched. See Figure 5.55.

Hip Flexor Stretch 2

Scoot to the bottom edge of the table so that the gluteals are at the edge. Lie back and bring the left knee to the chest by grabbing under the knee and hang the right leg with the knee extended over the edge of the table. Make sure the back stays flat against the table. This stretches the right iliopsoas. See Figure 5.56.

Hip Flexor Stretch 3

Start in the same initial position as Hip Flexor Stretch 2. The right, extended leg hanging over the table now can be bent at the knee to increase the length of the rectus femoris, the biarticular quadriceps muscle, which is a synergist for hip flexion. Don't let the back arch. The therapist may assist with this motion. See Figure 5.57.

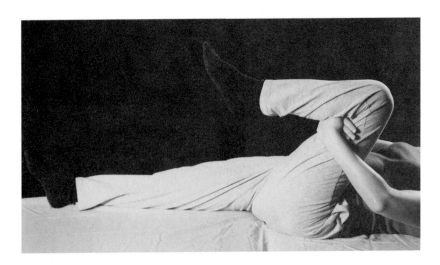

Figure 5.55

Hip flexor stretch 1

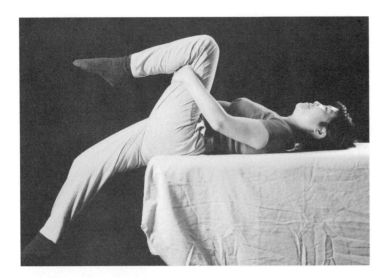

Figure 5.56

Hip flexor stretch 2

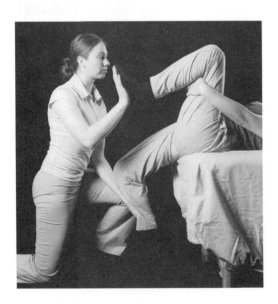

Figure 5.57

Hip flexor stretch 3

Hip Flexor Stretch 4

Have the client kneel on a mat or on a table and place both hands flat in front of him or her. Next have the client flex the right hip and knee and place the foot flat on the mat. Do not overflex the knee in this position; always keep the knee over the support foot. Thus, if you dropped a gravity line from the knee it should never fall in front of the toes. Then have the client bring the left hip back into extension as far as he or she comfortably can. After the client is in

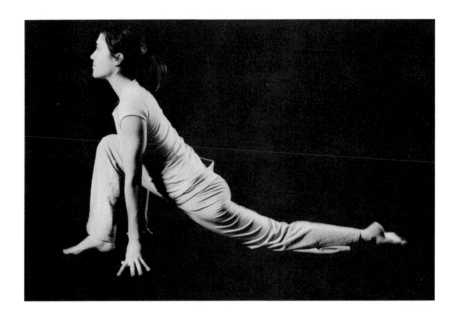

Figure 5.58

Hip flexor stretch 4

the proper position have him or her gently bring the hips forward and rotate the hips gently toward the forward knee (or in this case clockwise). Instruct the client to keep his or her head up so that the eyes are always level; also remind the client not to arch the lumbar spine during this stretch. See Figure 5.58.

Hip Flexor Stretch 5

Start in the same position as Hip Flexor Stretch 4, except the client now flexes the knee of extended leg to stretch out the rectus femoris. See Figure 5.59.

Hip Flexor Stretch 6

Position the client on his or her left side with the left hip and knee flexed for a stable base of support. The therapist stands with his or her right foot forward and the left foot back. The therapist then cradles the client's right leg under his or her right arm and supports the client's sacrum with his or her left hand. The therapist then switches feet so that the left foot is forward and the right foot is back, as he or she rotates the client's hip into extension and a stretch off the right hip flexors. See Figure 5.60.

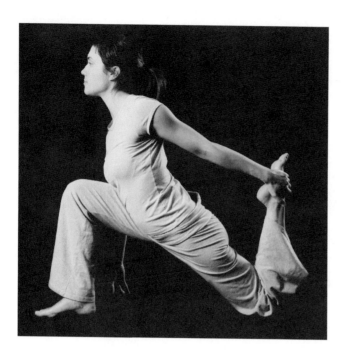

Figure 5.59

Hip flexor stretch 5

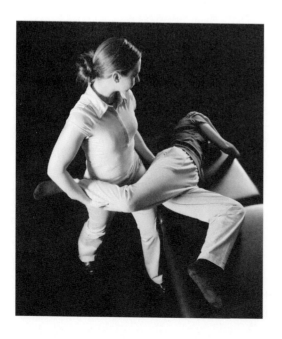

Figure 5.60

Hip flexor stretch 6

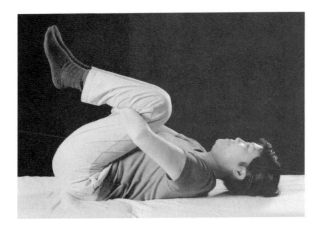

Figure 5.61

Lumbar extensor
stretch

Exercises to Stretch the Lumbar Extensors

If the client has anterior pelvic tilt, the low back muscles must be stretched to help the client achieve a neutral pelvic alignment.

Both Knees to the Chest
The client lies supine, bringing both knees to the chest and locking the hands under the knees, and lets the low back muscles lengthen and relax. See Figure 5.61.

Both Knees to the Chest While Rolling
The client lies supine, bringing both knees to the chest and locking the hands under the knees, and then adds a side-to-side roll.

Both Knees to the Chest While Rocking
The client lies supine, bringing both knees to the chest and locking the hands under the knees, and then rocks forward and back. Don't allow the client to rock back up on his or her neck, and encourage the client to tighten the abdominals when rocking forward.

Seated Trunk Flexion
With the client seated on the edge of a chair with the legs spread wide apart, about 130 degrees, feet flat on the ground, have him or her bend slowly forward, turning into and relaxing each

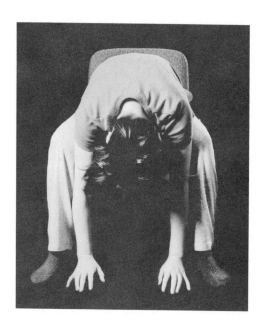

Figure 5.62

Seated trunk flexion

vertebral segment from the top of the cervical region down to the sacrum. The client should exhale slowly on the way down until the hands touch the ground as far in front of them as is comfortable. Do not let the client bounce or force excessive range; the goal is to be in control and let the muscles lengthen and relax. As the client bends forward the therapist can lightly touch the paraspinal muscles along the transverse processes of the vertebrae to help the client tune more effectively into his or her body and relax each segment in descending order. After the stretch is complete the client should take a big complete inhalation as he or she sits up, straightening each vertebral segment from the bottom to the top. See Figure 5.62.

Trunk Flexion over an Exercise Ball

Prone, the client places his or her abdomen over an exercise ball that is large enough for the client's body so that when the feet are touching the ground the hands are airborne. Let gravity relax the upper, middle, and lower back. The client may roll slightly forward and back or shift his or her weight from side to side. In addition, massage strokes can be combined with the ball and movements on the ball.

Exercises to Stretch the Trunk

When hypertonic, the deep trunk muscles can contribute to back pain and spasm and therefore must be addressed in a comprehensive treatment plan.

Quadratus Lumborum Stretch 1

Position the client sidelying on the left side with his or her back close to the side edge of the table. Have the client flex the left hip and knee to 90 degrees, grasp the top of the edge of the table with his or her right hand, and then let the extended right leg stretch to the table in a position of slight hip extension. Variations depend on the client's level of flexibility. A bolster can be placed under the client's left hip, or the client's right hip can be extended so that the right leg falls off the table, allowing gravity to help increase the stretch. You will see how this gravity-assisted position will separate the twelfth rib from the iliac crest and stretch the quadratus lumborum (QL). The therapist may also apply a myofascial release stretch to the QL by crossing his or her hands, placing one on the ribs and one on the iliac crest, and then leaning his or her weight in to lengthen the QL. Hold this stretch until the tissues release. See Figures 5.63 and 5.64.

Quadratus Lumborum Stretch 2

Position the client sidelying on his or her left side, left hip and knee flexed to 90 degrees, with the right hand grasping the top edge of the table and the right hip extended so the leg is hanging near

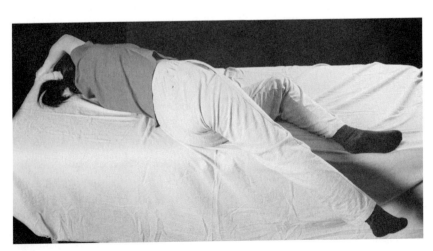

Figure 5.63

Quadratus lumborum
stretch 1

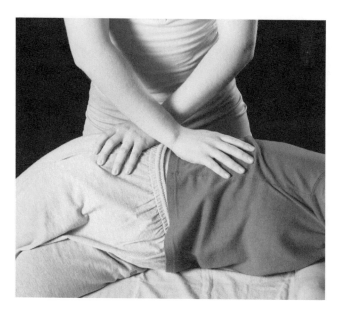

Figure 5.64

Myofascial release to the quadratus lumborum

the edge or just off the side edge of the table. The therapist folds his or her hands and grabs on to the client's right iliac crest. Instruct the client to hike the hip against your force for a 6 count and then instruct the client to relax. When he or she relaxes you lower your center of gravity and pull down on the iliac crest to stretch the QL. See Figure 5.65.

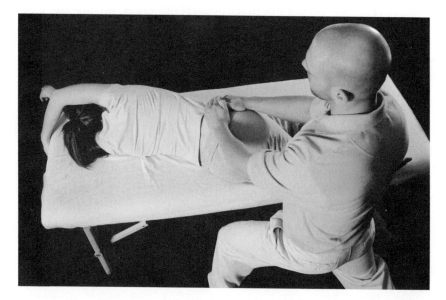

Figure 5.65

Quadratus lumborum stretch 2

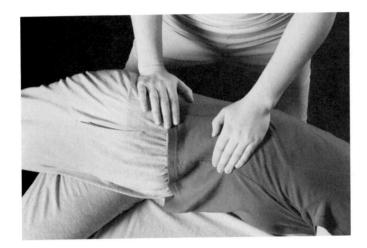

Figure 5.66

Pull and push
quadratus lumborum
(QL) stretch

Pull and Push Stretch

The pull and push stretch should be done sidelying on the left side, with the left hip and knee flexed slightly for a stable base of support, a bolster under the left hip, and the right leg extended and in line with the torso. The therapist places one hand on the client's posterior superior iliac spine and one on the anterior rib cage and then pulls with the hand on the ribs while pushing with the hand on the ilium. The opposite stretch is then performed by placing one hand on the ASIS and one on the posterior ribs and then pulling with the hand on the ilium while pushing with the hand on the ribs. The therapist may also direct some of the force from the hand on the pelvis in more of a diagonal direction, toward the feet, as opposed to a straight anterior posterior force application. The QL fibers wind in different directions, and the trunk rotation component of these stretches provides a different direction of stretch to help improve QL range. See Figure 5.66.

Trunk Twisting

Standing, shoulders flexed to 90 degrees and the elbows extended, rotate the neck and trunk in a clockwise direction as far as possible without straining the knees. This helps stretch the oblique abdominals and can also help stretch a tight QL. Another option for this stretch is to have the client stand with his or her back 10-12 inches from a wall and then have the client rotate in either direction until he or she can place his or her hands on the wall. The client should hold the stretch and then switch. See Figure 5.67.

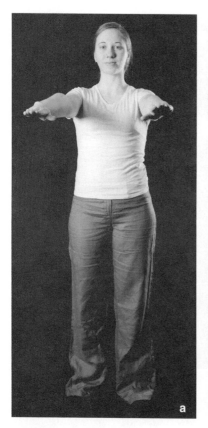 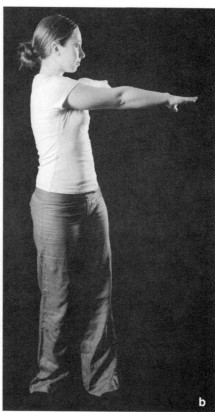

Figure 5.67

Trunk twisting.
a: Starting position;
b: Ending position

Side Bending

Standing, laterally flex the trunk to the left while bringing the right arm over the head. A variation of this stretch is to have the client stand facing a wall with arms above the head and fingertips facing each other. If the right QL is tight, have the client cross his or her left leg in front of the right, then shift his or her weight over the left leg as he or she laterally flexes the trunk to the left. To increase the stretch the hands can also be moved along the wall in the direction of the stretch. These exercises stretch out the QL, the latissimus dorsi, and the ITB. See Figure 5.68.

Sidelying on an Exercise Ball

Have the client lie on his or her right side on an exercise ball with the right leg (bottom leg) forward, the left leg back into extension beyond neutral, and the top arm over his or her head. This position can also be combined with massage strokes. See Figure 5.69.

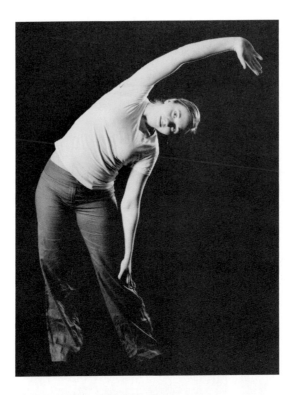

Figure 5.68

Side bending

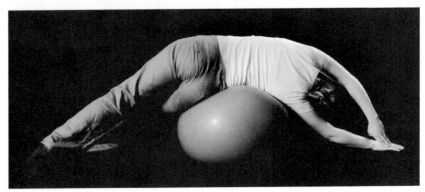

Figure 5.69

Side lying over an exercise ball

Core Strengthening

The core of the body refers to the deep musculature that attaches to the hips, pelvis, low back, and trunk. These muscles stabilize and support our body and absorb shock during movement. The abdominals, gluteals, hip flexors, lumbar extensors, and scapula stabilizers are included in this group of core muscles. Many individuals have weak core muscles, which contribute to their poor posture and pain. The following exercises will help strengthen the body's core musculature.

Abdominal Exercises

Abdominal strength is an essential component to help us prevent back injuries and pain.

Crunches

Have the client lie supine with hips and knees flexed, feet flat on the ground, or with the bottoms of the feet on a wall, or with the backs of the legs on a chair or on an exercise ball. When performing abdominal stretching exercises do not allow the client to brace his or her feet under an immovable object because this will shorten the hip flexor muscles, which we are trying to stretch in most cases. Beginners should fold their arms across their chest and then sit up without using their neck flexors. Have them sit up only as far as they comfortably can. They should feel the contraction in their rectus abdominus just below their sternum. For more resistance have clients practice more advanced crunches by placing the tips of their thumbs by their ears or behind them on their upper thoracic vertebrae—not behind their head. Clients can throw their neck vertebrae out of alignment if they pull themselves up with their hands behind their heads. See Figures 5.70 and 5.71.

Modified Situp

Have clients lie supine with their hips and knees flexed and the feet flat on the ground. Clients should tighten their transverse abdominus muscle and keep it contracted throughout all phases of this

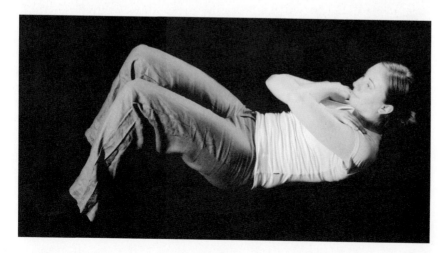

Figure 5.70

Crunches

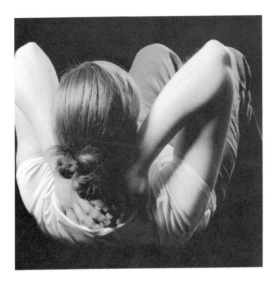

Figure 5.71

Advanced crunches

exercise. Have clients lift the right knee toward the chest as they sit up and then touch that knee with either hand, after which they return to the starting position while still maintaining an eccentric contraction of their abdominals. Clients can work one side first and then the other, they can alternate knees, or they can do both knees at the same time. Clients can also perform this exercise with the hips flexed, knees flexed to 90 degrees, and both feet elevated, so their feet are in the air for the whole exercise. See Figures 5.72 and 5.73.

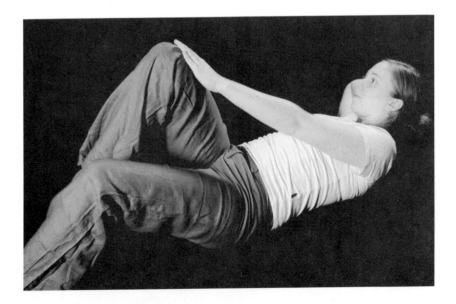

Figure 5.72

Modified situp

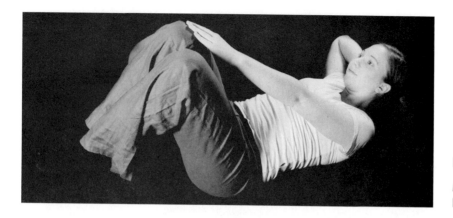

Figure 5.73

Modified situp with both knees elevated

Reverse Crunch

Have clients lie supine with hips and knees flexed and feet flat on the ground; then have them use their abdominals and their arms to push themselves into trunk flexion, so that the chest is as close to their knees as possible. The thighs and the trunk should resemble the letter V. Next, have clients push their feet into the ground and eccentrically contract their abdominal muscles as they lower themselves into as much trunk extension as possible. This is followed by a concentric contraction of the abdominals as the client returns to the V position. See Figure 5.74.

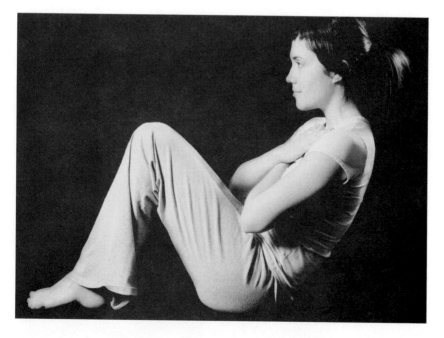

Figure 5.74

Reverse crunch

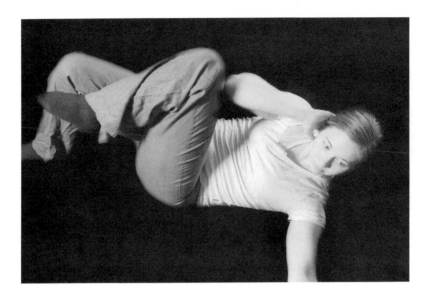

Figure 5.75

Twisting situp

Twisting Situp

Have the client lie supine with hips and knees flexed and feet flat on the ground. Instruct the client to contract the abdominals and sit up. When the client is at the peak of trunk flexion he or she should twist the trunk counterclockwise while flexing the left hip, moving the left knee toward the right shoulder. The client should have his or her right hand and his or her left knee meet halfway. Maintain contraction of the abdominals during the entire exercise. More advanced methods have the client sit up straight, with thumbs by ears, and then the client twists and touches the right elbow and left knee halfway between. This option can also be performed with the hips and knees flexed to 90 degrees and the feet off the ground. See Figure 5.75.

Advanced Twisting Situp

With legs elevated in a vertical position, twist the trunk to reach the left hand to the right toe. See Figure 5.76.

Belly Button to the Back Bone

With clients lying with hips and knees flexed and feet flat on the ground, have them suck in the abdominal contents, bringing the belly button toward the lumbar vertebrae. This is easy on the back. See Figure 5.77.

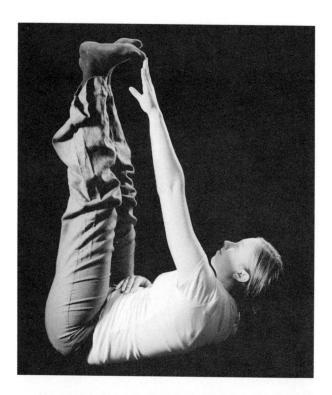

Figure 5.76

Advanced twisting situp

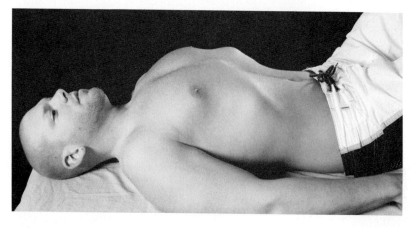

Figure 5.77

Belly button to the backbone

Bug on Its Back

With the client lying supine on a mat or table, have the client bring the right knee to the chest and extend the left leg so it is 6 inches off the table or mat, while raising the extended right arm overhead. Hold for 5 seconds and then switch, bringing the left knee to the chest, extending the right leg 6 inches off the ground, and raising the extended left arm overhead. Do not allow the arms or legs to

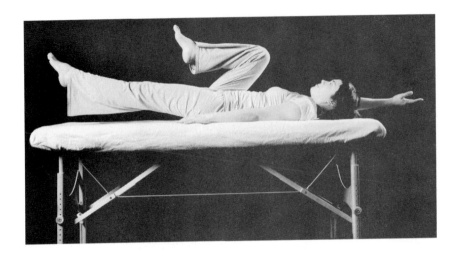

Figure 5.78

Bug on its back

touch the mat throughout this exercise. It is extremely important to contract the transverse abdominus and to keep the low back flat throughout the entire exercise, never letting the back arch off the ground. Also relax the neck muscles and always keep the head in contact with the mat. As the client gets stronger, dumbbells can be held in the hands or light weights can be strapped to the ankles. See Figure 5.78.

Pelvic Tilt

With the client lying supine, hips and knees flexed and feet flat on the ground, tighten the lower abdominals, rotate the pelvis posteriorly, and flatten the lower back to the ground. Bring the belly button toward the lumbar spine. See Figure 5.79.

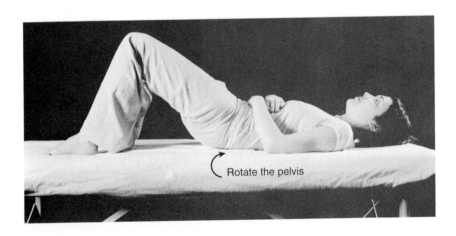

Rotate the pelvis

Figure 5.79

Pelvic tilt

Triple Abdominal Strengthener

With the client lying supine, hips and knees flexed and feet flat on the ground, instruct the client to take a deep breath and then exhale while he or she sucks in the entire abdominal region, rotates the pelvis posteriorly (flattening the lower back to the ground), and then compresses the lower ribs by tightening the oblique abdominals.

Cat Backs

Have the clients position themselves on their hands and knees with their neck extended so they are looking straight ahead. They should then suck in their abdomen while arching or rounding their back toward the ceiling. See Figure 5.80a and b.

Side Situp

Have clients sidelying, resting on their left side. They should pivot off their left elbow to sit up in a position of lateral flexion, strengthening their oblique abdominals. See Figure 5.81.

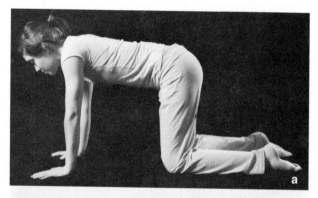

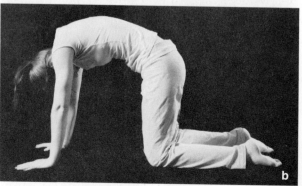

Figure 5.80

Catbacks. **a:** Starting position; **b:** Finishing position

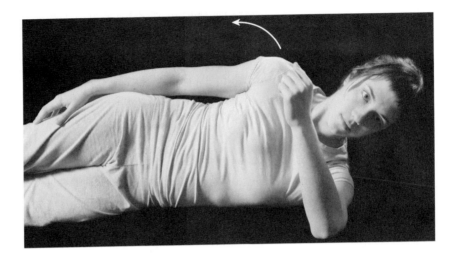

Figure 5.81

Side situp

Trunk Stabilizers

Have clients sidelying on their right side, with their weight resting on their right hand and forearm. Have clients raise their hips up, pivoting off their feet, to bring their torso and the legs in a straight line. This exercise strengthens the trunk-stabilizing musculature. When the client gets strong enough, this can also be performed with the right arm extended, the right hand being the only upper-extremity contact point with the ground. See Figure 5.82.

Abdominal Stretches

Have the client lie prone on his or her abdomen with elbows flexed, forearms on the ground, and hands under the face. Next have the client push up by slightly extending his or her arms, always keeping

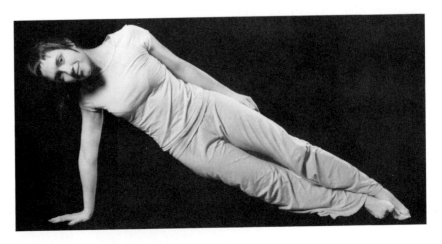

Figure 5.82

Trunk stabilizer

the abdomen in contact with the mat. More advanced clients will be able to straighten their arms. It is important not to contract the lumbar extensors while performing this exercise. See Figures 5.83 and 5.84.

Exercise Ball Supine Stretch

An additional way to stretch the chest and abdomen is achieved by having the client lie supine on an exercise ball. Have the client keep his or her feet on the ground for control and have the client lean back over the ball with arms comfortably out to the sides in shoulder horizontal abduction. They progress by bringing the arms over the head into shoulder flexion. See Figure 5.85.

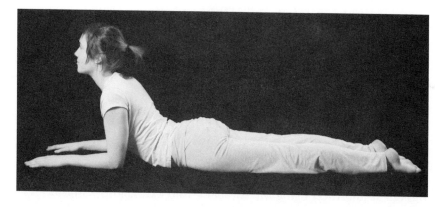

Figure 5.83

Abdominal stretch

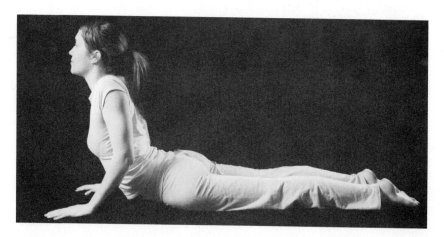

Figure 5.84

Advanced abdominal stretch

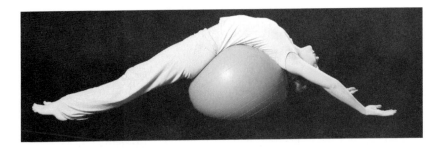

Figure 5.85

Exercise ball supine stretch

Gluteal Exercises

Adequate gluteal strength is needed to help us maintain a neutral pelvic alignment.

Hip Tilts

Have the client lying supine, with hips and knees flexed and feet flat on the ground. Squeeze the gluteals together, as if squeezing a dime between them, and raise the hips off the floor as high as possible. To increase the difficulty, straighten one leg and then the other while keeping the gluteals elevated and together. See Figure 5.86.

Knee Up Mule Kick

While on the hands and knees bring the right knee forward toward the chest and then bring the hip back into extension, without arching the lumbar spine. See Figure 5.87a and b.

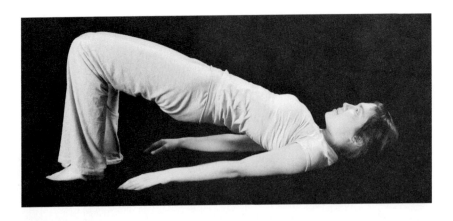

Figure 5.86

Hip tilts

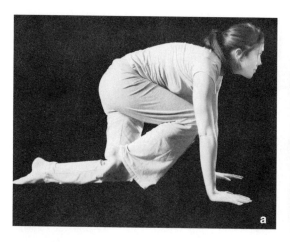

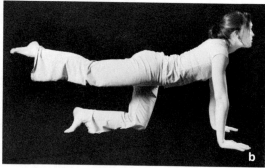

Figure 5.87

Knee up mule kick. **a:** Starting position; **b:** Ending position

Two-Point Alternate Balance

Starting from a hands-and-knees position, raise the opposite arm and leg in the air, keeping them in line with the torso. Keep the head up and don't let the lumbar spine arch. When extending the leg, tighten the gluteals, not the lumbar extensor muscles. See Figure 5.88.

Table Tops

Begin seated on a table or on a mat with the knees bent, feet flat on the ground, and the hands flat on the ground, just lateral to the gluteals. Squeeze the gluteals together and raise the hips and torso

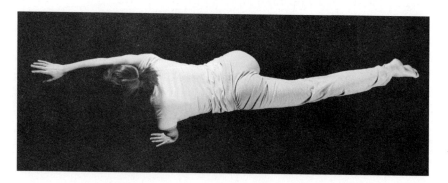

Figure 5.88

Two-point alternate balance

Figure 5.89

Table tops

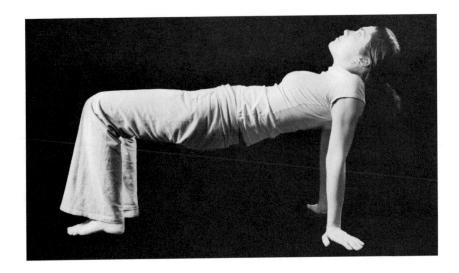

until the front of the body is as flat as the top of a table. Squeeze the scapulae together to strengthen the rhomboids and middle and lower trapezius. This exercise also strengthens the wrist extensors and the triceps. See Figure 5.89.

Side Leg Lift

To tone the gluteus medius and minimus muscles, the client should lie on his or her side and raise the leg up against gravity. As the client gets stronger light weights can be strapped to the ankles. This exercise can also be performed with the hip slightly flexed or extended.

Gluteal Stretches

Supine, with hips and knees flexed and feet flat, have the client raise the right leg over the top of the left leg. Grasp the right knee with the right hand and the right ankle with the left hand. Without straining the right knee bring the right leg toward the left shoulder. The angle of the stretch can be modified by simply adjusting the amount of external and internal hip rotation. Another option from the same starting position is to have the client grasp his or her left knee and bring it toward the chest; however, this does not afford control over the angle of the stretch. See Figure 5.90 and 5.91.

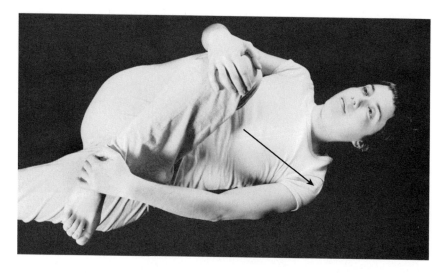

Figure 5.90

Gluteal stretch 1

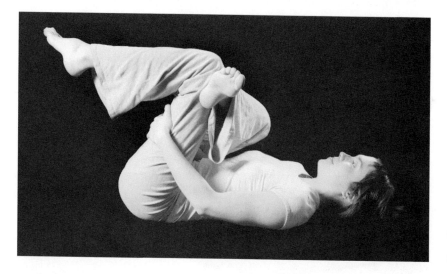

Figure 5.91

Gluteal stretch 2

Back and Gluteal Stretch

On the hands and knees with the toes plantar flexed and the instep on the mat, flex the trunk, bring the gluteals toward the heels, and let the head fall forward until it rests on the mat. Stretch the upper and mid back by walking the fingers along the mat as far as they can go in a superior direction. To stretch the gluteals, relax the shoulders and upper back, stretch by lifting the head slightly and then shifting the weight to each side by moving the hip first over one heel and then the other. See Figure 5.92.

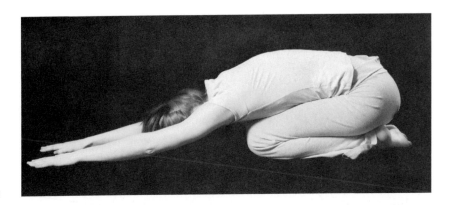

Figure 5.92

Back and gluteal stretch

Exercises for the Hip Lateral Rotators

The hip lateral rotators can contribute to gluteal and sciatic pain. Keeping these muscles flexible can reduce problems.

Windshield Wipers

To warm up the hip lateral rotators flex the hips and knees, place the feet flat on the mat, and move both knees in unison from one side to the other. See Figure 5.93.

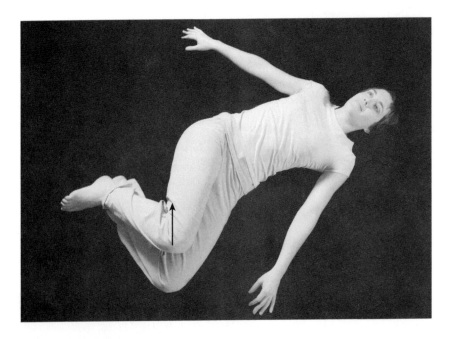

Figure 5.93

Windshield wipers

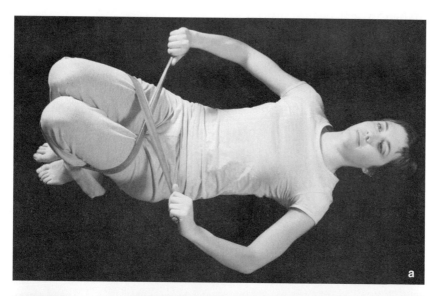

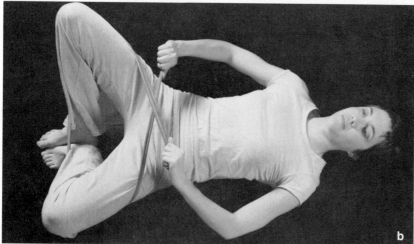

Figure 5.94

Butterflies with resistance. **a:** Starting position; **b:** Ending position

Butterflies with Resistance

Another warmup for the hip lateral rotators begins in the supine position, with hips and knees flexed and feet flat on the ground. Wrap some tubing or a therapeutic rubber band around the client's thighs, have the client spread the thighs apart and then slowly return the legs back together. This engages the hip lateral rotators and prepares them for stretching. See Figure 5.94a and b.

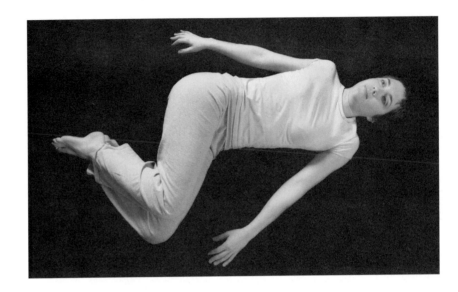

Figure 5.95

Supine hip lateral rotator stretch 1

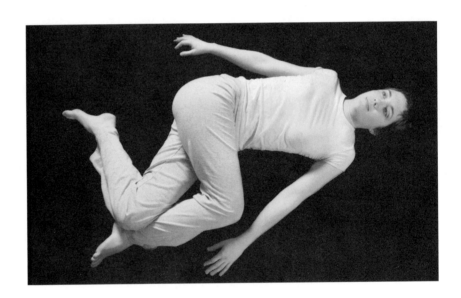

Figure 5.96

Supine hip lateral rotator stretch 2

Supine Hip Lateral Rotator Stretch

To stretch the hip lateral rotators, start in the supine position, with hips and knees flexed and feet flat on the ground. Let both knees fall to the same side while keeping the shoulders on the mat. For a more advanced stretch cross the right leg over the left and then, while keeping the shoulders on the mat, let both legs fall to the left. Then reverse sides. See Figures 5.95 and 5.96.

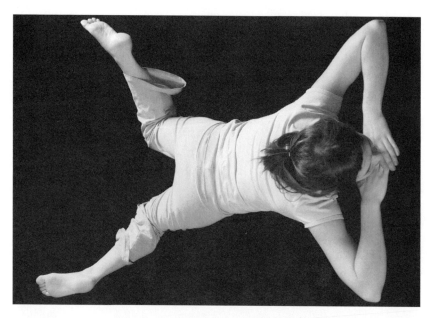

Figure 5.97

Prone hip lateral rotator stretch

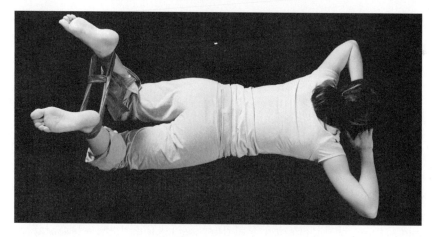

Figure 5.98

Prone hip lateral rotator stretch with resistance

Prone Hip Lateral Rotator Stretches

Have the client lie prone with the knees flexed to 90 degrees and the soles of the feet facing the ceiling. Have the client internally rotate the hips, which will move the feet laterally, and use reciprocal inhibition to relax and help stretch out tight hip lateral rotators. A rubber band can be used around the lower legs to provide resistance to internal rotation to help stretch and relax tight lateral rotators. This resistance technique can also be combined with friction applied with reinforced fingers, the palms, knuckles, forearm, or elbow to the gluteals and hip lateral rotators. See Figures 5.97 and 5.98.

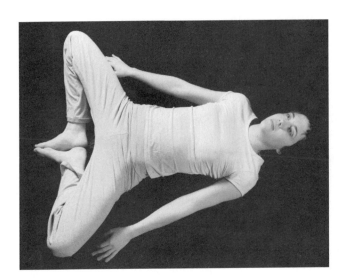

Figure 5.99

Butterflies

Exercises for the Hip Adductors

Try to achieve balance in the length of the hip adductors on both sides of the body.

Butterflies

To warm up the adductors, lie supine with the soles of the feet together, bring the heels toward the gluteals, gently spread the knees apart, and then bring them back together repeatedly. To stretch the adductors, stay in the externally rotated and abducted position with the knees spread apart and let gravity pull on the knees. Instruct the client to feel the muscles lengthen, relax, and let go to the pull of gravity. See Figure 5.99.

Side Lunge

Another warmup for the adductors is performed standing with the right foot forward, the left foot to the side, and the heels lined up about shoulder-width apart. Keeping the right foot flat on the ground gently lunge back and forth to the left 10-20 times without allowing the left knee to advance farther than the toes of the left foot. Then switch sides and repeat. See Figure 5.100a and b.

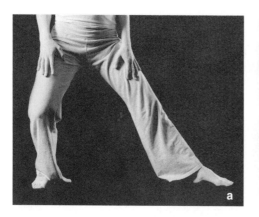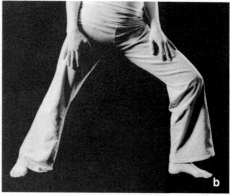

Figure 5.100

Side lunges. **a:** Starting position; **b:** Ending position

Seated Adductor Stretch

Place the soles of the feet together, grab the ankles, take a deep breath, straighten the spine, bring the heels toward the gluteals, and spread the knees as far apart as possible. The client can allow the force of gravity to perform the stretch, or he or she can place his or her forearms on the thighs, applying gentle force to help stretch the adductors. See Figure 5.101.

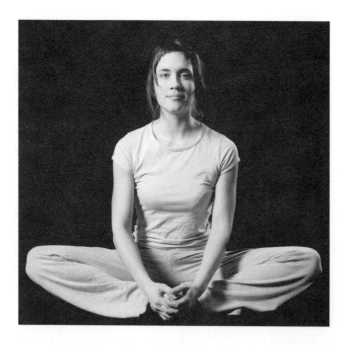

Figure 5.101

Seated hip adductor stretch

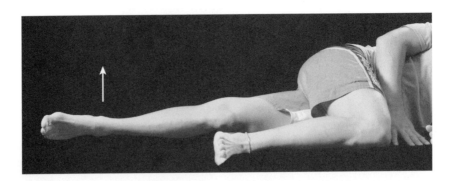

Figure 5.102

Seated hip adductor and medial hamstring stretch

Seated Adductor and Medial Hamstring Stretch

Long sitting, spread the extended legs as far apart as possible into abduction, keeping the toes pointed toward the ceiling, Next straighten the spine, place the hands at the sides by the gluteals, then push up on the fingertips to move the trunk forward into flexion to stretch the adductors and semimembranosus. It is important to keep the spine straight and the abdominals contracted throughout this exercise to prevent back strain. See Figure 5.102.

Hip Adductor Leg Lift

Start this exercise with the client lying on the left side with the right hip and knee flexed and as far forward as possible and the left leg hip and knee extended and in line with the torso. Contract the adductor muscles of the left leg, and raise the left leg toward the ceiling. This helps tone and strengthen the hip adductors. See Figure 5.103.

Figure 5.103

Hip adductor leg lift

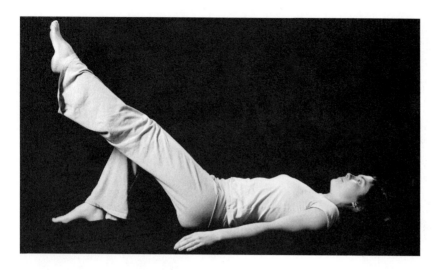

Figure 5.104

Knee extension

Exercises for the Quadriceps

Strengthening and stretching the quadriceps should be a part of everyone's exercise routine.

Knee Extension

Start with the client in the supine position, hips and knees flexed and feet flat on the ground. Straighten one leg and then lower it slowly; when the foot touches the ground lift the other, always keeping the thighs parallel. To prevent anterior cruciate ligament strain extend the knees without hyperextending them. Ankle weights can be added for more resistance. This is a good warmup to perform before stretching the quadriceps. See Figure 5.104.

Forward Lunge

Start with the client standing, left foot forward and the right foot back, and toes pointed straight ahead. Lunge forward by flexing the left knee and lowering the right knee toward the ground. Do not allow the knee of the front foot to go beyond the toes. This activity tones the quadriceps. See Figure 5.105.

Standing Quadriceps Stretch

Standing while balancing or holding on to a bar or a chair for support, grasp the right instep with the right hand and bring the right hip straight back into extension to stretch the quadriceps. Do not force

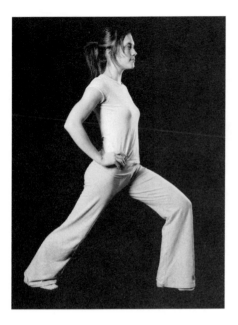

Figure 5.105

Forward lunge

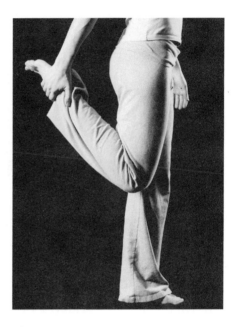

Figure 5.106

Standing quadriceps stretch

the heel to the gluteal; instead concentrate on bringing the hip into extension. If clients cannot grasp their instep, have them grasp their sock. The hip can also be slightly internally rotated or externally rotated to focus the stretch on different fibers of the quadriceps. In addition, the right instep can be grasped by the left hand to further change the angle of this stretch. The client must be careful not to torque and twist the knee joint. The stretch should be felt in the belly of the quadriceps muscle. This stretch can also be performed sidelying. See Figures 5.106 and 5.107.

Kneeling Quadriceps Stretch

Have clients kneel with their toes plantar flexed, and then instruct them to lean back as far as they comfortably can, placing their hands on the ground for support. Pillows can be placed between the gluteals and the backs of the legs so that clients can gradually let the quadriceps lengthen and relax. Remove layers of the pillows as their flexibility improves. This stretch is not recommended for individuals with knee problems or those who have had surgery recently. See Figure 5.108.

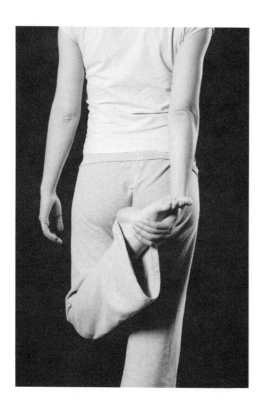

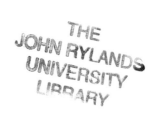
Figure 5.107

Opposite leg
quadriceps stretch

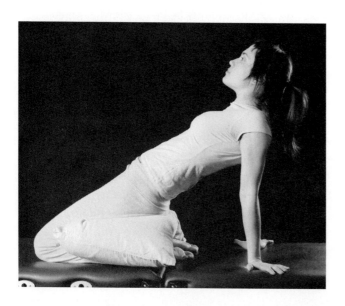

Figure 5.108

Kneeling quadriceps
stretch with a pillow

Hamstring Exercises

Maintaining hamstring flexibility prevents athletic injuries and should be included as part of a routine stretching program.

Hamstring Warmups

Standing, contract the right hamstring and touch the right hand to the right heel; then contract the left hamstring and touch the left hand to the left heel. Repeat 10-20 times on each side by alternating sides. Next, touch the right hand and left heel together behind the back, once again alternating sides, touching the opposite hand and heel. For the third part of this hamstring warmup have clients touch their right hand and their left heel or knee in front of their body, alternating sides and touching the opposite hand and lower extremity in front of them.

Seated Hamstring Stretch

Have clients sit with the left leg extended in front of them with their toes plantar flexed and their right knee flexed, the sole of their right foot resting against the inner part of their left thigh. Clients next should raise their arms over their head while inhaling a deep breath, straightening their spine, and contracting their abdominals. Clients then lower their arms and try to touch as far down their left leg as their flexibility will allow. If they dorsiflex their left ankle and grab on to their toes, this is also a calf stretch. Clients may use a strap or an old necktie to lasso their foot if they cannot grab it to help them stretch their hamstring and calf. From this position clients can also push down on their right thigh to add a stretch of their right adductor muscles. See Figures 5.109 and 5.110.

Straight Leg Lower Hamstring Stretch

If the client is older or has limited flexibility, have them, lying supine, flex the left hip and knee and rest the left foot flat on the ground to perform this exercise. If the client is reasonably flexible, he or she can start lying supine with both knees extended and legs resting on the ground. Next have the client raise the completely extended right leg as high as possible. Make sure that the right knee

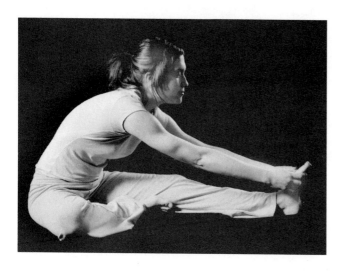

Figure 5.109

Seated hamstring stretch

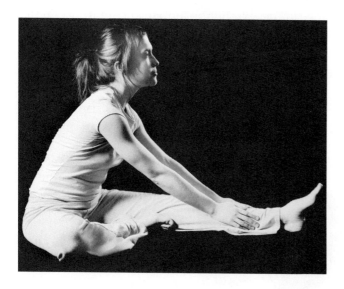

Figure 5.110

Seated hamstring stretch for tight muscles

does not flex. The client also can contract the right quadriceps, bring the toes toward the nose, and push the heel to the ceiling to help with the stretch. A belt or a strap can also be used to help the stretch. This stretches more of the lower fibers of the hamstrings. See Figure 5.111.

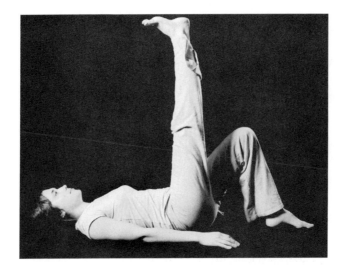

Figure 5.111

Straight leg lower
hamstring stretch

High Hamstring Stretch

With the client lying supine, extend the left leg and let it rest on the mat. Flex the right hip and knee and bring the flexed right knee to the chest. When the right knee is as far as it will travel toward the chest, have the client grasp the right calf and try to straighten the right leg while keeping the knee as close to the chest as possible. This stretches the upper part of the hamstrings. This stretch works even better with assistance from the therapist or a partner. See Figure 5.112.

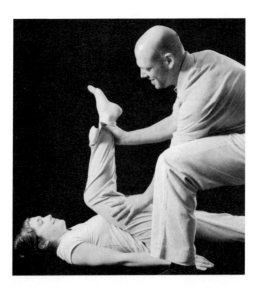

Figure 5.112

Assisted high
hamstring stretch

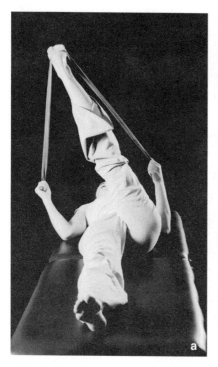
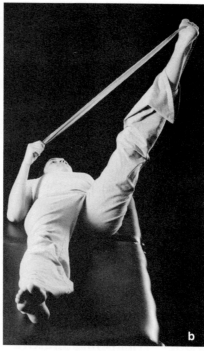

Figure 5.113

a: Lateral hamstring stretch; **b:** Medial hamstring stretch

Stretching the Lateral and Medial Hamstrings

With the client in the supine position, raise the extended left leg into hip flexion as far as it will comfortably move and then move it gently left across the body to help stretch out the left biceps femoris. Move the leg left laterally away from the body to stretch the medial hamstrings. A belt or assistance from the therapist or a stretching partner can greatly assist this stretch. See Figure 5.113a and b.

Contract-Relax-Antagonist-Contract Hamstring Stretch

Start with the client supine on the mat or table with both hips and knees extended. Have the client actively raise the straight right leg as far as possible into hip flexion. The therapist then kneels on the table and places his or her hand or shoulder on the client's calf and instructs the client to isometrically contract the hamstring enough to meet the resistance being provided. This is not a strength challenge;

the goal is to engage the hamstrings for 6 seconds to try to get the Golgi tendon organs to fire off. After 6 seconds of resistance the therapist instructs the client to relax, and after 2 seconds of post-isometric relaxation, the client is advised to contract the quadriceps to actively move into more hip flexion with the knee completely extended. Contracting the quadriceps reciprocally inhibits the hamstrings and allows the agonist (the quadriceps) to stretch the antagonist (the hamstrings).

Standing Hamstring Stretch

Stand with the left foot forward and the right foot to the side with the heels lined up and the feet spread apart at a comfortable distance. Bend the left knee, turn the hips clockwise, and then bend forward to stretch the right hamstrings. It is important to keep the left knee bent throughout this exercise so that no strain is put on the low back. See Figure 5.114.

Standing Hamstring Stretch 2

With the client standing, instruct him or her to carefully raise the right leg and place the heel over a stable object of a comfortable height. Always start with a low object and progress to higher challenges as flexibility increases. Have the client bend the left knee

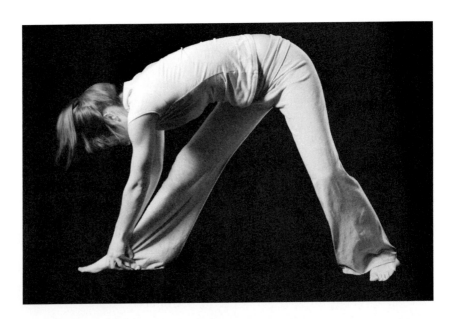

Figure 5.114

Standing hamstring stretch 1

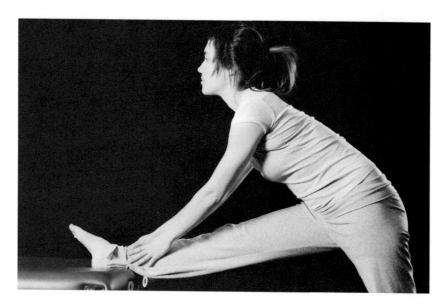

Figure 5.115

Standing hamstring stretch 2

slightly, to ease the strain on their low back, as he or she leans forward to stretch the right hamstrings. Never allow the knee of the leg being stretched to hyperextend. See Figure 5.115.

Exercises to Stretch the Tensor Fascia Latae and the Iliotibial Band

Athletes, particularly runners, need to perform these stretches on a regular basis.

Tensor Fascia Latae and the Iliotibial Band Stretch 1

Position the client lying on the left side with the back close to the side edge of the table. Have the client flex the left hip and knee to 90 degrees and extend the right hip back until the right leg hangs off the side edge of the table. Have the client externally or internally rotate the right hip to change the angle of the stretch until the optimal position is achieved. See Figure 5.116.

Tensor Fascia Latae and the Iliotibial Band Stretch 2

To stretch the left tensor fascia latae and the iliotibial tract, position the client's left side beside a chair or a wall. Instruct the client to rest his or her left arm on the wall or the chair for balance and

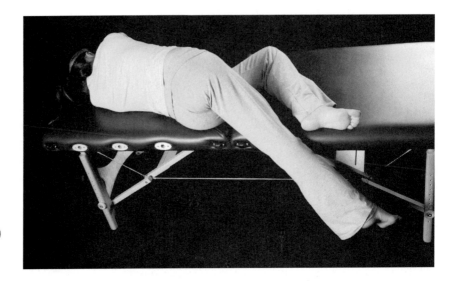

Figure 5.116

Tensor fascia latae (TFL) and iliotibial band (ITB) stretch 1

support. Next have the client place his or her right foot flat on the floor with the hip and knee flexed to 90 degree and cross the left leg behind his or her body as far as is comfortable in a lateral direction on the opposite side of the body. The client should allow his or her body to ease toward the floor as the stretch increases. See Figure 5.117.

Exercises for the Triceps Surae (Gastrocnemius and Soleus)

Lower leg flexibility can reduce significantly the incidence of muscle strain and nighttime cramping.

Heel Raises

To warm up the calves before stretching and for strength development, perform heel raises with the client freestanding or with the hands placed on a chair or a wall for support. Have the client raise his or her heels up as high as possible and then lower down slowly to benefit from the significant strength gains achieved during the eccentric or lengthening contractions of a muscle resisting gravity. Another calf-strengthening option that takes full advantage of the benefits of the eccentric training is to have clients raise up on the toes using both calves and, when at the peak of their elevation, instruct them to remove the weight from one foot and lower themselves using only the eccentric contraction of one calf.

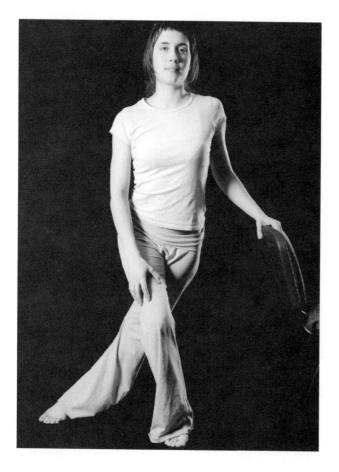

Figure 5.117

Tensor fascia latae (TFL) and iliotibial band (ITB) stretch 2

Toe Raises

The client should stand and use the tibialis anterior muscles to bring the toes to the nose. This strengthens the primary muscles of dorsi flexion and reciprocally inhibits and helps stretch out tight muscles of plantar flexion.

Gastrocnemius Stretch 1

Have the client stand facing a wall with the left foot forward and the right foot back, heel on the ground, with the right leg extended but the knee not locked, head up, and the eyes facing straight ahead. Next have the client bend his or her left knee, turn the toes of the right foot slightly inward, keeping the right heel on the ground, and then bring the hips toward the wall. The client should feel the stretch in the belly of the gastrocnemius and not in the calcaneus tendon. See Figure 5.118.

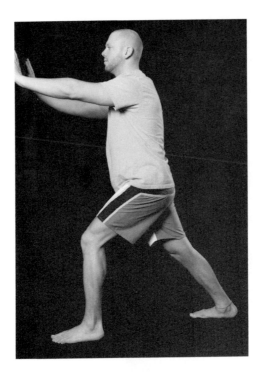

Figure 5.118

Gastrocnemius
stretch 1

Gastrocnemius Stretch 2

Have the client stand and place the toes of the left foot against the base of a wall with the left leg extended but not locked out. Next have the client bring the hips to the wall as he or she stretches the gastrocnemius and toe flexor muscles. See Figure 5.119.

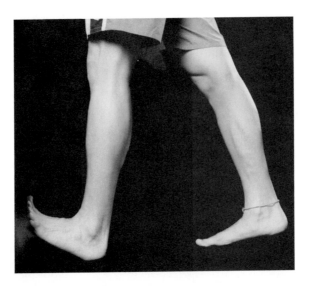

Figure 5.119

Gastrocnemius
stretch 2

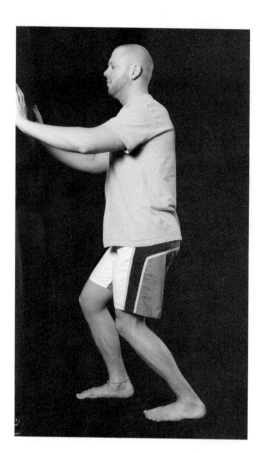

Figure 5.120

Soleus stretch 1

Soleus Stretch 1

Have the client stand facing a wall with the right foot forward and the left foot back about 6 inches and a few inches to the side of the front heel. Have the client bend both knees as far as is comfortable. The stretch should be felt in the lower, deeper calf muscle, the soleus. Bending the knee knocks out the biarticular gastrocnemius and focuses the stretch on the soleus. See Figure 5.120.

Soleus Stretch 2

Have the client stand and place the toes of the left foot against the base of a wall with the left knee bent. Next, while maintaining the knee flexion, have the client bring the patella toward the wall to stretch the soleus, toe flexors, and tibialis posterior. See Figure 5.121.

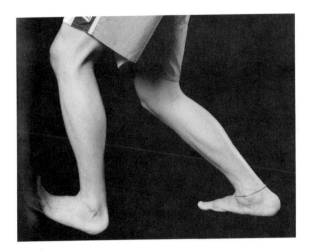

Figure 5.121

Soleus stretch 2

HOME EXERCISE PROGRAM

Now that we have completed our review of therapeutic exercises, the following sample 50-minute warmup, core strengthening, total-body stretching, and muscle-balancing program will help you design a home exercise program for your client or for your own use.

Sample Client Home Exercise Program

Warm Up the Whole Body for 10 Minutes

To begin have clients move their feet and shift their weight from foot to foot throughout the warmup. If any of these activities cause them pain, adapt it by making the movement smaller or selecting another exercise.

> Shoulder rolls: Raise both shoulders up, back, and down 10–20 times.
>
> Shoulder circles: 10 small, 10 medium, and 10 large circles with 5 of each from back to front and 5 from front to back.
>
> Single arm raise: Abduct one shoulder, raising one arm over the head while swinging the other arm behind the back. Have the client fully extend the wrist of the elevated hand and look at the hand for 2 seconds before switching. The client should alternate sides until he or she completes 10 times for each side.

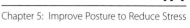

Chest stretches: Standing, cross the arms in front of the chest (shoulder horizontal adduction) and then bring the elbows back while squeezing the scapulae together in the rear. Alternate the arm on top every repetition until 10 cycles are completed.

Heel raises: Bend the knees while swinging the arms back into extension beyond neutral; then straighten the knees while raising the arms over the head, into shoulder flexion, and raising the heels up in the rear, plantar flexing the ankles. Repeat 10 times.

Toe raises: Raise the toes up in the front toward the nose, into ankle dorsiflexion, while swinging the arms forward in front of the chest. Lower the toes while swinging the arms back.

Hamstrings warmup: Touch the right hand to the right heel behind the gluteals and then the left hand to the left heel, alternating sides, 10 times on each side. Next touch the opposite hand and heel behind the gluteals, alternating sides, 10 times on each side. Now lift the right leg and then touch the left hand and heel or knee in front of the body, alternating sides, 10 times on each side.

Shoulder external and internal rotation: Start with both shoulders in the neutral position, and when externally rotating the right shoulder, internally rotate the left shoulder. Switch and repeat 10 times for each shoulder. Keep those feet moving.

Side lunge: With the left foot forward and the right to the side with the heels lined up and the legs spread as far as comfortable, lunge toward the right foot 10-20 times, then switch. When lunging, don't let the knee travel past the toes.

Forward lunge: Standing straight up, move the left foot forward and the right foot back. Then step forward with the left foot 6–12 inches, bend both knees, and move the right knee toward the floor. The client may also horizontally abduct the shoulders while lowering the knee to the floor. Repeat 5–10 times on each side. As the quadriceps gain strength the client will be able to lower the knee closer to the ground, eventually being able to lower the knee gently to the floor.

Clap front and back: Standing with the feet moving, clap the hands in front of the body and behind the back 10 times.

Clap behind and above: Keep the feet moving and clap the hands behind the back and above the head 10 times.

Hip flexion, external rotation, and abduction: If necessary, the client may hold on to a chair, an exercise bar, or the wall for balance. Have the client raise his or her right hip into flexion with the knee flexed and then externally rotate and abduct the right hip. The client then adducts the hip and extends the knee to return to the starting position, which is standing posture, without twisting the back. Repeat this exercise 10 times for each side.

Knee up mule kick: The client may once again hold on to a chair, an exercise bar, or the wall for balance. Lift the right knee into flexion and then tighten the gluteal to bring the hip into extension beyond neutral. Do not allow the back to arch. Complete 10 repetitions for each side.

Standing Stretches for 10 Minutes

Perform one of the variations of these stretches outlined in the text.

Chin down head back: Hold 30 seconds.

Neck lateral flexion: Hold 30 seconds and switch.

Neck rotation: Hold 30 seconds and switch.

Side bends: Bend to the left side with the left hand sliding down the side of the left leg and the right hand and arm reaching over the head as far as it can go. Hold 30 seconds each side.

Trunk twisting: Bend the knees slightly and flex the shoulders until the arms are parallel to the ground; then twist the trunk clockwise as far as comfortable without straining the knees. Hold for 30 seconds on each side.

Back and neck flat against the wall: Hold for 30 seconds.

Gastrocnemius stretch: Hold for 30 seconds and switch.

Soleus stretch: Hold for 30 seconds and switch.

Standing quadriceps: Stretch for 30–60 seconds and switch.

Standing tensor fascia latae and iliotibial tract: Stretch for 30–60 seconds and switch.

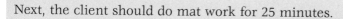

Next, the client should do mat work for 25 minutes.

Pelvic tilt hip tilt: Lying supine, hips and knees flexed and the feet flat on the ground, flatten the lower back toward the mat by tightening the lower abdominals. Next raise the hips up and hold for 5–10 seconds, and then slowly lower down. Repeat for 60 seconds.

Knee extensions: Lying supine, hips and knees flexed and feet flat on the ground, straighten one leg and then lower it while raising the other. Do not lock out the knees. Ankle weights can be added for increased resistance. Repeat for 60 seconds.

Butterflies: Lying supine, hips and knees flexed and feet flat on the ground and together, spread the knees apart and then back together, working the hip abductors and adductors. Repeat for 60 seconds.

Windshield wipers: The client should be supine, hips and knees flexed and feet flat on the ground and together. While keeping the shoulders on the mat and the knees together, let both legs fall to one side and then the other as if the legs were windshield wipers. Repeat for 60 seconds.

Core Strengthening

Crunches: Build up to 60 seconds.

Opposite elbow and knee: Build up to 60 seconds.

Bug on its back: Build up to 60 seconds.

Table tops: Build up to 60 seconds.

Cat backs: Build up to 60 seconds.

Two-point alternate balance: Build up to 60 seconds.

Mat Stretching Series

From the list of exercises select the stretches appropriate for the flexibility level of the client. Instruct him or her to breathe diaphragmatically and to slowly allow the muscles being stretched to lengthen and relax. Never force a stretch.

Hip flexor stretch: Hold for 60 seconds, or 3 sets of 20-second stretches.

Lumbar extensor stretch: Hold for 60 seconds, or 3 sets of 20-second stretches.

Hip adductor stretch: Hold for 60 seconds, or 3 sets of 20-second stretches.

Hip lateral rotator stretch: Hold for 60 seconds, or 3 sets of 20-second stretches.

Gluteal stretch: Hold for 60 seconds, or 3 sets of 20-second stretches.

Seated hamstring stretch: Hold for 60 seconds, or 3 sets of 20-second stretches.

Quadriceps stretch: Hold for 60 seconds, or 3 sets of 20-second stretches.

Back and gluteal stretch: Hold for 60 seconds, or 3 sets of 20-second stretches.

Next perform standing postural realignment and kinesthetic awareness training for 5 minutes.

Standing overhead arm raise 1 and 2: Repeat each twice, focusing on breath control.

Shoulder rolls: Slowly raise the shoulders up and back when breathing in and exhale when lowering the shoulders. Repeat 3 times.

Scapula squeeze: Hold for 30 seconds.

KINESTHETIC AWARENESS TRAINING

Complete the home exercise program with kinesthetic awareness training. Have the client practice finding, modeling, and feeling "the position." "The position" is the spot where the client's head is in balance over the neck and shoulders, the eyes are level, and there is no neck tension whatsoever. Instruct the client to stand tall and bring the chin down and head and shoulders back and down into normal posture. Clients should learn how good "the position" feels, and throughout each day, whenever they are feeling stress, strain, and tension, they should bring themselves to this spot. No

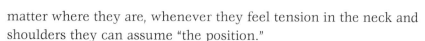

matter where they are, whenever they feel tension in the neck and shoulders they can assume "the position."

We have discussed how to improve static or stationary muscular balance and posture. For optimal physical stress management it is essential that the client also learn to feel when their muscular balance and posture are deviated when they are moving and to make the necessary adjustments. Dynamic Postural Alignment Training can be achieved through focused walking.

FOCUSED WALKING

Focused walking combines slow walking, postural realignment, and muscular relaxation. When walking the client tunes into his or her body, feeling for restrictions, limitations, and postural deviations. Have the client start walking at a nice slow pace and check in with his or her body. The client should try to smooth out his or her gait and eliminate any barriers toward smooth forward progression. The client should be aware of his or her feet, knees, hips, pelvis, shoulder, neck, and head position while moving. Relaxing away excess muscle tension in the body can be accomplished while walking. Most of us are not aware of our bodies, but by making changes based on areas that we feel are tight, we can optimize how our body functions.

For example, the other day I was walking and I tuned into my body because my knee hurt and my back felt stiff. When tuning into my body I realized that I was pointing my left toe out while walking, and when I corrected this my knee pain was reduced. I also felt as if the right side of my pelvis was higher when I walked and that my pelvis did not swing forward equally on both sides. I practiced relaxing my tight muscles and consciously was able to smooth out my gait. Now I have less back pain and stiffness. I was also carrying my shoulders too high and my head too far forward. I brought my head back and let gravity pull my shoulders down. When I finished my walk my body felt great and I felt as if I had just completed a session of relaxation.

The client should experiment with dynamic postural alignment during focused walks to determine if it can help relieve some negative effects of stress. It may also benefit the client to add other fitness training techniques such as aerobic exercise and weight training to his or her weekly stress reduction schedule.

SUMMARY

Before we elaborate on other exercises that can help reduce stress, let's review some important concepts:

- If your client demonstrated atypical posture and muscular imbalances on his or her Personal Stress Inventory, then therapeutic exercises can be an important addition to the personal stress reduction program.

- If it is out of your scope of practice or if you are not properly trained and qualified to make exercise recommendations to help your clients regain body balance, then refer them to appropriate professionals.

- Many postural faults are caused by muscular imbalances.

- The 10-minute quick body scan is another useful assessment tool.

- An imbalance in one part of the body can affect the bones, muscles, ligaments, and fascia in the rest of the body.

- Many clients need feedback from the therapist to correct posture and improve their kinesthetic sense or feeling of how their body parts are aligned.

- Upper and lower crossed syndromes are frequently seen combinations of myofascial imbalances.

- The rules for practicing therapeutic exercises are to warm up, stretch, strengthen, and stretch again.

- Postural realignment exercises can be practiced briefly every day, even at work.

- Total body stretching and strengthening activities should be practiced at least 3 days a week.

- Dynamic postural alignment can be achieved through focused walking.

Exercising to Reduce Stress

The human body is a sophisticated machine that works best when exercised on a consistent basis. Aerobic exercise and resistance training are essential components that clients should add to their personal stress reduction program and weekly schedule to help them achieve and maintain optimal physical and psychological health. Unfortunately, this area is out of the traditional scope of practice of massage therapy. If any of your clients have an inactive lifestyle and a job that keeps them sedentary, they will benefit greatly from the daily practice of exercises that condition their heart, lungs, and vascular system and tone their muscles. The information presented in this chapter is intended to improve the massage therapist's understanding of the body's requirement for aerobic and resistance training. Therapists can use this information to improve their own personal training programs, to share with clients, and to know when to refer clients to physical education classes or other professional fitness trainers. This chapter will discuss the potential dangers of not exercising, the benefits derived from fitness training, and how to safely use aerobic exercise and resistance training to combat the negative effects of stress. In addition, potentially dangerous exercises that must be avoided or used with caution and cross training will be discussed.

OUR BODIES ARE DESIGNED TO BE ACTIVE

Historically, people had to perform physical work to survive. Chopping wood, pitching hay, cultivating and planting the fields, hauling water from the well or pump, hunting, harvesting, churning butter, and milking cows were all part of a day's work. They even had to walk out back to go to the outhouse. They worked hard, ate natural unprocessed foods, and were not subjected to the fast pace and information overload of today's world. People living in this century have grown soft because in most instances their survival does not require physical exertion and for whatever reason they are not satisfying their body's need to be worked with daily exercise.

Many people today do not move and exercise enough. They drive their cars everywhere; spend too many hours in front of a computer working, playing games, or surfing the Internet; and avoid sports and active hobbies. They don't have to work to eat—they just have to drive to the store and open a package or buy fast, unhealthy, supersized food. Many would rather be spectators than participants. Obesity is now an epidemic plaguing our society. With current obesity trends, today's children may be the first generation that will not outlive their parents. There is no disputing that how someone looks and feels physically will have an impact on their self-image and psychological health. By encouraging sedentary clients to safely increase their activity level, the therapist can help them reduce this element of their stress.

To reduce stress, people must incorporate bouts of physical activity into their everyday lives. Being physically active is one behavior that contributes to a person's overall health and well-being, a state that some authors refer to as "wellness." In the book *Fit and Well*, Fahey and colleagues wrote:

> The human body is designed to work best when it is active. It readily adapts to nearly any level of activity and exertion; in fact, physical fitness is defined as a set of physical attributes that allow the body to respond or adapt to the demands and stress of physical effort. The more we ask of our bodies—our muscles, bones, heart, lungs—the stronger and more fit they become. However, the reverse is also true—the less we ask of them, the less they can do. When our bodies are not kept active, they begin to deteriorate. Bones lose their density, joints stiffen, muscles become weak, and cellular energy systems begin to degenerate. To be truly well, human beings must be active. Unfortunately, a sedentary lifestyle is common among Americans today. More than 60 percent of Americans are not regularly phys-

ically active, and more than 25 percent are not active at all (Fahey et al, 2005:4–5).

EFFECTS OF PHYSICAL INACTIVITY

A more comprehensive list of the physical symptoms that are frequently demonstrated by those who eat a poor diet and lead inactive lifestyles (smoking may further exacerbate these problems) includes the following:

- Poor circulation, reduced cardiorespiratory endurance, and diminished work capacity.
- Abnormal blood chemistry, clogged arteries, high blood pressure, and an increased chance of experiencing a heart attack, stroke, and diabetes.
- Because of disuse, muscle mass shrinks, and fat and useless **connective tissue** fill the void, resulting in a loss of strength, flexibility, and power.
- Decreased **metabolic rate** and the storage of body fat and excess weight, which can contribute to the wear and tear on the weightbearing joints (osteoarthritis).
- Aches and pains, muscle tension, spasms, and atypical posture.
- A poor self-image, anxiety, and depression.
- Sleeping difficulties.
- Low energy.

EFFECTS OF PHYSICAL ACTIVITY

Conversely, the routine practice of moderate exercise on a daily basis has been shown to have many positive effects on the human body. The Surgeon General's 1996 report on physical activity and health reported that regular physical activity improves health in the following ways:

- Reduces the risk of dying from heart disease.
- Reduces the risk of developing diabetes and colon cancer.
- Reduces the risk of developing high blood pressure and helps reduce high blood pressure in people who already have it.
- Reduces feelings of depression and anxiety.

- Helps control weight and helps build and maintain healthy bones, muscles, and joints.
- Helps improve the strength, balance, and mobility of older individuals.
- Promotes psychological well-being.

TAKE SMALL STEPS TO INCREASING ACTIVITY LEVEL

It's never too late to begin exercising. In fact, even individuals who have been sedentary for many years may achieve significant improvements in their strength, endurance, flexibility, coordination, balance, and posture after the practice of moderate exercise on a regular basis. Exercise can also help prevent injuries, increase breathing efficiency, elevate **HDL** (high-density lipoprotein) levels (good cholesterol), and help the client sleep better, reduce muscle tension, lose weight by burning calories, and think more clearly. The evidence is indisputable that if you keep your body strong and fit and your mind active you will prevent premature aging. Without a doubt exercise is good for the human mind and body, but it must be gradually incorporated into a person's lifestyle. The biggest mistake made by people reintroducing exercise into their lives is that they do too much activity too soon and end up hurting themselves. So advise your clients not to start with marathon training but to gradually add more physical activity into their daily schedule.

Sedentary clients should be encouraged to begin a fitness program by modifying their behavior so that more activity is added into their daily lives. They should be advised to park at the farthest end of the parking lot to increase the distance walked to their office or the store, to take the stairs instead of the elevator, to walk during breaks instead of eating fattening foods (such as doughnuts), and to take a brief walk after lunch and dinner. Or they can play some dance music that they enjoy and then dance their way through their dusting, vacuuming, laundry, or preparing dinner (although they must be careful when cutting up vegetables). They can also add a few of the warmup exercises listed in the previous chapter to increase their calorie burn as they glide through their chores. Jogging in place, doing calisthenics, or riding an exercise bicycle while watching television are other ways that a client can increase activity level and burn more calories without taking a lot of precious time away from other activities. You can also recommend that the client perform some core strengthening activities and stretching exercises every night while watching the evening news.

Monitoring Your Daily Steps

In 2001 the Surgeon General of the United States, Dr. David Satcher, recommended that to increase health and fight obesity, a person should strive to take 10,000 steps every day. Ten thousand is a lot of steps—in fact, it is about 5 miles for someone with an average stride. A sedentary client may take as few as 1,000–3,000 steps a day. For health it is recommended that a person walk at least 5,000 steps a day. To lose weight they should walk the 10,000 steps. Walking is a great activity that does not put as much stress on the joints and muscles as jogging. However, to prevent injury, sedentary clients should start with a low amount of steps and then gradually increase their steps to the desired amount.

The easiest way to obtain true data on the activity level of a person is to measure how many steps they take each day in the course of their daily lives. Interested individuals should purchase or borrow a **pedometer.** Some pedometers, which cost around $10 to $30, also convert the steps taken into the amount of calories burned while walking each day, a useful bit of information for those trying to balance their caloric intake with their energy expenditure. They should wear this small, unobtrusive, inconspicuous device every day for a week. They should record the results on the blank copy of the walking endurance improvement plan form located in Appendix 9. Table 6.1 provides an example of a completed form. These results will give a clear indication of their true activity level and how many steps that they take each day. Add all of the steps taken in 1 week (week 1) and divide by 7 to get the average daily steps. This average is a baseline or starting point. Let's say that the client averaged 3,000 steps each day for the trial week. For the second week the client should strive to walk 500 steps more each day or 3,500 every day. For the third week the client should add 500 more steps so that he or she walks 4,000 steps each day. The client should keep adding 500 steps to the daily exercise each week until he or she achieves the desired goal.

TABLE 6.1

Sample Walking Endurance Improvement Plan

Enter the number of steps that you take each day on the chart below. At the end of the week, tally the total number of steps taken and then divide by 7 to get the average steps taken per day.

	Monday	Tuesday	Wednesday	Thursday	Friday	Saturday	Sunday	Total # of Steps Per Week	Average # of Steps Per Day
Week 1	2,500	3,100	3,500	1,750	3,250	4,000	1,500	19,600	2,800
Week 2	3,100	3,400	4,000	2,750	3,050	3,500	2,500	22,300	3,186
Week 3	3,600	3,900	4,000	3,000	4,000	4,000	3,000	25,500	3,643
Week 4	4,000	4,500	4,500	3,500	4,500	4,250	3,750	29,000	4,143
Week 5	4,600	4,400	5,000	4,000	5,000	4,500	4,500	32,000	4,571

Planting the Seeds of Health

Gardening is another great activity to encourage the sedentary client to try to help reduce stress and improve health and fitness. Gardening provides walking; toning; and time for clients to smell the flowers, forget about problems, and think their own thoughts. Working the earth can be very relaxing and satisfying and helps ground a stressed person. Then there are the flowers and great tasting vegetables to enjoy from the harvest as an added benefit from all the hard work. Now that we have discussed ways clients can increase their activity level to improve health, we must talk about progressing to the next level, fitness training.

FITNESS TRAINING

Fitness training kicks it up a notch, but it doesn't have to be too strenuous to start. The major difference between activity and fitness training is that a person generally changes clothes before fitness training and probably sweats more. Yes, sweating is good for you. The following information is provided to help steer clients in the right direction when fitness training. The massage therapist is not expected to be a fitness expert, although combining massage therapy with a certificate in personal fitness training is becoming popular at some institutions. Massage therapists should encourage

Determine your target heart range.

Find activities that you enjoy.

Wear comfortable shoes that have good shock absorption, have adequate toe room and arch support, and resist pronation.

Warm up before exercising—move the joints through their normal range of motion 10–20 times.

Elevate your heart rate to its target range and keep it at that level for 20–50 minutes 3–5 times a week.

Periodically monitor the pulse to make sure that the appropriate intensity is maintained.

Cool down after exercise.

Stretch after cooling down.

Vary the length, frequency, and intensity of the training sessions.

Try different activities to prevent boredom and overtraining some muscle groups.

Figure 6.1

Summary of fitness training tips

their clients to take physical activity classes at their local community college, YMCA, or adult education program. Classes are fun, and they provide clients a chance to meet people. They also make them commit to a routine that will force them to get off the couch or away from their computers. Professional physical education teachers and fitness instructors should be able to help your clients design and implement a safe program according to their age, level of fitness, physical limitations, and abilities. Clients should start slowly and then gradually build up endurance. As their fitness increases they can exercise for longer, more frequently, and at a faster pace. If any client is considerably overweight or has a history of coronary problems, they should consult with their physician before beginning a cardiorespiratory training program. Figure 6.1 provides a summary of fitness training tips.

AEROBIC ENDURANCE TRAINING

Aerobic (cardiorespiratory) **endurance training** refers to exercises that develop the heart and lungs by keeping the body's major muscle groups moving for a prolonged period while elevating and maintaining the heart rate in a person's target range or zone. The **target heart range** (THR) or zone refers to a range of heart beats per minute that a person should try to stay within while exercising for safety and for beneficial training effects to occur. During bouts of aerobic activity clients should elevate their heart rate to at least the low end of their range and not let their heart rate fall below that number for the duration of the activity. In addition, to prevent injury clients should try to not let their heart rate exceed the high end of their range during exercise. The following simple formula can be used to determine the target heart range.

CALCULATING A TARGET HEART RANGE

One formula for calculating target heart range is 220 – AGE = Maximum Heart Rate (MHR). Then take the maximum heart rate and multiply it by the intensity of exercise to get the training heart range, or MHR × intensity = THR. The THR is determined by factoring in different intensities of exercise into the formula according to the level of fitness. An individual with poor fitness may begin the program factoring into the formula an intensity of 50–70 percent, whereas a person of average fitness will factor in an intensity level of 60–75 percent. A highly fit person will factor in 70–85 percent. Please note that this formula does not work for everyone, especially children and older adults. For more accurate results the client should have a stress test performed by a cardiologist or exercise physiologist or use the heart rate reserve formula:

$$
\begin{array}{c}
220 \\
\underline{- \text{ age}} \\
\text{Max Heart Rate} \\
\underline{\times \text{ \% Intensity Level Range}} \\
\text{Target Heart Range in beats per minute (BPM)}
\end{array}
$$

The heart rate reserve formula is more accurate, but it is also more complicated. To calculate the heart rate reserve formula, first take your resting pulse. (Directions on how to take a pulse measurement are provided later in this chapter in the section "Working in the Target Zone.") It is best to measure this right when you wake up in the morning. Next, take 220 and subtract your age to get your maximum heart rate. Now subtract the resting pulse from the maximum heart rate. This gives you your heart rate reserve. Next, multiply the appropriate intensity level range according to your level of fitness by the heart rate reserve. Finally, add back the resting pulse rate to get your target heart range.

$$
\begin{array}{r}
220 \\
\underline{- \text{ age}} \\
\text{Max Heart Rate} \\
\underline{-\text{Resting Pulse}} \\
\text{Heart Rate Reserve} \\
\times \% \text{ Intensity Level Range} \\
\underline{+ \text{ Resting Pulse}} \\
\text{Target Heart Range}
\end{array}
$$

Let's work through a few examples:

Client A is a sedentary 50-year-old male.

$$
\begin{array}{r}
\text{Step 1: } 220 \\
\underline{- 50} \\
170 \text{ BPM}
\end{array}
$$

Maximum heart rate is

$$
\begin{array}{cc}
\text{Step 2: } 170 & 170 \\
\underline{\times 50\%} & \underline{\times 70\%} \\
85 \text{ BPM} \quad \text{to} & 119 \text{ BPM}
\end{array}
$$

Target heart range

Client A's maximum heart rate is 170 beats per minute. When training it is recommended that this person elevates and maintains his or her heart rate above 85 and below 119 beats per minute. If the exercise range recommended by the formula is too hard or too easy, it should be adjusted accordingly by changing the intensity level factored into the formula.

Client B is a 28-year-old highly fit individual with a resting pulse of 54 beats per minute.

$$
\begin{array}{r}
\text{Step 1: } 220 \\
\underline{- 28} \\
192 \text{ BPM}
\end{array}
$$

Maximum heart rate is

$$
\begin{array}{r}
\text{Step 2: } 192 \\
\underline{- 54 \text{ (Resting pulse)}} \\
138 \text{ (Heart rate reserve)}
\end{array}
$$

$$
\begin{array}{cc}
\text{Step 3: } 138 & 138 \\
\underline{\times 70\%} & \underline{\times 85\%}
\end{array}
$$

	Step 4:	96.6		117.3
	Step 5:	+54		+54
Target heart range		151 BPM	to	171 BPM

Client B's maximum heart rate is 192 beats per minute and he or she should train somewhere in the safe zone, between 151 and 171 beats per minute.

WORKING IN THE TARGET ZONE

To ensure that a person is working at the proper intensity when training, a wireless heart rate monitor can be used or he or she periodically can measure the heart rate by taking his or her **pulse.** The carotid artery and the radial artery are two areas used to measure the pulse. Always use the fingertips, not the thumb, because it has a pulse of its own. Find the carotid pulse on the neck just beneath the angle of the jaw. The radial pulse is found on the anterior wrist fold just on the outside of the large tendon below the thumb. Once you have located the pulse, simply count the number of beats in 10 seconds and then multiply by 6.

The therapist should practice taking his or her own radial and carotid pulses and then use the formulas to figure out his or her training heart rate. It's also a good idea to practice finding the radial and carotid pulse on another human.

BEGINNING YOUR FITNESS TRAINING SESSION

To begin a fitness training session a person should first warm up to prevent injury. A proper warmup elevates the body's temperature and prepares it for activity by moving blood to the working muscle and connective tissue (see the sample warmup outlined in Chapter 5). After the body is adequately warmed up, about 10 minutes, clients can perform a few stretches to further prepare themselves for action (never stretch without warming up first). After the warmup and stretching, begin an aerobic training session to elevate the heart rate to the target range—do not start the timer until the target zone is reached.

When concluding an aerobic exercise session participants should never abruptly stop moving. Instead, they should keep the legs moving at a reduced pace, slowing the pace more every minute, for 5 minutes or longer or until the heart rate drops below 100 beats per minute. During the cool down the constant movement of the leg muscles acts like a pump to assist with the venous return of blood to the heart. An adequate cool down prevents post-exercise drops in blood pressure and dizziness. After cooling down clients should stretch while they are still warm.

Beginners should start a program slowly and then gradually build up endurance. You must remind beginners not to overdo it at first because they may feel good while working out, but 2 days later they will discover aches and pains in muscles that they didn't know they had.

They should try to find activities that are fun and that they are able to enjoy. Brisk walking, hiking, jogging, cycling, cross-country skiing, dancing, kick boxing, swimming, and using the treadmill and elliptical striders are all good aerobic activities. Golf, tennis (for most of us), weightlifting, bowling, and other start-and-stop activities do not help train the heart and lungs because the necessary intensity of exercise is not maintained for a long enough time.

Individuals with very low levels of fitness should start by exercising 3 days a week for 12–15 nonstop minutes with their heart rate elevated in the target range. As their endurance and conditioning increase, they should increase the length or duration of their activity to 20 minutes and then keep progressing until they can exercise in their target range for 30, 40, or even 50 minutes. As they progress they can also increase the frequency of their training to 4 or 5 days a week. In addition, they can increase the difficulty or intensity of their workouts by doing things such as adding an uphill run or ride or going a farther distance or at a faster speed. Now that we understand how to safely get an aerobic exercise program going, it will greatly benefit us to review the principles of **resistance training** to comprehend how it can be a valuable addition to personal stress reduction programs.

RESISTANCE TRAINING

Progressive resistance exercise training is a great way to improve muscle tone and strength, burn more calories, prevent injuries, and improve self-image. Resistance training helps increase muscle mass, and larger, more toned muscles act like a furnace, burning more calories even when at rest. Increasing muscle tone and strength will help stressed clients feel better about their bodies, reducing that aspect of their stress.

Resistance Training for Stress Reduction

There are different ways to do resistance training; however, for stress reduction the client should focus on **isotonic** progressive resistance exercises—lifting light weights through their full range of motion. This type of lifting will not build a person up like a body-builder but will help them gradually increase their strength and tone and stabilize their lax joints. Isotonic training means that a person moves a constant weight through the full range of motion. It is comprised of concentric or shortening muscle contractions, where the distal attachment moves closer to the proximal attachment and eccentric or lengthening muscle contractions, which occur when a muscle lengthens as it lowers a weight, slowly resisting the pull of gravity. As clients become stronger, they will progressively add more weight to their workout.

Always start slowly with weightlifting because although it may feel great when lifting the first day, the true test comes 48 hours later when the delayed muscle soreness kicks in. Everyone usually experiences some soreness when they start a program. Ideally, clients will add three resistance sessions to their weekly personal stress reduction plan with a day off in between each session to give their body a chance to recover.

Start a program by selecting weights that can be moved 8 times or repetitions (reps) through the full range of motion. On the first day, start with 1 set of 8 reps for each exercise. As strength is gained, increase the number of reps to 12, and if time permits add more sets. When one can easily lift a weight for a set of 12 reps, increase the weight by 10–15 percent.

Breathing and speed of movement are important aspects of a proper progressive resistance exercise training program. The breath should never be held when lifting weights; instead try to breathe normally, exhaling when lifting against gravity (concentric contraction) and then inhaling on the recovery (eccentric braking, resisting against the pull of gravity). In addition, weightlifting should be performed slowly. One should take 2 seconds to perform

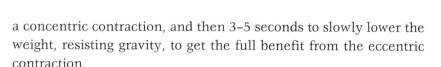

a concentric contraction, and then 3–5 seconds to slowly lower the weight, resisting gravity, to get the full benefit from the eccentric contraction.

Before lifting, a person should warm up thoroughly. Aerobic exercise can be a good warmup for weightlifting. If the client does not have dumbbells or access to gym equipment, books or large cans of food can be used for resistance. Although they may eventually progress to free weights if they are just starting out at a gym, recommend that they use the weight machines at first to develop a base of tone, strength, and proper body positioning while lifting. Free weights are more difficult because balancing a weight bar requires the recruitment of more motor units and core muscles for stabilization. In addition, for safety, a partner will be needed for spotting when lifting free weights.

Resistance Training for the Massage Therapist

To have a long and successful career, a massage student must become a massage athlete. To avoid and prevent injuries massage therapists must be physically fit. They must have enough muscular strength and endurance and flexibility to meet the demands of this profession. This author encourages all massage therapists to routinely participate in a resistance exercise program that works both their upper and lower extremities.

CONTROVERSIAL EXERCISES

Before embarking on an exercise regimen, consider the following controversial exercises and activities that are potentially dangerous and should be avoided or used with caution. Please share this information with your clients so that they do not sustain injuries while training. Figure 6.2 provides a summary of these controversial and potentially dangerous exercises.

Rolling the Neck in Full Circles

The grating sound that is heard when the head rolls back into extension beyond neutral is actually bone rubbing on bone. This exercise will lead to wear and tear on the facet joints, and if continued on a regular basis, it may lead to degenerative changes in the cervical

Rolling the neck in full circles

Lat pulls behind the head

Straight leg trunk flexion against gravity

Bending and twisting while lifting

Improper situps and leg lifts

Pulling heavy objects

Hurdler's stretch

Ballistic or bounce stretching

Poor wrist positioning

Holding the breath while exercising

Isometric exercises

Very deep squats

Open chain knee extension

Back extensions with weights

Hip internal rotation and adduction across the midline

Excessively repeating the same exercise

Exercising with improper footwear

Figure 6.2

Summary of controversial and potentially dangerous exercises and activities

vertebrae. Instead of performing full neck circles, use the safe neck stretching exercises outlined in Chapter 5.

Lat Pulls Behind the Head

Proper lat pulls are performed in front of the head and chest while sitting in erect posture. Behind-the-head lat pulls contribute to forward head posture and neck strains. So, always maintain good posture when working the lats—chin down, eyes level, head and shoulders back, and the bar out in front of the head and chest.

Straight Leg Trunk Flexion Against Gravity

Bending forward to touch the toes with the knees locked and bending and twisting to touch the opposite hand to the toes can cause back injuries. Combining gravity and limited hamstring and lumbar spine flexion flexibility with the weight of the skull, thorax, and upper extremities can overstretch, strain, and injure the muscles, fascia, ligaments, and discs of the lumbar region. Eliminate the danger imposed by the force of gravity by performing these activities while sitting.

Bending and Twisting While Lifting

Improper lifting technique puts severe strain on the muscles, fascia, ligaments, and intervertebral discs of the lumbar region. Never use your back to lift. Instead, bring the object being lifted directly in front of the feet, bend the knees, and keep the head up and the back straight. Then lift with the legs and gluteals as the object is brought in as close to the body as possible.

Improper Situps and Leg Lifts

Situps should not be done with the knees extended and the feet locked under an object for support because these actions will overstrengthen the hip flexor muscles (iliopsoas) and contribute to anterior pelvic tilt, hyperlordosis, back pain, and possibly even sciatica. Double-leg leg lifts also overstrengthen the iliopsoas. When doing situps and leg lifts, always keep the pelvis neutral, don't let the back arch, and focus the exercise on the abdominals and not the hip flexors. For proper technique refer to the safe abdominal strengthening exercises outlined in Chapter 5.

Pulling Heavy Objects

When trying to move heavy objects, don't pull them toward you. This can strain the back and throw the vertebrae out of alignment. The human body is built to be much stronger at pushing an object using the strong gluteals, quadriceps, and calves than pulling with the back musculature. So when moving heavy objects, always push—don't pull.

Hurdler's Stretch

Sitting on the ground with the left leg extended out in front of the body, the right leg back with the hip internally rotated and the medial aspect of the knee on the ground as the torso is moved forward or back can damage the medial meniscus of the right knee. Instead use the safer hamstring and quadriceps stretches listed in Chapter 5.

Ballistic or Bounce Stretching

Rapidly moving a joint through its range of motion by bouncing can exceed the limits of the joint and lead to injury. Rapid stretch fires the muscle spindle, which contracts the muscle to prevent the joint from going too far and can actually inhibit gains in flexibility and cause injury. The client should not try to force the muscles to stretch abruptly; it is safer and more effective to perform slow, relaxed, smooth, steady, controlled stretches, allowing the muscles to lengthen and relax. Using the antagonistic muscle to stretch with a little pressure assisting the movement is another safer alternative.

Poor Wrist Positioning

Whether lifting weights, performing a massage, or typing, maintaining the wrists in the extended or neutral position prevents injuries. Avoid activities that place and maintain the wrists in flexion, extension beyond neutral, and radial or ulna deviation.

Holding the Breath While Exercising

Particularly when doing resistance exercises, holding the breath can raise the blood pressure and lead to decreased blood flow to the heart and subsequently the brain. This can cause dizziness and even loss of consciousness (blackouts). So keep breathing as normally as possible when working out aerobically and when lifting weights; exhale when lifting, and inhale on the recovery. A person with high blood pressure should not lift heavy weights.

Isometric Exercises

Isometric exercises can raise the blood pressure and inhibit blood flow to the heart, brain, and general circulation. They should be avoided by older clients and those with high blood pressure. To gain strength and tone, these clients are better off lifting light weights through the full range of motion.

Very Deep Squats

When squatting don't let the angle between the upper and lower leg drop to less than 90 degrees. Deep squatting places a great deal of strain on the posterior cruciate ligament and the patella. Also, when doing lunging exercises do not allow the knee to move in front of the toes.

Open Chain Knee Extension

A person with knee pain should avoid open chain knee extension exercises in which the feet are not touching anything and the pads of the machine are against the shins. It is easier on the knee joint to perform leg exercises in which the feet are pushing against a plate (i.e., closed chain exercises). Straighten the legs but do not allow the knees to lock out when performing knee extension exercises.

Back Extensions with Weights

Back extensions with weights exercises consist of hanging the upper body over a bench, face down, and rising up with a weight behind the head. These exercises can overstrengthen the lumbar extensor muscles and contribute to an anterior tilt of the pelvis. Generally these muscles are strong enough, so avoid this type of activity.

Hip Internal Rotation and Adduction Across the Midline

A person who has a shallow hip socket, indicated by a clicking sound when the hip is moved, should avoid internally rotating and adducting the hip across the midline because it may pop the head of the femur out of the acetabulum. Also be cautious performing passive range of motion on someone with a hip replacement. Although there are different types of hip replacements, the general rule post-surgery is to avoid hip flexion beyond 90 degrees and internal rotation and adduction across the midline.

Excessively Repeating the Same Exercise

Performing the same exercises all the time is boring and monotonous and can overtrain the same muscle groups, which can lead to poor flexibility and repetitive strain injuries. Instead, try to vary activities by cross training. Cross training simply means alternating and diversifying your training regimen. For example, on Monday run, Wednesday cycle, Friday swim, and Sunday hike. Also if finger-, hand-, or wrist-intensive activities are part of the client's job, then try to persuade him or her to avoid these sorts of activities for hobbies.

Exercising with Improper Footwear

It is important to select the proper footwear for the type of training being done. A good pair of running shoes should provide excellent shock absorption, have a well-defined arch, have a wide base of support to prevent rolling the ankle, and be wide and long enough for the specific shape of the foot. Cross-training shoes are a little heavier than running shoes and will work well in the gym but are not as good on the track or trail. Don't skimp on shoes and socks—your feet will thank you.

SENSITIVELY COMMUNICATING WITH YOUR CLIENT

Now we must tackle the tough issue. How does the stress reduction massage therapist gently persuade already-stressed and overloaded individuals to change their behavior and incorporate fitness into their lives? The best way is to show them the facts and help them realize that exercise is a different type of food for their body that will help them age more slowly and help combat stress. Exercise does not require all-out effort and lots of pain; people show benefits from even modest increases in their activity level.

Some highly stressed individuals don't respond well to the gymnasium or health club environment, so encourage your clients to start their program by walking during work breaks, to take the stairs instead of the escalator or elevator, and to try to increase their energy expenditure during their activities of daily living. Encourage them to do calisthenics while watching television and to walk to the store rather than drive whenever possible. It is also useful to review with the client some of the common excuses for not exercising, such as no time; no energy; too old; too out of shape; the weather is too hot, too cold, too rainy, or too snowy; just can't get around to it; friends aren't into it; and it's not cool. It's a beneficial homework assignment for clients to list their reasons for exercising, their excuses for not, and then their plan for fitting three to four aerobic exercise and three resistance exercise sessions or simply just more activity into their weekly schedule.

SUMMARY

Now we have a better appreciation of the importance of aerobic and resistive exercise stress as stress reduction tools. Before we move on to the next chapter on stretching, some important concepts to remember follow:

- Aerobic exercise and resistance training can help reduce stress.

- The human body requires exercise, and a lack of exercise can lead to a variety of physical problems and diseases.

- Obesity is an epidemic plaguing our society.

- Moderate exercise on a regular basis can help improve the strength, endurance, flexibility, coordination, balance, and posture of individuals, even if they have been sedentary for many years.

- Walking and gardening are great fitness activities.

- Aerobic endurance training and resistance exercise instruction is out of the scope of practice for many massage therapists. If not qualified, refer your clients who need these elements added to their stress reduction programs to appropriate classes and professionals.

- For the training effect for the heart and lungs to occur, a person must elevate and maintain his or her heart rate in his or her target zone for 20–50 minutes.

- Progressive resistance exercises can improve muscle tone, increase muscular strength and endurance, burn calories, help improve self-image, and help prevent injuries.

- Massage therapists are athletes who need to stay fit and can benefit from the routine practice of aerobic and resistance exercise training.

- Inform clients to try to avoid potentially dangerous exercises.

- Cross training involves altering and diversifying a training regimen.

- Convince your clients that exercise is another type of food for their bodies that will help them age more slowly and help them naturally combat stress.

Stretching Your Client

At times clients need help stretching out their tight musculature to rebalance and realign their posture. No matter how hard they try, active stretching just does not produce the desired flexibility results. This chapter outlines norms for human **range of motion** (ROM), explains current ROM terminology, and provides some tips for safely stretching out your clients. Discussion includes performing active assistive stretching, using neurological reflexes to aid stretching, determining end feel, and performing passive ROM.

NORMAL JOINT RANGE OF MOTION

What are the normal ranges of motion for human joints? This is a great question with no definitive answer; if you look in six different textbooks, you'll most likely find six different responses. Genetics, age, activity level, accidents, injuries, and lack of proper exercise all can affect joint range, and the disparities in normal joint range numbers in the literature may be attributed to the population used for the measurements and how the measurements were obtained. It stands to reason that young athletes will demonstrate greater joint flexibility than sedentary 60-year-olds.

There is also a lack of agreement in ROM terminology between the massage therapy profession and the medical profession. Specifically, the term **hyperextension** is frequently used in massage therapy textbooks and literature to describe normal ROM of the wrist, hip, and shoulder, which the medical profession calls extension beyond the anatomical position or extension beyond neutral. The American Physical Therapy Association, the American Medical Association, and the American Academy of Orthopedic Surgeons only use the term hyperextension to describe atypical injurious motions that extend a joint beyond its normal range. To ensure accurate communication between massage therapists and medical professionals, it behooves the massage therapy industry to adopt and use the standardized terminology accepted by the medical community.

In the following descriptions of the normal ROM of the major joints of the body, the anatomical position is the starting point used for each motion unless otherwise noted. Remember that the numbers posted are averages and merely guidelines to respect when passively stretching a client, so to prevent injury and the discomfort of your clients always take into account their age, fitness level, and physical limitations. For your convenience Table 7.1 summarizes the ROM norms for upper- and lower-extremity joints in a quick reference chart.

Ranges of Human Joint Movements

Neck

The anatomical position is considered zero and is the starting position for all movements of the neck. The neck can bend forward into 0–85 degrees of flexion in the sagittal plane and move back into 0–70 degrees of extension. The neck also laterally flexes (side bending) from 0 degrees to 45 degrees in the coronal plane on each side. The neck rotates around a vertical longitudinal axis from the anatomical position to 0–80 degrees of rotation on each side.

Shoulder

From the anatomical position the shoulder can flex forward in the sagittal plane from 0 degrees to 180 degrees and extend backward in the same plane from 0 degrees to 60 degrees. The shoulder can also abduct from 0 degrees to 180 degrees in the coronal plane and adduct to 0 degrees as the shoulder returns to the anatomical position from an abducted position. Some authors profess that the shoulder can adduct across the midline up to 45 degrees (McAtee and Charland, 1999); however, this author lumps this movement of the shoulder across the midline with shoulder horizontal adduction.

External rotation (lateral rotation) 0–90 degrees and internal rotation (medial rotation) 0–70 degrees of the shoulder are measured from a different starting position. The starting position (0) for measuring external and internal rotation of the shoulder is called

TABLE 7.1

Upper- and Lower-Extremity Range of Motion Reference Chart

Upper Extremity		Lower Extremity	
Shoulder	**Degrees**	**Hip**	**Degrees**
Extension	60	Extension	10
Flexion	180	Flexion	125
Abduction	180	Abduction	45
Adduction	0	Adduction	10
Lateral Rotation	90	Lateral Rotation	45
Medial Rotation	70	Medial Rotation	45
Horizontal Abduction	30		
Horizontal Adduction	135		
Elbow	**Degrees**	**Knee**	**Degrees**
Extension	0	Extension	0
Flexion	145	Flexion	140
Forearm	**Degrees**	**Ankle**	**Degrees**
Supination	90	Plantar Flexion	45
Pronation	90	Dorsiflexion	20
Wrist	**Degrees**	**Foot**	**Degrees**
Extension	70	Inversion	40
Flexion	80	Eversion	20
Ulnar Deviation	45		
Radial Deviation	20		

the neutral position, which is approximated by abducting the shoulder to 90 degrees and in line with the torso and then positioning the forearm and wrist at a 90-degree angle to the upper arm and parallel to the ground. To perform external rotation, from the neutral position rotate the fingertips toward the ceiling without dropping the upper arm. To perform internal rotation, from the neutral position rotate the fingertips toward the ground without dropping the upper arm.

The shoulder can horizontally adduct from 0 degrees to 135 degrees or move 45 degrees past the midsagittal line. The starting position for measuring shoulder horizontal adduction is approximated by abducting the shoulder to 90 degrees, in line with the coronal (frontal) plane and parallel to the ground. To horizontally adduct, move the arm parallel to the ground across the chest as far as possible. The shoulder can horizontally abduct from 0 degrees to 30 degrees. Perform shoulder horizontal abduction by starting from the same position as shoulder horizontal adduction and moving the shoulder in a posterior direction horizontal to the ground.

There are no norms for shoulder elevation, depression, protraction, retraction, and circumduction. Just compare one side of the client's body to the other and try to balance both sides in the course of the treatments.

Elbow

In the anatomical position the elbow is extended to 180 degrees, or 0 degrees if it is the starting position for another movement, such as elbow flexion. For a small percentage of the population the elbow normally extends beyond 180 degrees. The elbow can flex forward in the sagittal plane from 0 degrees to 145 degrees.

Radioulnar Joint

The radioulnar joint is where supination and pronation occur. From the anatomical position rotate the forearms so the thumbs are facing forward in the sagittal plane; this is called mid position. Supination and pronation are measured from mid position. From mid position rotate the forearms medially so the thumbs point toward the body into 0–90 degrees of pronation. Rotate the forearms laterally from mid position into 0–90 degrees of supination, which is back to the anatomical position.

Wrist

All movements of the wrist start from the anatomical position. The wrists bend forward into flexion in the sagittal plane from 0 degrees to 80 degrees. The wrist moves backward 0–70 degrees into extension. The wrist moves into radial deviation by laterally flexing in the coronal plane toward the thumb and radius from 0 degrees to 20 degrees. The wrist moves into 0–45 degrees of ulnar

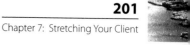

deviation by bending in the coronal plane toward the pinky finger and the ulna.

Trunk

The anatomical position is considered 0 (zero). From the anatomical position the trunk can bend forward into 0–90 degrees of flexion in the sagittal plane and move back into 0–30 degrees of extension. The trunk also laterally flexes (side bending) from 0 degrees to 30 degrees in the coronal plane on each side and rotates around a vertical longitudinal axis from the anatomical position to 0–45 degrees on each side.

Hip

All movements of the hip start from the anatomical position. From this position the hip can flex forward in the sagittal plane into 0–125 degrees of hip flexion (with the knee flexed) and only 0–90 degrees of flexion (with the knee extended). The knee-flexed position gives a more accurate appraisal of true hip flexion range because bending the knee eliminates restrictions caused by the hamstrings. The hip can extend backward in the same plane from 0 degrees to 10 degrees. The hip can also abduct from 0 degrees to 45 degrees in the coronal plane and adduct 0–10 degrees across the midline. If you add some hip flexion, the hip can adduct up to 30 degrees across the midline. The hip can medially rotate from 0 degrees to 45 degrees and laterally rotate from 0 degrees to 45 degrees.

Knee

In the anatomical position the knee is in 180 degrees of extension, or 0 degrees if it is the starting position for other movements. Knee extension more than a few degrees beyond 180 degrees is considered atypical and problematic. The knee will bend in a posterior direction into 0–140 degrees of knee flexion.

Ankle

From the anatomical position, pointing the toes away from the nose will cause the ankle to plantar flex from 0 degrees to 45 degrees. With the knee flexed and bringing the toes toward the nose, the ankle will dorsiflex from 0 degrees to 20 degrees. With the knee extended, the gastrocnemius will limit dorsiflexion to about 10 degrees.

Foot

Inversion is a combination of slight ankle plantar flexion, foot adduction, and supination. From the anatomical position, slightly plantar flex the ankle and rotate the sole of the foot medially (supination) and slightly adduct the forefoot into 0–40 degrees of inversion. Eversion is the combination of slight dorsiflexion of the ankle, foot pronation, and forefoot abduction. From the anatomical position, slightly dorsiflex the ankle and rotate the sole of the foot in a lateral direction (pronation) and abduct the forefoot into 0–20 degrees of eversion.

Now that we have completed our review of which directions and on average how far human joints move, we must now focus our attention on how the nervous system can help us stretch our clients more effectively.

NEUROLOGICAL REFLEXES

In addition to understanding the normal limits of joint flexibility, it is important that massage therapists understand how the body's **mechanoreceptors** and neurological reflexes can be used to help safely stretch a client. The body has a variety of mechanoreceptors, which are sensory feedback organs that provide the central nervous system feedback from the skin, muscles, connective tissue, tendons, joints, and fascia. A class of the body's mechanoreceptors, the muscle spindles, are proprioceptive organs, which provide feedback on the internal state of a muscle. These sensory nerve endings are made up of intrafusal fibers that are located in the belly of the muscles and that run the length of the muscle. Annulospiral fibers and flower-type receptors surround these intrafusal fibers, and together they provide feedback about the muscle to the spinal cord. These structures constantly monitor the muscle fibers, detect the rate of stretch in a muscle, and determine how fast and far it is moving (Beck, 2006). When a muscle is stretched too far or too quickly, the spindle cells fire off, contracting the muscle to prevent more stretch that may result in injury. This involuntary automatic reflex that prevents overstretching of the muscle tissue is called the myotatic stretch reflex. An example of this reflex occurs when a physician taps with a rubber hammer on the patella tendon and the knee jerks involuntarily. To prevent this reflex from interfering with a stretch, it is important to stretch slowly and not to bounce while stretching.

The **Golgi tendon organs** (GTOs) are another type of proprioceptive organ located in the tendons and at the musculotendinous junction. The GTOs work with other mechanoreceptors to provide information to the nervous system on muscle tension, how hard a muscle is working, and the amount of force pulling on the bone to which it is attached. There has been much controversy about the role of the GTO in stretching, and contrary to popular belief it is now postulated to have only a weak inhibitory function and is not much of a factor in strength development and stretching. **Reciprocal inhibition** plays a much more important role in stretching than the GTOs.

Reciprocal inhibition refers to the reflex mechanism that shuts down the antagonist when an agonist contracts. Therefore, when the quadriceps muscles contract, the hamstrings are automatically relaxed by reciprocal inhibition to allow movement to occur at the knee joint. Reciprocal inhibition and postisometric contraction relaxation are both used in **contract-relax-antagonist-contract** (CRAC) stretching to improve flexibility. CRAC is a type of proprioceptive neuromuscular facilitation (PNF) stretching that is safe and very effective at increasing flexibility. To stretch the hamstrings using CRAC the client lies supine and raises his or her extended right leg into hip flexion, contracting the quadriceps to do the work. The leg should be raised slowly, so that the spindles of the right hamstrings do not fire, and it should be raised as far as the hamstrings comfortably allow. The therapist places his or her hand or shoulder against the client's gastrocnemius and tells the client to resist their force, not to try to knock them over. Hold this contraction of the hamstring for a slow 6 or 10 count. Pause for a few seconds after the contraction to allow time for the postisometric relaxation to occur. After this brief delay instruct the client to contract the quadriceps to reciprocally inhibit his or her hamstrings and to bring the extended leg into more hip flexion, increasing the hamstring length. Thus when the **agonist** (the quadriceps) contracts, the **antagonist** (the hamstrings) relaxes and can be stretched further. After the quadriceps are contracted for 3 seconds, stretching the hamstrings, the therapist adjusts his or her position forward to take up the slack created by the increased flexibility. Repeat the whole sequence 3 or 4 times. These techniques should be used as part of treatments when needed and in conjunction with the active stretching exercises outlined in Chapter 5, which should be assigned as homework for the client. Let's now focus our attention on passive stretching.

PASSIVE STRETCHING

When a massage therapist performs passive ROM, the client is totally passive and does nothing at all. The muscle being stretched should be thoroughly warmed up before attempting to passively stretch it. The client should be placed in a position that is comfortable for him or her and for the therapist. The joint being stretched must be isolated and then slowly moved through the range, trying to approximate the client's full range without injury or undue pain or discomfort. The therapist should learn to stretch opposite the line of muscle pull using varied angles to effectively stretch the muscle fibers that run in different directions. Stretch the client until mild tension, but not pain, is felt in the muscle. If the client experiences pain, tingling or numbness, or spasm, or the therapist feels a hard bony feel from a stretch, back off immediately. When performing passive ROM, the therapist must be an effective communicator. The client must be instructed to keep breathing while being stretched because muscles require a constant supply of oxygen; the client also should be instructed to inform the therapist when a stretch is too uncomfortable. The therapist must also be a capable observer of the client being stretched, always looking for grimacing, crying, panting, holding of the breath, and compensation (the substitution of other joint movements to try to achieve the desired range).

It's essential that therapists always use proper body mechanics to avoid injuring themselves while performing passive stretching and myofascial releases. Sometimes when performing these techniques a therapist has to wait quite a while for the muscle and the connective tissue to release. Therefore, therapists must always use gravity to their advantage. It is important that they keep a dual awareness between the client's body and of the condition of their own body. Constant readjustments in the therapist's body positioning may be needed when performing these procedures.

The therapist must also learn to distinguish among the different qualities of movement that they may feel when they approach the end of a client's range. The texture of the resistance felt when a joint reaches its end of range is known as **end feel.** Therapists must tune in to the client and learn to feel the difference between soft

- Warm up the muscle and joint thoroughly before stretching.
- Position the client in a posture that will be comfortable for both of you.
- Always maintain proper body mechanics and use gravity to your advantage.
- Stretch a muscle slowly and use different angles to stretch the muscle fibers that run in different directions.
- Never bounce stretch.
- If the client feels pain or tingling or if you feel a bony end feel back off immediately.
- Maintain effective communication with the client throughout a stretching session.
- Make sure the client keeps breathing.
- Constantly monitor the client for signs of pain, discomfort, and the substitution of other joints to achieve a target range.
- Keep a dual awareness of your body and your client's.

Figure 7.1

Tips for safely stretching your client

end feel, which is the normal soft, springy end feel of a healthy muscle's range, and pathological end feels, such as protective muscle spasm, scarred tissue, grating bones, or the boggy, squishy sensation caused by **edema.** The feeling felt when bone contacts with bone is called hard end feel, whereas pain that abruptly stops a joint movement well before the end of a normal range is called empty end feel. Figure 7.1 summarizes some tips for safely stretching your client.

ACTIVE ASSISTIVE STRETCHING

Active assistive stretching is a combination of active movement by the client and an assist by the therapist. The client moves a joint through his or her ROM as far as possible, and then the therapist assists the client to complete or improve the ROM. This can help a client's body get used to once again experiencing normal range in a joint that has restrictions. Clients can also be instructed to use one arm to assist their other arm through a restricted portion in their range. For example, a client who has limited right shoulder flexion can interlace his or her fingers and then flex his or her shoulders as far as possible with no restriction. When the restriction is reached, the client can use the left arm to help raise the right overhead.

A more advanced version of active assistive exercise is called active isolated stretching, or the Mattes Method. In the Mattes

Method of stretching the client actively contracts the muscle or group of muscles antagonistic to the muscle that needs to be stretched. They continue this contraction of the antagonist, moving the joint as far as they can go, through their ROM. When they reach the limits of their range they continue the contraction and the therapist applies 1 or 2 pounds of pressure, helping them stretch in the desired direction. After 2 seconds of pressure, the therapist relaxes and the client returns actively to the starting position. The movement is slow and steady; 8–10 repetitions should be done in this fashion. For example, using this method to stretch the hamstrings, the client will contract the quadriceps, raising his or her extended leg into hip flexion. When the client reaches the end of his or her range, the massage therapist will assist the client further through the normal range by adding 1 or 2 pounds of pressure in the desired direction. After 2 seconds of pressure the therapist relaxes and the client actively returns to the starting position. The direction of stretch can be modified to achieve the optimal angle desired for the stretch.

The massage therapist also can try to loosen tight joints by performing some gentle friction all around the joint, on the joint capsule, and on the tendons, before stretching. Vibration and heat or ice also can be used to desensitize an area that is painful to allow for a greater stretch. Gross and specific myofascial releases also can be used to help relieve fascial restriction and improve pain-free ROM. Experiment with the aforementioned techniques until you find the ones that work for the specific problems presented by your clients.

SUMMARY

Before we move on to outline some techniques to help you deeply relax your client, some concepts to remember from this chapter are as follows:

- Muscle spindles constantly monitor muscle fibers and detect the rate of stretch in a muscle, along with how fast and far it moves.

- When a muscle is stretched too far too fast, the muscle spindles cause the muscle to contract to prevent further stretch. To avoid this response, stretch a muscle slowly.

- Reciprocal inhibition refers to when an agonist contracts and inhibits the antagonist.

- CRAC stands for contract-relax-agonist-relax. It is a type of PNF stretching that uses the agonist to stretch the antagonist.

- During passive ROM, a client does nothing except relax and give feedback.

- Stretch the client's tight muscles and joints in a variety of angles to isolate different fibers that may be tight.

- End feel refers to the texture of resistance felt when a joint reaches its end of range.

Deep Relaxation: The Art of Doing Nothing

The regular practice of deep relaxation is the next component to add to your client's personal stress reduction program. Routine relaxation practice is an essential coping strategy that should be used by everyone to help reduce the stresses and strains of life. The physiological changes induced by relaxation are exactly opposite to the body's stress response, reducing sympathetic nervous system arousal and helping the body return to homeostasis. This chapter discusses the physical and mental changes produced by the relaxation response. In addition, general relaxation tips, muscular relaxation, autogenic training, visual imagery, auditory relaxation, and how to relax a client are outlined. Combining deep relaxation with massage treatments and a sample relaxation session also are discussed.

THE ANCIENT ART OF RELAXATION

Long ago, people realized that the regular practice of deep relaxation produced important physiological, psychological, and spiritual benefits. Many of the relaxation techniques developed by ancient cultures were often associated with religious lifestyles, such as yoga and Zen. The ancient Hebrews, Christians, and Egyptians also practiced deep relaxation. Our ancestors realized that setting aside some time each day to deeply rest was essential for the well-being of their spirits, minds, and bodies. Until recently, this practice was all but abandoned by our fast-paced society that traditionally sees relaxation as a waste of time.

Reading, watching television, and watching sporting events are very popular forms of relaxation but, unfortunately, do not provide the deep relaxation necessary to combat stress. In fact, these forms of relaxation bombard the central nervous system with stimulation that actually adds to your stress level. Quality relaxation comes from the quiet times when you think your own thoughts, relax your tight muscles, calm your emotions, rest your mind, and do absolutely nothing.

Deep relaxation or meditation has gotten a lot of bad press. Too often associated with "alternative lifestyles," meditation has gained the unfair reputation of being slightly out of the mainstream and therefore suspect. The word "meditation" bothers some people because they falsely assume that it is something mystical or magical. One should not worry because meditation will not make you shave your head, contort like a pretzel, kiss cobras, walk on hot coals, or don orange robes and sell books at the airport; however, it will, after 20 minutes, relax your body as deeply as 8 hours of sleep can. Meditation is a completely natural physiological phenomenon that everyone can learn to control and use to their advantage.

THE PHYSIOLOGY OF RELAXATION

Research has indicated that meditation fosters a physiological state that is opposite to the stress response. When a person meditates, breathing and heart rate decrease, blood pressure lowers or stabilizes, oxygen consumption declines, and brain-wave activity slows to a more restful state. The sympathetic nervous system appears to be inhibited when a person meditates. Bloomfield and colleagues (1975:231) reported that if transcendental meditation is practiced regularly it has a tendency to "reduce stress, anxiety, and tension; synchronize brainwave patterns; improve learning ability, perceptual motor performance and reaction time; reduce depression and neuroticism; increase self-actualization; decrease cardiac output and heart rate, improve organization of memory, reduce oxygen consumption and breathing rate; increase speed of problem solving, foster creativity, and provide the body with as deep a state of rest as eight hours of sleep in only twenty minutes."

RELAXATION METHODS

There are many ways to deeply relax; some people take naps, some sit quietly and reflect on their own thoughts, whereas others practice focused breathing or transcendental meditation. As long as the technique is natural and doesn't involve drugs, routinely practicing deep relaxation effectively reverses the negative effects of stress. Which technique is best for your client? You won't know until you try a variety and find the deep relaxation method optimal for his or her body, mind, and state of stress. Then, after you've found the proper one, making it part of your client's comprehensive stress reduction plan will improve his or her health immensely. Try to encourage your client to practice relaxation 3 times a week for 15–20 minutes. The client must find the time to do nothing, to turn off worries, to abandon the senses, to stop negative thoughts, and to pause and refresh. Use relaxation techniques in a session and teach your clients to do it at home.

GENERAL RELAXATION TIPS

Use the following list of general relaxation tips to help your client begin to establish good relaxation practices.

Begin with the Proper Attitude

Have an open mind and no anxiety about possible success or failure. Everyone succeeds because relaxation is simply doing nothing. To succeed, all a person has to do is passively will relaxation to occur. This "can't fail" attitude is one of the most important elements for learning how to relax.

Create the Proper Environment

A quiet, softly lit, comfortable place with a moderate temperature is the best place for relaxing. Disconnect the phone and hang up a "do not disturb" sign. A mat or a comfortable chair and soothing music or a prerecorded relaxation session is also helpful. Create a special place where it is OK to just be and do nothing.

Stick to a Routine

Reduced stress and improved health comes when you to practice 15-20 minutes of deep relaxation at least 3 times a week. Find a convenient time and set it aside for the sole purpose of deep relaxation. Some possibilities are before you go to work, coffee breaks, lunch time, or just after work. If your office isn't suitable, try lying or sitting in your car while listening to a prepared recording.

Expect to Relax

Everyone experiences relaxation in his or her own special way. Some people explain the sensation as a tingling, followed by numbness and a sense of well-being; others experience warmth, heaviness, and peacefulness. Don't try to steer and rationalize your experience; expect relaxation to happen and then just passively let it happen and enjoy.

RELAXATION TECHNIQUES

Use the following list of relaxation tips to help your client achieve a state of relaxation at any time they desire.

Focused Breathing

As described in Chapter 4, controlled breathing is the key to relaxation. Begin each relaxation session with some long, slow, deep, diaphragmatic breaths, while focusing the entire awareness on the breathing process. Deep relaxation naturally occurs with focused breathing. Refer back to the breathing exercises in Chapter 4.

Muscular Relaxation Techniques

The following muscle relaxation techniques can be used to help your clients recognize and relax their hypertonic muscles. These techniques also increase body awareness and, ultimately, help to deeply relax the mind and body.

Progressive Muscle Relaxation

Instruct clients to passively will all of their muscles to relax, from the top of their head down to the tips of their toes. If you prefer you may work from their toes up; it doesn't matter. For example, instruct the client to relax all the muscles of their forehead and scalp and then to let this wave of relaxation spread down their eyebrows, eyelids, and eyes. Then instruct them to relax the muscles of their cheeks, jaw, mouth, lips, and tongue. You get the idea. Be as specific with your commands as you want, but use terms that clients will understand as you progressively relax from one end of their body to the other.

Contract-Relax

For muscles that a client just can't seem to relax, the contract-relax technique works well. Contract one muscle or a group of muscles for 5 or 6 seconds (without holding the breath) and then relax the muscle by doing the opposite of contracting it (doing nothing). For those hard-to-relax clients you can exercise every muscle or muscle group in the body this way. Work from head to toes or toes to head.

Contract-Relax with Resistance

The contract-relax with resistance technique is particularly useful for clients who do not have good body awareness because the muscular contractions will increase their ability to feel the difference between the contracted and relaxed states. Have the client contract a muscle or muscle group for 6 seconds while pushing or pulling against an immovable object or an opposing body part and then relax it. For instance, push down on a desktop with your palms to contract the triceps and latissimus dorsi for 6 seconds and then relax the contraction. Or place your right hand against your left and provide resistance to left elbow flexion for 6 seconds and then relax the muscle you have just tightened. As before—make sure the client does not hold his or her breath while doing this exercise.

Diminishing Tensions

Accountants and engineers really respond well to this technique in which we put numbers on their muscle tension and relaxation. While contracting a muscle (with or without extra resistance), slowly and incrementally count to 6 and then relax it bit by bit while counting backward from 6. Thus, have a client contract a muscle for 6 seconds, counting 1–2–3–4–5–6, and then relax it a little bit more on each descending number 6–5–4–3–2–1; after 1 the muscle is completely relaxed.

Biofeedback

Biofeedback is another possible course of action for those individuals who don't respond to the previously outlined techniques. The use of an electromyograph or electromyometer provides a reading (in microvolts) or a sound representing a muscle's actual tension. Biofeedback may be useful for clients who experience muscle spasms that just won't quit. Clients can use the feedback from the machine to learn how to relax because it lets them see how the microvolt readout changes or listen to how the sound elicited changes as their muscle relax. This will improve their ability to feel their muscle tension and relaxation and gain greater control over their body areas that are tense. They also make biofeedback equipment that helps individuals control their skin temperature, brain waves (electroencephalogram), and galvanic skin response (GSR; the minute amounts of perspiration in the skin). A stress reduction massage therapist should find and develop a professional relationship with a qualified biofeedback practitioner in the area to make referrals to when needed. They may also be a great source of referral to your practice. Biofeedback frequently is used with the next relaxation technique to be discussed, autogenic training.

Autogenic Training

Autogenic training is a relaxation technique that effectively reduces blood pressure, improves circulation to the hands and feet, and promotes an overall feeling of deep relaxation. It also has proved useful in relieving migraine headaches. It is a great, easy-to-use technique that will help relax your clients during a treatment session or for use as relaxation homework. To experience autogenic training, sit or lie down in your quiet relaxation place. Close your eyes and relax by focusing on your breathing or by doing some of the muscular relaxation exercises previously outlined. Then, silently and slowly repeat suggestions of warmth, heaviness, and deep relaxation to yourself. Don't try to force these suggestions to come true; just passively will them to occur. Silently repeat each phrase for up to 30 seconds.

Examples of self-relaxation phrases follow (substitute right and left and hands, legs, and feet where appropriate):

My right arm and hand are growing warm and heavy.

My right hand is growing warmer and warmer.

Warmth is flowing into my hand(s).

My arms and hands feel heavy and warm.

My arms and hands feel warm, comfortable, and completely relaxed.

I feel quiet and warm.

I feel relaxed, comfortable, and peaceful.

My whole body is completely relaxed.

My chest and abdomen are completely relaxed.

I feel warm, heavy, and deeply relaxed.

My thoughts are calm and peaceful.

My whole body feels relaxed, comfortable, and peaceful.

My body feels limp and loose like a rag doll.

I feel all my tension melting away.

Another effective relaxation technique to use with your clients involves developing their ability to daydream.

Visual Imagery

Most people practice deep relaxation without even knowing it. Daydreaming is essentially a form of deeply relaxing meditation, although it's not as deep, controlled, or relaxing as a planned meditation experience. When you daydream, your eyes roll up into their sockets, pointing at a spot above and between the eyebrows. Your whole body relaxes, brain waves slow, and you see a mental picture from what is commonly called "the mind's eye," "third eye," or "mirror of the mind." Improving the client's ability to daydream through the practice of guided **visual imagery** experiences is beneficial because the slowing of the brain waves that occurs during a daydream and any deep relaxation or meditation session can help unlock the relaxation response of the mind and body.

When you're aware and alert and have all senses functioning, your brain-wave rate will be 13 cycles per second or above.

This is known as the beta level of consciousness and is associated with being attentive, oriented, and anxious. While daydreaming or mediating, the brain-wave rate slows down to the alpha level, or between 8 and 13 cycles per second. Alpha brain waves represent a state of rest, relaxation, and relief from attention and concentration. The five senses are abandoned and the external world is "turned off." In addition to providing deep physiologic rest, the alpha state allows a person to momentarily change his or her mental perspective. During relaxation sessions clients can clear their minds and distance themselves from their thoughts. The result is an altered viewpoint that opens their minds to new thoughts and unleashes their full measure of creative intelligence. After 20 minutes in the alpha state, the brain is far more efficient in carrying out its normal beta activities with increased clarity and renewed vigor. Consequently, your clients' ability to reduce their brain-wave rates to alpha at will improves the ability to relax on demand.

Following are some imagery examples that you can use with your clients and some directions on how to improve their ability to voluntarily produce alpha brain-wave rates and to deeply relax. First, have the client read through the list and pick an image that seems pleasant for him or her. Then, position him or her in a comfortable, quiet, isolated location, free from distractions. Instruct your client to close his or her eyes and talk him or her through some of the focused breathing and muscle relaxation exercises that were previously presented. Then when your client is in a relaxed state, instruct him or her to passively envision the relaxing image he or she has selected. As your client passively thinks about the image, his or her brain will enter the alpha level of consciousness, just as if your client were daydreaming. The images are as follows:

> In your mind picture your perfect place of relaxation. This is a place that you can mentally travel to whenever you are stressed. Think about mountains, waterfalls, tropical islands, the ocean, the desert, or whatever place relaxes you the most.

> Picture fond childhood memories. Relive a picnic with your parents, the holiday season with your family, your favorite birthday party, or your first bicycle.

Picture a field of beautiful flowers fluttering in the soft warm breeze. Notice the kinds and colors of flowers. Try to develop a sense of color in your mind's eye. Think about lying back in a hammock and letting the warm gentle breeze rock you into a deep state of relaxation.

Imagine you are floating on a raft on a clear, warm ocean. The waves are gently rocking you underneath a blue sky dotted with large white puffy clouds. The sea air smells of salt and you can hear the gulls in the air as the relaxed pitch of the waves gently rocks you into a deep state of relaxation.

Picture yourself as a bird gliding on a warm breeze. See through the bird's eyes and watch the ground pass slowly beneath you. Notice what kind of bird you've become.

Picture white healing light surrounding you, your loved ones, or anyone who needs some positive energy. This light charges you with energy; you feel strong, confident, and deeply relaxed.

Let whatever thoughts that come into your mind flow freely. Just watch the pictures and let your imagination run wild.

Picture a pebble dropping into the still surface of a pond. Notice the concentric ripples, and then watch them disappear as the surface turns into a mirror once again.

Picture your own mental TV set or movie screen on which you can view anything you desire. Ask your subconscious for answers to questions or problems that you have and watch the answers on the screen.

In your mind, create your perfect chair. When you sit in this chair all of your troubles leave, your health improves, and you instantly become deeply relaxed.

Picture the most tense part of your body. Picture the muscle fibers and watch them lengthen as they grow more and more relaxed. Feel all physical sensation leave this muscle as a wave of relaxation takes it over. Then spread this sensation to the rest of your body.

Picture yourself floating through a rainbow of colors, each color adding to your relaxation, vitality, health, confidence, and self-actualization. Picture yourself becoming the person you want to be.

Picture yourself piloting an old wooden sailboat that is heading out on the cool, blue, calm ocean. Envision the boat's billowing sails, the blue horizon, the golden sunshine, and white froth breaking across the bow. Listen to the sounds of the wooden hull and mast creaking and straining as you glide across the glistening surface. Relax to the songs of the gulls and the gentle tones of the far-off bells ringing their melodious messages. You are in total control of your destiny. Feel the euphoria, confidence, and peacefulness of this adventure.

Picture yourself walking down an ancient marble staircase as you listen to the faint sounds of a flutist playing in the distance. When you reach the bottom you find that you are in a beautiful courtyard full of artistic treasures. You are surrounded by bronze, gold, and marble statues and the fragrant smell of exotic flowers in bloom. It is dark and the only light comes from the dancing flames of many candles burning. You come to a beautiful pool full of very warm, but not too hot, water. You take off your robe and descend into the water and find a lounge chair made precisely for you. You lie back with your head comfortably out of the water. You take a deep breath, deeply relax, and enjoy the peaceful sounds of the flute.

If you have a medical problem picture the affected organ, gland, body part, or system as being dark and then see it surrounded by white light until it returns to its natural healthy appearance.

Create your own relaxing visual experiences. Try to think of peaceful, harmonious, positive, or inspiring thoughts. Or picture yourself in the future having successfully changed your life for the better, so that you have become the person that you want to be.

Another visualization technique for deep relaxation is to have clients focus all of their awareness on a body part, such as their hand or their tan tien, the energetic and geographical center of their body. Instruct them that if their thoughts wander, they should immediately refocus and return their concentration to the body part. If visual detachment exercises sound like "contemplating your navel," that's because they are traditionally used as beginning exercises for people learning meditation. As it happens, some highly respected and widely admired people drew their energy from meditation and deep relaxation. For instance, former U.S. President John F. Kennedy developed the ability to will himself to sleep almost instantly and was able to grab a few minutes of refreshing rest between meetings. Whether he called it meditation or some other name, this ability to powernap is one tool that can help a stressed individual survive on too little sleep and rest.

Auditory Relaxation

Another way to enter a state of relaxation is through auditory detachment in which sounds, rather than visualization, bring on a relaxed state. Using key words or sounds (called a **mantra** in meditation), your client can will his or her body and mind to relax. Ultimately, the goal of meditation is to create a completely restful void in the mind, uncluttered by any sights or sounds. In this deeply restful state, the thoughts and internal dialogue are completely still and a person becomes totally relaxed.

Auditory relaxation for deep relaxation uses a mellifluous, easily recited word that is said over and over again silently, quietly, or aloud. The sound helps your client to focus his or her concentration and awareness. A common keyword is OM, composed of three sounds: A, U, M. To begin, instruct the client to inhale deeply and slowly. Then have the client say "aah" in a low, steady, controlled voice. The client should make the sound come from the back of the throat. Have the client hold the sound until one-third of his or her air is gone. Then, without stopping, have the client transform the "aah" into an "oh" sound produced at the front of the mouth, giving it a nasal character. The client should hold the "oh" sound for the second one-third of the breath. Again without stopping, instruct the client to transform the "oh" into the "mmm" sound. Tell him or her to press the lips together and make the sound loud enough to vibrate strongly through the head and chest. Have the client hold the sound until the breath is finished. Then he or she should inhale to fill the lungs and try to still his or her body and mind by thinking peaceful thoughts. The client should spend 10–20 seconds in silence before repeating the whole procedure. The whole process can be repeated 7 times.

Other sounds besides OM can be used. They can be either natural or imagined. When you hear a natural source of repetitive sound, such as a waterfall, the ocean surf, wind, or the humming of bees, simply listen and focus your awareness on the sound. You can also use artificial sound sources to relax. Music profoundly relaxes many people, so experiment with different types of music and various sound effects to determine those that soothe each client the most. Classical music is the best for some, the flute for others, whereas other people prefer recordings of only nature sounds. Combining the auditory methods with other relaxation techniques can be especially effective. Tell your clients that when they feel tense, they can easily relax by repeating a keyword, listening to music, breathing diaphragmatically, slowing their brain to its alpha state, and then trying a visual imagery exercise or just simply letting their thoughts flow freely.

SAMPLE RELAXATION SESSION

To conduct a relaxation session for your client, play some relaxing background music and then begin with 5 minutes of focused breathing work as previously outlined. After the breathing, perform 5 minutes of muscular relaxation, relaxing each part of the client's body starting at the top of the head and working down to the tips of the toes. It also helps to repeat autogenic suggestions of warmth and heaviness while relaxing the musculature. Following is a sample of how to use the autogenic suggestions in a relaxation session. You can slowly read the sample relaxation script to your client, relaxing his or her entire body in this fashion. Ad lib by placing extra focus on the muscle groups that the client needs to release:

> Relax the muscles of your forehead and scalp. Let this wave of deep relaxation flow down your face to your eyebrows, eyelids, and the muscles of your eyes. Relax the muscles of your cheeks, jaw, mouth, lips, and tongue. Let this wave of relaxation spread down, relaxing the muscles of the front, side, and back of your neck where so much tension accrues. Go deeper and deeper into this tranquil state of deep relaxation. Relax your shoulders and allow this feeling of relaxation to spread down to the biceps and triceps of your upper arms, your forearms, hands, and fingers. Now repeat the following phrases silently to yourself: "My right arm and

hand feels warm and heavy, warmth is flowing into my fingers. My right hand and arm is feeling warmer and warmer. Warmth and relaxation are flowing into my fingers." Let this wave of relaxation now spread down to the muscles of the chest and abdomen. Let your breathing grow relaxed, yet full and satisfying. Now relax all the muscles of the back from the back of your neck all the way down to your hips.

Let this wave of relaxation take over your entire body. Feel the muscles of the front, side, and back of your hips totally relax as this wonderful relaxed feeling spreads down to the front, back, and sides of your thighs. Totally relax your upper legs, your legs growing warm and heavy, as this relaxed feeling spreads down to your calves, relaxing all the muscles of your lower legs, letting all the tension and tightness flow out, replaced by a warm feeling of relaxation. Now repeat the following phrases silently to yourself: "My right leg and foot are growing warm and heavy. Warmth is flowing into my toes. My left leg and foot are growing warm and heavy. Warmth is flowing into my toes. My right leg and foot are growing warmer and warmer. My left leg and foot are growing warmer and warmer. My legs and feet are warm, heavy, and completely relaxed. My mind and body are completely relaxed. My whole body feels relaxed, comfortable, and peaceful."

Next, perform 5–10 minutes of visual imagery or detachment exercises.

At the end of the relaxation period bring clients back to their awake level of consciousness by making some positive statement to them, such as, "You are slowly coming out of this deeply relaxed healthy state. You will be feeling much better than before. Your muscle tension, heart rate, and blood pressure will be reduced, and your ability to use oxygen will be improved. You will still be relaxed but awake and alert. On the count of three open your eyes, feeling much more relaxed than before." Count one, coming up slowly. Then count two and say "When you open your eyes you will feel deeply rested, as if you had full night's sleep." Then count three and say, "Open your eyes, feeling much, much better than before."

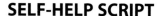

SELF-HELP SCRIPT

Give your clients a fun homework assignment. Instruct them to write a self-help relaxation script including elements that they find relaxing. Have them include the changes that they feel that they need to make in their lives or lifestyle to reduce their stress. It could include suggestions to stop smoking, to push away from the refrigerator, to control their temper, or to stop procrastinating. Have them bring it to their next appointment, and you can practice these positive affirmations after relaxing them.

COMBINING RELAXATION WITH MASSAGE TREATMENTS

To many, the concept of combining relaxation with massage treatments does not make sense. However, during relaxation the client is not asleep; clients are still alert and can be trained to function in this state to help reduce or eliminate their physical problems. It is better described as a state of relaxed concentration or relaxed focus. When in a relaxed state, clients can be trained to use the feedback from the heat and touch of the therapist's hands to pinpoint their areas of hypertonicity and melt them away with their minds. When a therapist uncovers an area that needs to be released, he or she presses gently on it and instructs the client to focus on the spot and try to breathe through it. Many times when the client tunes into the spot the therapeutic pulse is felt. The therapist works the spot until it releases, when the muscles fibers relax and the pulse slows, and synchronizes with the contralateral side. The client often may let loose a deep breath or sigh as the tension releases. This technique is most effective in the supine position. With this technique the therapist and clients work together to relieve stress and tension and counteract the body's physiological and mental response to their sympathetic nervous system arousal.

SUMMARY

Sleep improvement is our next topic; however, before we proceed review the following concepts:

- The routine practice of deep relaxation is beneficial for everyone to help reduce the stresses and strains of life.

- Deep relaxation can help people cope during times when they aren't getting enough rest and sleep.

- Deep relaxation fosters a physiological state that is opposite to the stress response.

- General relaxation tips include passively willing relaxation to occur, having a quiet comfortable place to practice, and trying to stick to a routine of practicing for 15–20 minutes 3 days a week.

- Natural relaxation techniques include focused breathing, muscular relaxation, autogenic training, visual imagery, music, sound effects, and auditory relaxation.

- Relaxed focus (relaxed concentration) can be used during massage treatments to help clients tune into and melt away areas of hypertonicity.

Helping Your Client Sleep

A relaxing, refreshing, full night's sleep is one of the greatest contributions that a massage therapist can make to help reduce stress and improve the quality of a client's life. If your client's stress profile indicated that he or she frequently was tired and lacked energy and had difficulty falling and remaining asleep, then sleep-improving strategies are the next element to consider adding to the client's personal stress reduction program. This chapter reviews the stages of a normal night's sleep, abnormal sleep patterns, the varying sleep requirements of different ages, commonly seen sleep-related problems, the effects of sleep debt, a sleep questionnaire/log, when to refer a client to a sleep clinic, natural sleep-improving strategies, and a sequence of massage techniques to help a client sleep more soundly.

EFFECTS OF SLEEP DEPRIVATION

Good-quality sleep is essential for successfully managing stress and maintaining health. Unfortunately, many people have lost the ability to effortlessly fall and remain asleep. Some go to bed and toss and turn, can't turn off their minds, or their legs just won't stop moving and they can't get comfortable. Frequent bouts of sleeplessness may lead to fatigue, anxiety, panic, and fear. Some people actually stop breathing temporarily when sleeping, which can be upsetting to both the sleeper and his or her bed partner. Sleep deprivation also can lead to cloudy thinking, impaired memory, reduced creativity, poor job performance, low energy, lack of motivation, irritability, impaired driving, and more injuries and accidents. It is estimated that 60 million Americans suffer from **insomnia**. Studies have linked immune system problems, diabetes, hypertension, obesity, and depression to poor-quality and insufficient sleep.

The massage therapist can help clients attempt to find out what is causing their problem and then develop a plan of action to resolve it. Because many factors influence sleep, there's no single magic cure-all that works for everyone. An individualized sleep improvement plan may require that the client visit a sleep clinic for diagnostic testing to determine if medication and treatment are necessary or if something as simple as making changes to their eating habits, living conditions, and lifestyle can make a difference. Before developing a sleep improvement plan, a therapist must first understand what happens during a night's sleep.

THE STAGES OF SLEEP

A normal night's sleep consists of four distinct non-rapid eye movement stages and a fifth stage known as **rapid eye movement** (REM). Sleep stages can be measured on an electroencephalogram (EEG), which records brain-wave activity and patterns by measuring the frequency and amplitude of its electrical impulses, and an electrooculogram (EOG) and electromyogram (EMG), which respectively identify eye and skeletal muscle activity. When people fall asleep their brain is still active but they are not conscious of the world around them. During this unconscious state of sleep the brain tunes into the body's internal environment rather than external stimuli. When a person goes to sleep they progress from the state of being awake, through stage 1 (light sleep), into stage 2 (moderate sleep), and then into stages 3 and 4, the deepest stages of sleep. In terms of brain-wave rates, beta waves are associated with being awake and alert, alpha waves are associated with relaxation with the eyes closed, theta waves are associated with the beginning stages of sleep, and delta waves are associated with the deepest sleep, seen in stages 3 and 4. After his or her time in stage 3 and 4 sleep, a person retreats through the stages backward, progressing from stage 4 to 3 to 2 to 1, which is then followed by time in the REM stage. In the REM stage the eyes move quickly around, the brain becomes more active, the blood pressure rises, and the breathing and heart rate become irregular. Dreaming is experienced during the REM stage. Figure 9.1 provides a look at the stages an adult sleeper goes through during a normal night's sleep.

Each complete sleep cycle takes roughly 90 minutes. People usually experience 4–5 sleep cycles per night. Most of a person's

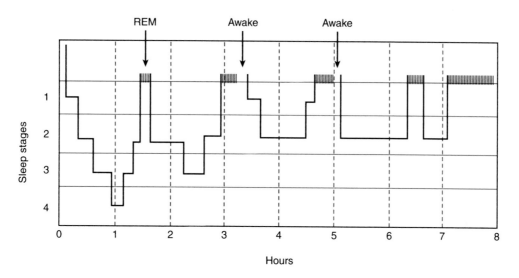

Figure 9.1

The stages of a normal night's sleep

stage 3 and 4 sleep is experienced in the first two sleep cycles. The amount of time spent in REM gets progressively longer as the night progresses; the least amount of REM sleep occurs in the first sleep cycle, about 10 minutes, whereas a person at the end of the last cycle may experience from 40 to 60 minutes of REM. The amount of time that a person spends in each stage during a normal night's sleep varies greatly because there are considerable differences between the sexes and between sleepers of different ages and different cultures. An average adult sleeper spends about 5 percent of the 8–9-hour sleep period in stage 1, 45–55 percent of the night in stage 2, 15–20 percent of the night in stages 3 and 4, and 20–25 percent of the night in REM. In a normal night's sleep no more than 5 percent of the time after sleep onset is spent awake. Elderly people spend less time in stage 3 and 4 and more time in stage 2.

HOW MUCH SLEEP DO WE NEED?

Depending on age, overall health, and stress level different people require different amounts of sleep. To stay healthy a person must get the proper amount of stage 3 and 4 and REM to replenish and repair the brain and bodies. Babies need about 16 hours, teenagers need 9 hours, and an average adult needs 7–8 hours of sleep each night. Not getting enough sleep takes a toll on the human mind and body. It is similar to writing a check with insufficient funds. Being overdrawn at the sleep bank has been termed **"sleep debt,"** and, just like a bank, the body demands to be paid back. The only way to eradicate a sleep debt is to get extra sleep. Teenagers need more stage 4 sleep to stimulate the release of growth hormone, which is important for brain development and physical growth. As we get older the amount of stage 3 and 4 sleep experienced diminishes. Older people also sleep more lightly and for shorter periods. Pain, alcohol intake, and nicotine use can all decrease the quality of sleep experienced. People with insomnia may experience the same sleep stages and body changes as a normal sleeper, but they spend less time in the deeper stages of sleep and REM. A long-term sleep debt may impair the immune system and inhibit the endocrine system's ability to produce and deliver the hormones needed to repair and regenerate the body.

An adult spends from 90 to 120 minutes of each night's sleep in the REM state. During REM the eyelids remain shut but the eyeballs move back and forth rapidly, in reaction to visual dream stimuli as dreaming occurs. Some psychologists believe that dreaming is a way of subconsciously resolving conflicts and finding solutions to problems. Others theorize that our thoughts and memories are consolidated during REM sleep. Experiencing enough REM sleep may be an important contributor to maintaining a healthy psyche. Although a multitude of sleep-related disorders have been documented in the literature, this chapter will focus on the three most prevalent disorders: insomnia, restless legs syndrome, and sleep apnea.

COMMONLY SEEN SLEEP-RELATED PROBLEMS

Insomnia, or the inability to sleep, appears in different forms. A person may have trouble falling asleep, or sleep-onset insomnia. It takes a normal sleeper a few minutes to fall asleep, whereas an individual with sleep-onset insomnia may spend 45–50 restless minutes trying to turn off their mind so they can fall asleep. Others may fall asleep soundly but wake up prematurely, whereas others don't feel rested after a full night's sleep. Things such as the environment, diet, lack of exercise, travel, social events, emotional situations, work overload, and psychological problems can all contribute to insomnia. To sometimes experience insomnia is normal. To often or always have difficulty sleeping indicates that it is a chronic problem that must be dealt with. In the United States, roughly 14 percent of the population has chronic insomnia. Insomnia is challenging to treat because sometimes it is a primary sleep problem but it can also be a symptom of another underlying sleep disorder. Once it is determined that the cause of the insomnia is not a serious medical problem, then the behavioral changes and techniques described in this chapter may be of benefit to your client. If the tips provided in this chapter do not help the client, he or she may need to visit the doctor. Sometimes the short-term use of hypnotics or sleeping pills may be the only way a person can break the cycle of insomnia and the anxiety experienced by not being able to fall asleep.

Restless legs syndrome (RLS) is a central nervous system disorder that leads to stress and chronic sleep loss. A person with RLS experiences what has been described as an itching, restless, tingling, jumpy, crawling, uncomfortable sensation in the legs that occurs during periods of inactivity or when trying to sleep. This disorder should not be confused with nocturnal muscle cramps. The individual with RLS just cannot seem to get comfortable, with the only relief coming from rubbing or moving the legs. Primary RLS is diagnosed when a person has a familial history of the disorder. Secondary RLS has been attributed to iron deficiencies, drug reactions, spinal cord and peripheral nerve lesions, kidney failure, pregnancy, and vertebral disc disease. About 10 percent of the general population and 19 percent of pregnant women are affected by RLS. A client with RLS symptoms should see his or her primary care physician to determine if prescribed medications will help relieve symptoms. Warm baths, massage, deep relaxation, and stretching can be useful adjuncts to medical treatment that may help a client cope with this disorder.

Obstructive sleep apnea is a condition in which the airway is restricted or completely collapsed, which causes a person to actually stop breathing for a time while sleeping. The sufferer will wake up repeatedly throughout the night, gasping for air, which fragments sleep and can result in anxiety from the fear of not being able to breathe. Loud snoring and constant fatigue are common symptoms of this disorder, which affects up to 30 million Americans. Sleep apnea frequently is caused by obesity, although many thin people also suffer from this disorder. A client with the aforementioned symptoms should be referred to a sleep center for testing, diagnosis, and treatments, which may include **CPAP** (continuous positive airflow pressure) **therapy,** surgery, or an oral appliance. CPAP therapy involves wearing a mask over the nose that supplies a positive air pressure to support the airway while a person sleeps. Surgery is another treatment option, and there are several different procedures available to prevent the airway from collapsing. A consultation with a sleep surgeon should be scheduled to determine whether surgery is an option and which procedure is most likely to obtain the desired results. Eating a healthy, low-calorie diet; performing aerobic exercises; diaphragmatic breathing training; and practicing relaxation are proactive measures a client with sleep apnea can take. Behavioral changes also can be effective for people who are only symptomatic when sleeping on the back. This involves developing a strategy to eliminate supine sleep—for example, sewing tennis balls to the back of the client's pajama tops.

SLEEP LOG

If the client experiences more than an occasional bout of sleeplessness, have him or her complete a sleep log for 1 week to determine if there are any patterns to his or her behavior or controllable factors that are contributing to the sleeping woes. Once uncovered, the therapist then should advise the client of some natural strategies to change the elements in his or her lifestyle and habits that are interfering with sleep. Table 9.1 provides a blank sample sleep log. Some pertinent questions to ask the client with sleep problems follow:

How long did it take to fall asleep?

What time (or times) did you awaken?

How much caffeine do you ingest every day?

What time do you eat dinner each night?

Do any foods you eat cause bloating, gas, indigestion, or acid reflux?

How much alcohol, if any, do you drink each night?

What activities do you perform the hour before retiring?

What nonprescription medications or drugs do you take that may interfere with your sleep?

How many cigarettes, if any, do you smoke each day?

TABLE 9.1

One-Week Sleep Log

Question	Mon	Tues	Wed	Thurs	Fri	Sat	Sun
How long to fall asleep							
Times you woke up							
Total daily caffeine intake							
Daily alcohol intake							
Dinner time							
Foods that upset your digestion							
Woke up gasping for air or short of breath							
Nightmares or recurring dreams							
Activities performed before retiring							
Nonprescription medications or drugs taken							
Number of cigarettes smoked							
Anxiety about sleeping							
Other info or factors interrupting sleep							

Did you awaken because you were short of breath?

Has a significant other ever mentioned that you seem to stop breathing or gasp for breaths of air at times each night when sleeping?

Do you have any thoughts or recurring dreams that keep you up?

Are there any other factors that might be interfering with your sleep?

CONTROLLABLE FACTORS THAT INTERRUPT SLEEP

The next step in a sleep improvement plan requires that the client evaluate the following environmental, dietary, physical, and mental aspects of his or her stress to see if they are affecting sleep quality.

Environmental

- Noise level
- Room temperature
- Dust
- Light level
- Uncomfortable bed and pillow
- Covers that are too restricting

Dietary

- Caffeine intake
- Eating heavy meals close to bedtime
- Eating foods that upset the digestive tract
- Taking medications that cause excitability
- Drug abuse
- Excessive alcohol intake

Physical

- Inconsistent bedtime
- Not enough exercise or exercising too close to bedtime
- Muscle twitches or cramps
- Pain
- Breathing difficulties

Mind

- Can't turn off the thoughts that keep them awake
- Stressful dreams
- Fear and anxiety about not being able to sleep

Now let's discuss how to help our clients reduce or eliminate the negative impact of these factors in our review of sleep-improving strategies.

SLEEP-IMPROVING STRATEGIES

The therapist should share the following list of natural sleep-improving strategies and practical tips with clients. Clients should experiment with the following suggestions to see if they help improve the quality of their sleep.

Set the Mood for Sleep

The quest for a good night's sleep begins where it all starts—in the bedroom. The bedroom is a place to sleep, rest, and have fun; it is not a place to work, eat, or worry. The ideal mood for a bedroom is one of comfort, security, and relaxation. The bedroom most conducive to sleep is quiet, dark, dust-free, and moderately cool (about 60–65°F). If allergies and a stuffy nose are frequent problems, clients should thoroughly dust their room; have their heating ducts, furnace filter, and drapes cleaned; and use an air purifier.

Consistent Sleep Schedule

Maintaining a consistent bedtime and rising schedule is critical. Retiring at about the same time each night programs the body's internal biological clock or circadian rhythm into a regular sleep pattern. Basking in 15–30 minutes of early morning sunshine everyday is also a good way to help program the body's natural sleep rhythm if the client has difficulty falling asleep at his or her desired bedtime.

Relax the Mind

Avoid highly stimulating activities, such as watching a violent movie or reading a mystery novel, close to bedtime or while attempting to get back to sleep when you've prematurely awakened. Also avoid reading about sleep problems before bed because you may subconsciously think you have the problem when you don't. Instead read a boring, dry book about subjects that you don't understand or that are of little interest. Of course, this book doesn't count.

Reduce Sleeping Anxiety

Don't go to bed worrying about sleeping. Try to go to sleep with a clear, calm, self-confident mind. To help relax the mind, silently repeat positive suggestions such as, "I'm going to sleep deeply and soundly the whole night through." "I will awaken in 8 hours completely relaxed, refreshed, and invigorated." "I will sleep deeply all night long." Or try repeating a short phrase silently to yourself, like repeating a mantra for meditation, such as "deep sleep," "calm and peaceful," or "rest easy."

Reduce Noise and Light

Fix that leaky faucet or noisy gutter downspout. Listen to soft music; sleep improvement CDs; or recordings of peaceful outdoor sounds such as rain, wind, or surf to mask out disturbing sounds. If unable to alter the environment, wearing earplugs and an eye mask can also reduce external stimuli. If a significant other's snoring is a problem, recommend a visit to a sleep disorder clinic to determine whether the snoring is a sign of obstructive sleep apnea. A short-term solution is to move to a separate room or buy some foam earplugs. Install room-darkening shades and lined curtains or wear eyeshades while sleeping to shut out excess light.

Comfortable, Supportive Bed

A comfortable bed is an absolute necessity. An old mattress, the wrong type of pillow, and uncomfortable bedding can be major contributors to sleep problems. A mattress and boxspring should be replaced every 10–15 years. If your clients wake up every morning with a stiff back, neck, or shoulders, ask them how old their mattress is, what kind of pillow they use, and what their regular sleep positions are. A mattress should be firm enough to provide those who sleep on their backs enough low back support to keep the spine in alignment. A mattress that is too soft does not give the back ligaments a chance to relax and can exacerbate the normal lordotic curve and back pain. A person should buy the best mattress that they can afford. They should try out different types of mattresses, pillows, and covers until they find the right combination. Mattresses come in many degrees of firmness, number and thickness of coils, and cover softness. It is important to find a mattress that provides enough support for the low back and neck yet is soft enough so that too much pressure is not placed on the shoulders and hips when sidelying. Firm mattresses help a bad back, but the right balance between comfort and firmness is strictly an individual preference. Don't be shy when shopping for a mattress. Lie down, relax, and try it out for at least 20 minutes before buying. Like a new pair of shoes, a new mattress may have a slight break-in period before a person gets used to it. Many mattress stores are now giving a free 30-day return policy to ensure that the firmness is right for the customer.

Comfortable, Supportive Pillow

A good pillow can be almost as important as a good mattress. If a person frequently gets up in the morning with a stiff neck and sore shoulders and upper arms, his or her pillow is possibly the blame. Advise clients who sleep on the back not to sleep on two pillows because this can contribute to forward head, neck pain, and headaches and actually can restrict airflow. A pillow should be comfortable, nonallergenic, cool, light, and designed to follow the normal curves of the neck. A natural curve neck pillow has two different heights to help the client sleep in proper alignment whether sleeping on the back or side. These pillows will ease neck pain and tension of the clients who sleep on the back by properly aligning the cervical vertebrae. The position in which the modern neck pillows place the head and neck can relax the anterior neck muscles and actually help open the air passageways, helping the client breathe easier. These pillows will also keep the side-sleeping client's neck parallel to the mattress, which reduces the neck pain and tension that results from having the neck crooked to one side all night long.

Appropriate Sheets and Covers

Comfortable sheets and covers are another part of the good night's sleep equation. Advise clients to use light blankets and only the amount that they need to keep warm because heavy covers can restrict the client's movements or cause feelings of claustrophobia, which can interrupt sleep. Use sheets that are cool, smooth, and clean and try blue or green sheets and covers because these tend to have a sedating effect. It also helps to leave enough room under the bed covers so the feet can move freely with no restrictions.

Sleeping Position

The client's sleeping position is another important element to consider. The best positions to sleep are on the back and the side. Back sleeping with a neck pillow and a good mattress that provides low back support is a good sleeping position for the client. If the client wakes up every morning with back pain, have him or her try sleeping with a pillow or bolster under the knees or a rolled-up towel under the low back for additional support. Side-sleeping clients should use a neck pillow to keep their spine in a straight line, and they should flex their hips and knees and place a pillow between their knees. If they wake up with shoulder pain or numbness (paresthesia) they also can hug a large pillow or soft bolster for relief. Whenever possible a person should avoid sleeping on the abdomen because it strains the neck and increases the lumbar lordotic curve. If the client cannot break the abdominal sleeping habit, the only way to partially reduce the strain it places on the back is to place a flat pillow under the pelvis and lower abdomen.

Regular Exercise

If the client has a high energy level and a sedentary job, he or she may not be physically tired at bedtime. Exercising during the day, preferably 4–5 hours before bed, will help tire the client. Participating in a regular routine of exercise, such as brisk walking, jogging, swimming, or cycling, and total body stretching may help the client sleep better.

Focused Breathing and Deep Relaxation

Focused breathing and deep relaxation can help clients calm their mind, turn off their internal voice, stop their negative thoughts, deeply relax their body, and bring on sleep. Start a relaxation for sleep session with long, slow, deep breaths; muscle relaxation; visual and auditory detachment exercises; and silent, positive statements of how the night's sleep is going to be deep, restful, and healthy. The client also may benefit from listening to a recording that induces relaxation and a deep natural state of sleep.

Warm Water

Warm water can relieve pain, reduce muscle spasms and tension, and produce an overall feeling of relaxation that can help a client sleep. Advise the client to take a warm bath and perhaps light a scented candle or add relaxing herbal oils, such as lavender, chamomile, or linden flowers, or infusions of herbs to the water to help him or her relax and unwind. Clients can also try to use a shower massage or sit in a hot tub before retiring for the evening. To increase their relaxation when they get out, they can give themselves a relaxing self-massage with a towel as they dry off.

Self-Massage

Clients can do basic self-massage to their feet, legs, neck, shoulders, chest, and abdomen to help them relax and unwind before sleep. They also can press the following acupressure points that traditionally have been used to treat insomnia.

Acupressure Points

Pericardium-6 (P-6) is located on the forearm two chun above the ventral wrist fold. A chun is the width of the client's thumb. Starting from the anatomical position the client should flex the right wrist and then press with the thumb of the left hand two chun above the crease between the tendons of the palmaris longus and the flexor carpi radialis. The pressure should be firm but not too hard. You can also flex the wrist and hold the point until it relaxes.

To find spleen-6 (Sp-6) the client should press and hold the point located three chun above the medial malleolus just behind the edge of the tibia. The massage therapist can gently rock the leg side to side while pressing this spot.

Diet

A client's diet may cause sleeping problems. What they eat, when they eat, and how they eat can all be significant. This is particularly true for people who suffer from RLS; even small amounts of caffeine can dramatically increase symptoms. Have clients keep track of their eating habits in their sleep log, and then see if their sleepless nights match a pattern in their eating behavior. For example, they may find that drinking a glass of wine before bed actually may be the cause of periods of wakefulness. Although diet, like so much else related to stress, affects each person differently, there are some general practices that help clients sleep better:

- Eat a moderate evening meal because overeating disturbs sleep.
- Eat as early in the evening as possible.
- Chew food slowly and thoroughly.
- Avoid evening meals that include heavy, spicy, or greasy foods or any foods that cause gas or indigestion.
- Avoid all caffeine (coffee, tea, and soft drinks).
- Avoid foods with high amounts of sugar, salt, and starch. Particularly stay away from foods with artificial flavors and colors and those considered junk food.
- Limit alcohol intake; too much alcohol disrupts the normal sleep cycle.
- Drink a glass of warm milk before bed.
- Eat a light, high-carbohydrate, low-protein snack an hour or two before bed. This will help the body use the essential amino acid tryptophan to produce melatonin, a drowsiness-inducing neurohormone secreted by the pineal gland when it is dark, and serotonin, a neurotransmitter that has a calming effect on the body.
- Don't eat high-protein foods shortly before bedtime because the large variety of amino acids present competes with the tryptophan available in the body, inhibiting the production of melatonin and serotonin.

Medications

Have clients check the side effects of all the prescription, dietary supplements, and over-the-counter medications that they are taking. If insomnia or excitability is listed, have them ask the doctor if there is an alternative prescription medication, or, if an over-the-counter medication is implicated, try to find an alternative remedy.

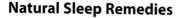

Natural Sleep Remedies

Many flowers, roots, leaves, fruits, and oils have a sedative and tranquilizing effect. Used in place of sleeping pills or other artificial drugs, these natural products can help a client get a deep, relaxing night's sleep. Please note that all supplements should be used with the same caution that is used with any other drug and should be avoided by pregnant and nursing clients.

Herbs have been used for centuries to help people relax and sleep. Herbs should be used cautiously because they affect people in different ways and some people experience allergic reactions to them. Brewing herbal teas using single herbs or combinations is a simple way for clients to see if they work for them. Try teas containing chamomile, skullcap, passionflower (Passiflora), primrose, hops, or valerian root. One popular combination mixes a spoonful of valerian root, catnip, skullcap, and hops steeped in a pint of boiling water for 15 minutes. You also can buy ready-mixed teas such as Nighty Night, Easy Now, and Sleepy Time. Drink your favorite sleep-inducing tea 30–60 minutes before bedtime. Herbs such as lavender, Jamaica dogwood, and St. John's wort also can be rubbed on the body or bathed in. Aromatherapy uses the smell of herbs to relax and calm the mind and body. Herb tablets, essential oils, and liquid extracts are other natural remedies for relaxation and aiding sleep and are available in health food stores.

Tryptophan

Tryptophan is an amino acid that is found plentifully in turkey, meat, fish, milk, cottage cheese, peanuts, oats, bananas, and even chocolate. The client should try to ingest some of these foods every day to ensure that the body has an adequate supply of this essential amino acid so that their body can produce melatonin and serotonin. Tryptophan was a popular dietary sleep aid supplement until it was taken off the market in 1989, when a bad batch from Japan caused a major outbreak of a serious bacterial infection. It is now marketed as a pet supplement, and a prescription form is being used to treat depression.

Melatonin

Melatonin is a naturally occurring hormone, produced in the pineal gland in the center of the brain and secreted when it is dark to help us fall asleep. A synthetic version is sold in health food stores as a dietary supplement that comes in capsules or tablets that are placed under the tongue. It is popular among air travelers to ease the burden of jet lag caused by changing time zones. As a sleep aid, take 3–6 mg of melatonin 30–60 minutes before bedtime. Although it appears to be safe, use this sleep aid sparingly because not enough research has been performed to determine if taking this supplement inhibits the pineal gland's ability to naturally produce and secrete melatonin. Because it is considered a supplement, the U.S. Food and Drug Administration does not regulate the side effects.

Supplements

Calcium complex (375 mg) and magnesium (150 mg) combine to act as a natural muscle relaxant. One to four of these tablets taken daily with or after meals reduces muscle spasms and helps a person sleep.

Vitamin supplements of B_3, B_6, and B_{12} help combat insomnia. The recommended daily dosage is 50 mg of niacinamide (B_3), 50 mg of B_6, and 100 mg of B_{12}.

Potassium relieves muscle cramps. If a person is deficient in potassium he or she may awaken frequently with muscle cramps, twitches, or both. Eating more bananas or cantaloupe (both are excellent sources of potassium) or taking a potassium supplement may help. Also try massage, muscle relaxation, hot water soaks, and stretching out the cramping muscles.

Lifestyle Changes

If clients' personal stress inventories clearly show that the stresses in their life come from their lifestyle, chances are that their sleep problems stem from the same sources. Changing one's lifestyle may be all it takes to get a good night's sleep, but for many this is easier said than done. Habits and a person's circle of friends may have to be changed to successfully reduce this element of stress.

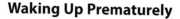

Waking Up Prematurely

If clients prematurely wake up from slumber, they should calm themselves immediately by thinking thoughts of warmth, heaviness, peacefulness, and relaxation. They should think about scenes that deeply relax them to help them fall gently back into a deep sleep. They must try to keep a positive attitude, believing that they will fall back to sleep and they will feel totally rested when they complete their night's slumber. They must try to avoid negative thoughts, such as "I'm not going to be able to fall back asleep and I'm going to feel terrible tomorrow," because once these thoughts creep in they are too often a self-fulfilling prophecy. If that doesn't work, they should get out of bed and leave the bedroom without putting a robe on. When they get cold enough, they should get back into bed, and the warmth of the covers should soon help them drift off into slumber. Avoid watching TV, working on the computer, and turning on bright lights.

Frequent Trips to the Toilet

If the client is plagued by pressure on the bladder and the frequent urge to urinate while trying to sleep, then have them avoid drinking any liquids after dinner. If their mouth is dry, they can chew on some crushed ice or humidify the air in their bedroom. If they still feel the urge to go to the bathroom, they should get up and go with a positive attitude. They should not toss and turn and prolong the agony; they should get up relaxed and happy because they have more time to sleep. They should tell themselves that once they have relieved themselves and returned to bed they will fall deeply asleep immediately. When getting up, try to use only a nightlight because bright lights may awaken them. Frequent nocturnal urination also can be symptomatic of prostate problems in men; diabetes; or, surprisingly, obstructive sleep apnea, so a trip to the doctor may be required for evaluation.

Work Stress

Many people lose sleep thinking about their job and work-related problems. If at all possible, don't bring work home, which, unfortunately, may not always be an option, particularly for those who work from home. The sleep problems caused by work worries manifest themselves differently. Sometimes people have difficulty falling asleep because their mind can't stop replaying a problem, a conversation, a stressful encounter, negativity, or an important decision. Sometimes our minds blow things out of proportion and we worry about things that in the whole scheme of things really aren't that important. If these types of thoughts are keeping any of your clients awake, teach them the thought-stopping technique, which simply requires them to yell "stop" when their mind is racing. They don't have to yell out loud, but a loud gasp or release of air while vocalizing the word "stop" can jar the mind enough to drop the negative thoughts from surfacing. These thoughts then should be replaced by imagining a relaxing scenario or using a mantra, such as the word "sleep." When other thoughts begin to encroach, repeat the exercise and return to the mantra.

Another way that work stress impairs sleep occurs when a person wakes up in the middle of the night after dreaming about a problem, a new assignment, or a big project and their mind comes up with a great idea. The person does not want to forget the idea so he or she lies half awake and tense for the rest of the night. If any of your clients experience this type of work-related sleeplessness, have them put a mini voice recorder on their nightstand. As soon as the ideas arrive, they should turn on the tape recorder, without turning on the light, and record their ideas. Then they can lie back, take a deep breath, and give a sigh of relief as they fall back asleep, content and assured that their wisdom is safely recorded. They should try not to wake up completely while recording because it will be more difficult to fall back into their natural sleep cycle. Work-related sleeplessness is a common problem that occurs to most people now and then. If it becomes a chronic problem, however, they might consider changing their job. A U.S. senator once remarked "I never met a man on his death bed that said, 'I should have spent more time at my job.'"

Day Organizer

Clients who lose sleep worrying that they will forget something important that they need to do the next day should keep a personal electronic organizer device or an old-fashioned weekly or daily appointment book on their nightstand. Once everything is recorded, they can go to sleep assured that all is safely planned and that they won't forget anything.

Muscle Cramps

Muscle cramps can wake a person out of a sound sleep. The client who has nocturnal muscle cramps should try eating more bananas and foods rich in calcium and magnesium. They may also try more daily exercise, self-massage, and stretching exercises. If none of these suggestions help, they should see a doctor.

Fear, Anxiety, and Nightmares

Fear, anxiety, and nightmares are psychological disturbances and emotional upsets that can interfere with a person's ability to sleep. If your client reports fear of sleeping, reports waking up in the middle of the night anxious, or frequently experiences reoccurring bad dreams, he or she should first try to pinpoint the cause of these problems. After the cause is determined behavioral changes can be implemented to try to relieve the symptoms. If the symptoms persist, then it might greatly benefit the client to seek the services of a professionally trained counselor or psychiatrist to help understand and resolve these issues; there could be an underlying psychological disorder present, such as posttraumatic stress disorder.

MASSAGE TREATMENTS FOR SLEEP IMPROVEMENT

A relaxation massage helps reverse the body's physical and mental reaction to stress and strain. It calms the mind and helps satisfy the basic human need to be touched in a caring, nurturing fashion. Massage is also one of the finest natural tools against insomnia that exists. A sleep-improvement treatment is more than just a massage because it combines the use of relaxing and soothing sounds, penetrating moist heat, diaphragmatic breathing, deep relaxation, and focused muscle relaxation in addition to the application of strokes. The massage techniques used are not designed to force the body of the client to change; they are designed to reeducate the client's body to naturally relax, unwind, rest, and assume its proper alignment. During these treatments the client and therapist both get into a relaxed state. Together they perform focused muscle relaxation in which the client and therapist work together to melt away areas of hypertonicity. The therapist searches the client's body for areas of tension, and when one is found the client uses the heat and energy from the therapist's hands to pinpoint its precise location. The client then breathes through the spot and uses his or her mind to relax it. The therapist does not stay in an area too long; he or she moves on to other areas of the body to prepare it for rest and sleep.

Massage Sequence for Relaxation and Sleep Improvement

The following sequence of techniques is offered as a guideline for relaxing the client and helping him or her sleep more soundly. Therapists should feel free to adapt it to suit their needs; however, therapists should avoid very hard friction and stick more to effleurage, compression, rocking, shaking and rolling, breathing and releasing tension, gentle pétrissage, and light friction. With this type of massage remember that less is more. The therapist must be well-grounded to perform this type of treatment. The therapist should practice moving heat through his or her hands. It helps therapists to picture energy or light entering them, through the area just above the center of their eyebrows, which some call the third eye. Then they should feel the energy flow to their heart and from their heart to their hands. Touch stressed clients with compassion and they will relax, unwind, and let go of their strain and tension. They will feel as if a weight has been lifted off of their shoulders after this type of treatment.

Start the treatment in the prone position with a bolster under the ankles; if the client has a bad back, place a pillow under the abdomen. If the client does not like the prone position, begin with them sidelying. Ask clients for their preference for relaxing music, such as classical, new age, or nature's sounds, and have their selection playing softly in the background. Unless contraindicated apply moist heat to the client's neck, shoulders, and back. The safe use of hydrocollators and Thera beads are explained in Chapter 10. After the heat is applied, the therapist should place his or her hands on the client's feet to ground the client to begin the treatment. Instruct the client to take 10 long, slow, deep, complete full breaths through the nose. For the first few breaths while holding the feet the therapist should tune into the client's body rhythm. The therapist should talk the client into a relaxed state using muscular relaxation and autogenic training passive suggestions of warmth, heaviness, and relaxation.

After the four or five breathing cycles have been completed begin the massage by working the way up the back of one of the legs with some soft compressions. Work right through the draping and perform one pass up the back of the leg, up to the ischial tuberosity, then glide the hands gently back down to the calcaneus, after which the therapist presses up the lateral aspect of the leg up to the ilium. Return to start once again, and then press up the medial aspect of the leg, up the adductors, avoiding contact with the client's private parts. Then cup the sides of the sacrum with the hands and rock it five times in a circular fashion, working from the center, observing how the client's body moves. Next continue up the back, compressing on the erector spinae up one side of the back to shoulders, right through the heat packs, all the while trying to calm and soothe the client. When at the shoulders place one hand on each shoulder and alternately press one then the other, three times, in an inferior and lateral direction using a slow, relaxed rhythm. Continue by pressing down the other side of the back until reaching the gluteals, where once again some more sacral rocks are performed. Proceed by gliding down the second leg to the foot and then repeat the compression passes, to the back, lateral, and medial aspects. After the third pass is completed, glide the hands back down to the foot and then undrape one of the client's legs.

The massage continues at one foot; the therapist presses the soles of the feet with his or her flat knuckles from base of the toes to the heels, just doing one pass at this time. Next, squeeze the heels and then glide the fingers along the sides of the calcaneal tendon. Continue by performing effleurage to the entire lower extremity, gliding over the medial, lateral, and posterior surfaces. The forearms work great for this. Next perform some pétrissage and some gentle friction to tense areas of the calves and hamstrings. Then flex the knee, grasp the foot and ankle, lift the leg slightly off the table, and shake it side to side in a pendulum fashion, relaxing the whole leg and hip; after a few shakes gently pound the thigh on the table (the poi pounder). Finish the leg with a whole-leg effleurage. Redrape and then rock the body as you move to the other side of the table to repeat the foot and legwork. Both lower extremities should take about 10 minutes. Don't linger on tender points too long; make note of them and you can return to them in the supine position. After you redrape the second leg, continue with gluteal and hip work. The gluteal and hip strokes performed can be administered right through the linens because the client should feel safe, secure, and comfortable. Baring the gluteals makes some feel very vulnerable, and this should not add to the client's stress. Discuss this with the client and use your best judgment.

Start the 5 minutes of gluteals and hip work by doing a compression pattern to the gluteals. This stroke is performed with the therapist on the side of the table, and the force is directed in an inferior direction to provide a gentle stretch to the lumbar region. Place the one hand on top of the other with the heel of the hand by the top of the ilium and the fingers facing inferior. Using a relaxed rhythm, compress the hands into the gluteals, using just the body weight, and then after the muscle rebounds slide the hands inferiorly, with the heel of the hand next to the sacrum. Continue down this line to the base of the gluteal, then slide the hands back up, move them slightly laterally, and then do the second line of compressions directed toward and over the ischial tuberosity. The therapist must not forget to readjust foot position when changing the angle of the compressions. After the second line is completed slide the hands back up and complete the third line of gluteal compressions directed toward the greater trochanter. If the gluteal were a piece of pie, we have just taken three slices. Figure 9.2 shows how to perform the three lines of compression to the gluteals. The first line is directed along the edge of the sacrum, the second is toward the ischial tuberosity, and the third is down to the greater trochanter. The therapist should follow each line three times, after which he or she should do some gentle friction circles right over the sacrum.

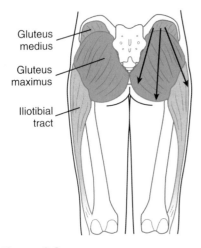

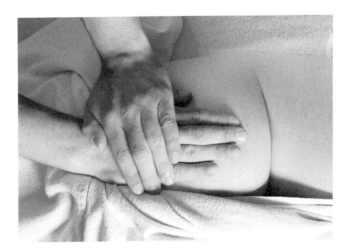

Figure 9.2

Compression pattern to the gluteals

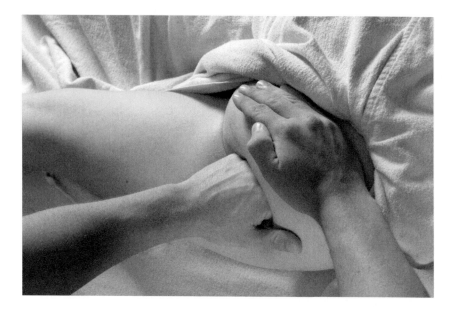

Figure 9.3

Pacman

The Pacman pétrissage is performed next. Figure 9.3 demonstrates the Pacman, which is performed by pushing tissue with the fist of one hand into the other hand, which is held flat. The wrist of the hand that is a fist is held as straight or neutral as possible, and the fist actually can be twisted as the therapist kneads the gluteal tissue. Travel along the gluteal from the medial to lateral and then press with the fist on the gluteus medius below the ilium and down to the top edge of the trochanter. Now circle around the trochanter with the flat palm or reinforced finger tips twice, after which you flex the knee and press the forearm gently down on the piriformis, while passively internally and externally rotating the client's hip joint.

This piriformis release is pictured in Figure 9.4. Now rock the client as you change sides of the table to work the other gluteus maximus and hip.

After the other gluteal is released, remove the heat packs, and, if still warm, place them on tight areas on the legs. Undrape the back and then effleurage the client's whole back and both sides of his or her body, including the lats, the obliques, the deltoids, trapezius, and the serratus anterior. This is followed by circular pétrissage up the back. Then flick the paraspinals away from the spinous processes, relaxing the muscles along the spine from the lumbar region up. Glide around the scapula with the forearm and circle with flat palms over the infraspinatus teres minor and teres major. Do some light

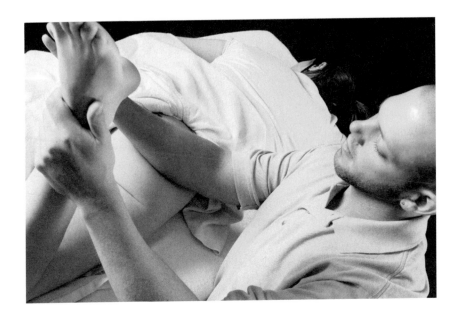

Figure 9.4

Piriformis release

friction to the rhomboids and levator scapula. Next move to the head of the table and perform a few two-handed effleurages to the neck and shoulders; then press down on the shoulders in an inferior and lateral direction. Check for tender spots on each side of the upper trapezius, working from the neck out to the acromion process, and try to release them with some circular friction. Now use the thumbs or fingers to glide longitudinally along the cervical spinous processes and then do some gentle flicking or use little friction circles along the cervical paraspinals. Do some friction circles to the occipital ridge and the external occipital protuberance. Then do some effleurage and light friction to the upper trapezius and the sternocleidomastoid. Now remove the packs and turn the client over.

Supine whole-leg effleurage is followed by some foot effleurage, foot squeeze, knuckling, separating the bones, and pressure to the entire sole of the foot. Work around the malleoli and then slide the thumb along the tibia from medial malleolus up to the knee. Then roll the leg gently side to side while pressing on spleen-6 and any other tender points on this inside lower leg line. Use reinforced thumbs to slide up the tibialis anterior muscle and do some easy cross-fiber or circular friction to any tender points. Next use the knuckles to glide up the lateral aspect of the lower leg along the peroneals or fibularis muscles. After gliding perform some friction to the tense areas located just under the head of the fibula. Next place the upward-facing knuckles under the calf, above the calcaneal tendon, and with the other hand roll the lower leg from side to side. Work your way up the calf from inferior to superior. For more pressure, the bolster can be moved out from under the leg being worked on to the other side. The hamstrings also can be worked with this type of knuckles-up, leg-rocking technique. Next perform some compression to the tensor fasciae latae, the iliotibial band (ITB), and the gluteus medius and minimus. Follow this with some forearm circles to the vastus lateralis and the ITB. Figure 9.5 demonstrates forearm circles to the ITB. Then perform some deeper forearm effleurage and pétrissage to the quadriceps. Now flex, externally rotate, and abduct the hip and work the adductors with some compression in a racetrack pattern, followed by some forearm gliding. Then give the whole leg a gentle pull and a shake if you desire, and then switch to the other side to massage the other leg.

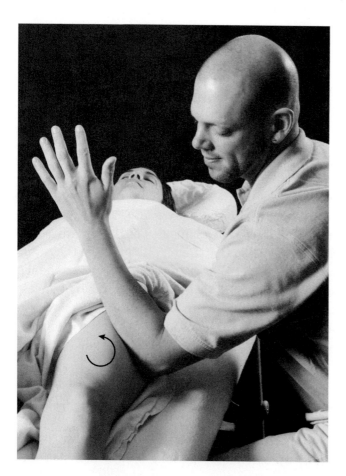

Figure 9.5

Forearm circles to the iliotibial band (ITB)

After the second leg is completed move up to the client's abdomen unless he or she prefers not to have it touched. Perform some gentle effleurage and pétrissage and project warmth and relaxation from your hands to the client's tan tien region. Next move on to the oblique abdominals and work the obliques on both sides with some effleurage and some gentle friction to the muscles attaching to the top of the iliac crests. Now move on to massage the tips of the ribs and then perform the diaphragm release that was outlined in Chapter 4. Follow this with some gentle gliding and friction to the serratus anterior and the intercostals working between the ribs. Work the muscles attaching to the sternum area in the same fashion.

Continue this massage by working some effleurage and gentle pétrissage and friction to the client's pectoralis major. Try to release any areas of hypertonicity not through force; instead have the client tune into these areas that you are touching and try to consciously relax them. Don't forget to release the muscles attaching to the anterior, inferior aspect of the clavicle. Then release the tension in the client's pectoralis minor working from the coracoid processes down to ribs 3,4, and 5, where they attach. Next perform some gentle gliding strokes to the top inside edge of the clavicles, without pressing into the posterior triangle of the neck. When you find a sore spot, have the client elevate his or her shoulders while you still maintain contact. At this time, perform the thoracic release that was outlined in Chapter 4.

Next perform some work to the client's hands, fingers, and arms. After a whole-arm effleurage, apply gliding knuckles to the client's palm and then stretch the fingers and the palm. Rub between the web of each finger and stretch and massage the flexor retinaculum (transverse carpal ligament) by extending the client's wrist and separating the muscles at the base of the hand eminences. After working the hands and fingers, use your forearm to glide up the client's forearm. Then do a more focused glide and friction circles with the thumb or reinforced fingers along the radius and ulna, working all the forearm flexors and extensors. Next press P-6, and if it is tender you can flex the wrist and hold the point until it relaxes. Spend some extra time on the medial epicondyle area of the humerus, the proximal attachment of many of the hand and wrist flexors muscles, and by the lateral epicondyle where many extensors originate. Move up to the biceps and triceps and perform effleurage, pétrissage, and some gentle friction. You can hold the client's wrist, flex the elbow, and place the knuckles of your other hand under the client's triceps, using gravity for force as you move the arm side to side, much like you did under the calves. Now, while still holding the wrist, abduct the shoulder and swing the arm and shoulder in a pendulum-type fashion. Finish the arm and shoulder by doing some light friction circles to the anterior middle and posterior deltoids and gently circle around the head of the humerus. Now switch arms.

After finishing the second arm and shoulder, it's time to move up to the neck. Sit on a stool at the head of the table and do a few two-handed effleurages to the neck and shoulders. Follow the effleurage with some gentle pressure to the client's upper trapezius tender points, working from the neck to the acromion process. Instruct the client to tune in to these points, and then take some deep breaths and relax them away. Next perform some gentle friction to the clavicular and sternal attachments of the sternocleido-mastoid and work your way up the muscle to the mastoid process. If you find an area that is very sensitive, apply some soft vibration to desensitize it and then instruct the client to breathe through the points you are touching and to try to consciously relax them. You can work the scalenes in the same fashion. If you get to an extremely tender point, you also can try positional release techniques to relieve them. To use these positional release techniques, maintain contact on the painful area while shortening the muscle, using all planes of motion until you find a position in which the pain is gone. Hold the head in that position for 90 seconds and then slowly move the neck back to the anatomical position. If you were working on the right side of the neck, rotate the head to the left (counterclockwise) and do a few head-turned, one-handed effleurages to the right neck and shoulder muscles. Return to the anatomical position and do the other side of the neck. After finishing the other side of the neck do some gentle friction circles to the occipital ridge and the base of the skull from the mastoid process to the foramen magnum. Next perform some longitudinal and cross-fiber gliding to the cervical paraspinal muscles, followed by either some flicking or gentle friction circles to the muscles attaching to each segment of the cervical vertebrae. After these strokes, perform some overlapping cupping effleurages to the back of the neck. Next perform some gliding or gentle friction circles to the muscles of the forehead, cheeks, jaw, temporal mandibular joint (TMJ), temples, and scalp.

After completing this work, continue the massage by releasing the suboccipital muscles. The therapist should extend his or her fingers and flex the hands at the metacarpal–phalangeal joint and then place the fingertips at the base of the client's skull. Next raise the client's head up off the table, resting only on your fingertips and instruct the client to breathe, relax, let his or her neck muscles relax, and let the head fall back toward the table. If this position is too painful for the client, lower the head down immediately. If the client is comfortable with this position, stay there until the head lowers down into your palms. When the head is completely lowered move your thumb and index fingers around the outside edge of the client's ears and place the tips of your middle fingers on the base of the client's skull on each side of the foramen magnum. With gentle force bring the fingertips toward you, just enough for the client's head to nod slightly forward and the chin to go down. Hold this position for a few seconds and then release it and do some soothing circles to the musculature at the base of the skull and the back of the neck.

To complete this massage for sleep improvement, place the tips of the middle fingers back on the base of the skull by the foramen magnum. Touch this spot gently and instruct the client to breathe and focus all awareness on this point. The therapist projects caring, warmth, heaviness, and relaxation to this spot, and the client tries to tune in and relax this point with all of his or her awareness. The therapist should feel for a pulsation emanating from this spot on the client. This therapeutic pulse indicates that the client and therapist are making contact and the therapist should stay there until the pulses on each side synchronize and slow. Now that the massage is completed, let the client rest for a while. When the client is ready, help him or her from the table. Figure 9.6 outlines a sample time breakdown for performing this sleep-improvement massage.

Massage Sequence Timeline

The 60-minute timeline for a sleep improvement massage outlined previously is to help the therapist gauge his or her time when trying this sequence. Add and delete strokes according to

Prone

Body area	Time per body area	Total time
Feet and legs	5 min each	10 min
Gluteals and hips	5 min	15 min
Back and sides	10 min	25 min
Neck and shoulders	5 min	30 min

Supine

Supine legs	5 min each	40 min
Chest and abdomen	5 min	45 min
Arms and hands	3 min each	51 min
Neck and shoulders	5 min	56 min
Head and face	4 min	60 min

Figure 9.6

Time breakdown for a sleep improvement massage

the specific needs of your clients. Don't fret if you go over or under a little time in one area or another. Keep the massage at less than an hour and figure out a way to allow your client some time to rest after this type of work that won't affect your next appointment. If the client falls asleep, it is ideal to let him or her sleep as long as possible until you must get ready for your next client.

SUMMARY

Before we move on to discuss techniques for pain control, some important concepts to remember about sleep are as follows:

- A normal night's sleep consists of four to five 90-minute cycles that are made up of four distinct stages and a state known as rapid eye movement.

- Sleep debt occurs when a person does not get as much sleep as his or her body needs. This can lead to illness and injury.

- The only way to eliminate a sleep debt is to get extra sleep.

- Age and sex influence how much time a person spends in each sleep cycle.

- Insomnia refers to the inability of a person to fall and remain asleep.

- Roughly 14 percent of the American public suffers from chronic insomnia.

- Restless legs syndrome is a central nervous system disorder that affects 10 percent of the general population and 19 percent of pregnant women. RLS manifests itself as an itchy, restless, tingling, or jumpy sensation in the legs that occurs during periods of inactivity and can lead to chronic sleep loss.

- Obstructive sleep apnea is a medical condition in which the airway is restricted or completely collapsed, causing a person to stop breathing while sleeping. A client with this disorder should get checked out at a sleep clinic.

- Keeping a sleep log is useful for someone who often or always suffers from sleeplessness.

- Clients with insomnia should consider changing aspects of their environment, diet, physical habits, and mental outlook to improve the quality of their sleep.

- A relaxation massage can help reverse the body's physical and mental reaction to stress and can help a person sleep more soundly.

Relieving the Pains of Stress

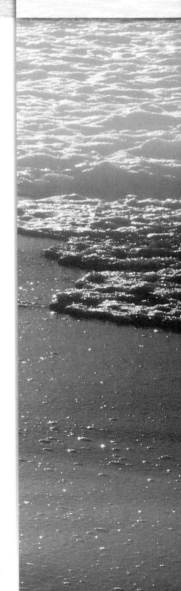

Although stress affects everyone differently, pain is one of the most common consequences. Pain can detract from the quality of a person's life, reducing concentration, preventing sleep, and impairing the ability to work and participate in routine activities. Pain also serves a valuable purpose. It is the body's way of reporting an important message: "We have a problem that has to be taken care of before it gets worse." If a person ignores this important message and takes medications that merely suppress the symptoms, he or she may exacerbate the original problem while creating secondary problems. Drugs and alcohol are the worst possible methods for coping with pain. They dull the senses, interfere with mental functions, create dependence, and may eventually damage health while doing nothing to get rid of the original source of pain. Aside from addiction, prolonged use of commonly used drugs to control pain may lead to gastric irritation and ulcers, liver damage, abdominal pain, bleeding, diarrhea, nausea, jaundice, kidney damage, heart attacks, and other cardiovascular problems. A wiser choice for coping with pain is to find its cause and then try to eliminate it at its source with safe, effective, natural techniques. This chapter outlines a variety of pain-control techniques that can be incorporated into a treatment plan and can be given to the client to perform as homework. The physiology of pain; kinesthetic awareness training; and modalities, massage techniques, self-massage, and indirect techniques that can be used to relieve pain are discussed.

PHYSIOLOGY OF PAIN

Soft-tissue damage releases chemicals that stimulate the body's **nociceptors,** which are peripheral nerve receptors located in the skin and other tissues. These sensory receptors receive and transmit information on painful stimuli through the spinal cord to the brain, which acknowledges this sensation as pain. The brain then stimulates the spinal reflexes to contract the musculature around the injury in an attempt to splint the area to prevent further movement and injury. The resultant increased muscle tone and spasm decreases the circulation to the area, preventing the exchange of oxygen and nutrients and the removal of the waste products of metabolism. After an injury the blood vessels become more permeable, which allows fluid to leak out, and the resultant edema (swelling) places pressure on sensory nerve endings, resulting in more pain. The resultant ischemic pain is sometimes worse than the original pain. This pain-spasm-pain cycle may continue until interrupted by the use of modalities, heat and ice, and the skilful application of massage techniques.

GETTING TO THE ROOT OF THE PROBLEM

The first step to eliminating pain is to isolate where it originates in the body and determine its causes. Try to uncover any patterns of pain caused by the client's daily activities, such as neck pain every time he or she rides in the car or back pain after sitting in a particular chair. Some factors that may contribute to pain are poor posture; excess muscle tension; vertebral misalignment; not using both straps of a backpack; sitting at a work station that is not ergonomically correct; laterally flexing the neck while on the telephone (not using a headset); lack of proper exercise; and using a chair, mattress, or a car seat that doesn't provide adequate back support. Once you know the type of pain and its causes, you can begin your campaign against it.

RELIEVING PAIN

The following recommendations for reducing pain are not intended to take the place of proper medical diagnosis and treatment. If any of your clients are experiencing severe pain, have them consult with a physician to ensure that their problem is not life threatening—for example, headaches caused by a brain tumor. Early diagnosis and treatment of such cases may mean the difference between life and death. Before you proceed with treatments, make sure that massage is not contraindicated for the client's particular condition. If any of your clients are under the care of a physician, chiropractor, osteopath, or physical therapist to help them relieve their pain, it is prudent to consult with these professionals regarding your treatment plan. Once it has been determined that massage is indicated, try some of the following suggestions for reducing their pain.

IMPROVING KINESTHETIC AWARENESS

Habitually poor posture can lead to pain, excess muscle tension, breathing difficulties, and headaches. The first step in reducing pain is to help clients improve their ability to recognize when their postural alignment is out of balance while sitting, standing, and moving, and then learn to self-correct it throughout the day. Kinesthetic awareness, sometimes called conscious proprioception, refers to this internal feeling of the position of the body and its parts in space. The police test for drunk driving by seeing if a person's ability to sense where the body is and how the parts line up is impaired. Touching the tip of the nose with the eyes closed, standing on one foot, and walking a straight line all test a person's conscious proprioception or kinesthetic sense.

For a few minutes at the end of a massage treatment have the client sit on the side edge of the table with the feet supported on a stool. Instruct the client to take a deep breath in through the nose and then exhale through the nose as he or she relaxes the shoulders and lets gravity pull the arms and shoulders toward the floor. Give the client feedback to correct the head, neck, and shoulder posture. The client's head should be balanced over his or her neck and shoulders, the chin should be tucked, and the eyes should be straight ahead; the client should try to find a spot where there is no neck tension. The shoulders should be retracted and neutral, not depressed or elevated. The client should be breathing diaphragmatically. Use whatever movements, pressure, or strokes are needed to help the client mold his or her posture into an improved alignment. Try raising the shoulders up, back, and down; reinforced thumb flicking or knuckling to the paraspinals; forearms to the upper trapezius; gentle friction to the levator scapulae and around the scapulae; and an elbow to the rhomboids. For some, pulling back on one shoulder while pressing the points between the scapula and the vertebral column is useful. Many individuals have a point on the back that when pressed will straighten the posture. For women many times that point is underneath the bra clasp. Try to find and relax that spot on female clients.

Once discovered the therapist should press it with a reinforced thumb, knuckles, or an elbow while in a comfortable, stable posture and have the client lean back as hard or as soft as desired as he or she lets the posture rebalance. When the client is as close as possible to the appropriate position instruct him or her to close the eyes and feel how great this position feels. Call this relaxed balanced posture "the position" and inform the client that whenever he or she feels neck and shoulder strain and tension throughout the day, he or she should assume it. To reinforce "the position" have clients open their eyes and then walk them to a mirror. Instruct clients to look in the mirror at their head, neck, shoulder, and eye alignment and how their shoulders are relaxed and do not move when they are breathing. Clients can use a mirror for feedback throughout the day to help them realign and rebalance themselves, and eventually they will feel that the balanced position is the correct position to maintain. Clients also can perform some of the simple stretching and postural realignment exercises recommended in Chapter 5 throughout the day to keep their joints mobile, muscles relaxed and flexible, and vertebral column properly aligned. Sometimes pain and stiffness are simply the result of inactivity.

GATE CONTROL THEORY OF PAIN

The **gate control theory of pain,** proposed by pioneering pain researchers Melzack and Wall in the 1960s, is based on the premise that nonpain signals can interrupt pain signals. The body has different types of sensory receptors that can be stimulated to override or interfere with pain signals. By stimulating the area where pain originates with nonpain type of stimulation, such as the application of heat, cold, and acupressure, we create a traffic jam of sensory impulses that can interrupt pain messages. Essentially the pain signals are interrupted because the brain is tricked, or distracted, to change its focus from the source of the pain to the other sources of stimulation. The brain responds to the sensations from heat and ice and the pressure of massage strokes by closing the neural gate and effectively suppressing the route that pain sensations travel. The same principle applies to the person who has pain but experiences less of it when busily engaged in activities. When the person has no task at hand, the pain becomes the focus and it grows in intensity. Taking the mind off the pain by occupying it with other stimulation reduces the amount of pain perceived. Using relaxation, visualization, and autogenic training to passively warm the hands and feet to fend off a headache is another example of occupying the brain and neural pathways to close the gate to the pain response. This theory provides some insight as to why modalities and massage effectively interrupt the pain-spasm-pain cycle.

MODALITIES

A **modality** is a type of therapeutic agent or treatment that can be applied to reduce the incidence or severity of physical problems. Heat and ice are two examples of modalities that have proved effective to interrupt the pain-spasm-pain cycle. These modalities can be integrated into a client's treatment program or recommended for home use when indicated. Table 10.1 compares the effects of ice and heat applications.

TABLE 10.1

Comparing the Effects of Ice and Heat Applications

	Ice	Heat
Reduces pain perceived	Yes	Yes
Increases circulation	No	Yes
Decreases circulation	Yes	No
Relieves muscle spasms	Yes	Yes
Decreases swelling (edema)	Yes	No
Increases swelling (edema)	No	Yes
Relaxing	No	Yes
Increases metabolism	No	Yes
Decreases metabolism	Yes	No
Increases tissue stiffness	Yes	No
Decreases tissue stiffness	No	Yes
Increases collagen flexibility	No	Yes
Decreases nerve conduction velocity	Yes	No

Heat Applications

Heat improves circulation to the soft tissues, increases muscle metabolism, reduces spasms and tone, decreases pain and stiffness, and can produce an all-over feeling of relaxation. The application of heat to a body part results in the **vasodilation** (relaxation of an artery's muscular wall and widening of the passageway) of the arteries and increased blood flow to the area. When heat is applied to the entire body, while taking a whirlpool or hot bath for example, the core temperature of the body will increase and produce a body-wide vasodilation. The increased circulation produced by heat applications will help the importation of oxygen and nutrients and assist in the removal of the waste products of cellular metabolism and nociceptive pain-producing chemicals. The application of heat also will increase the flexibility of collagen fibers, allowing the therapist to achieve more effective stretching and release of myofascial restrictions.

Precautions for Heat

The following are precautions for the use of heat:

- Fresh injury: Avoid using heat on a fresh injury or bruise for 48–72 hours because it will increase swelling and add to the time it takes to heal. Always wait to apply heat until the swelling goes down and temperature of the area subsides to normal.
- Pregnancy: Do not apply a heat source to the abdomen of pregnant women, and avoid total body submersion in hot water because of potential damage to the developing baby.
- Heart disease, uncontrolled high blood pressure, obesity, and circulatory problems: Avoid using heat over a large area with individuals with these problems because, as the body attempts to cool itself from elevated temperatures, the blood is shifted to the skin-surface capillaries and there may not be sufficient supply for general circulation and to feed the coronary arteries.
- Multiple sclerosis (MS): Many individuals with MS are heat intolerant, and heat has a tendency to exacerbate their symptoms and therefore should be avoided.
- Anorexia and the frail elderly: Be careful using heat sources on individuals with thin, brittle skin and limited muscle mass because the potential for burns is much greater.

- Diabetes and diminished sensation: Avoid using heat in this population because the client actually may be burned before he or she senses any discomfort.
- Intoxication: Heat can intensify the effects of alcohol, and the potential for passing out increases significantly, particularly in a hot tub.
- Open wounds, skin rashes, and infections: Avoid using heat with these conditions.

Procedures for Using Hot Water

There are different types of heat applications that are within the scope of massage therapy practice. The following section outlines how to safely use and apply heat in the form of hot water.

The ideal temperature for a hot tub is 104–106° F. Submerging the body for 8–10 minutes before a treatment can help clients relax their mind and their body. For lounging around the hot tub with friends, 100–102° F is the right temperature. Some spas set their tub temperature to 110° F, which is too hot for many. These treatments raise the core temperature of the body, so if the client feels feel faint, have him or her get out immediately. If client's heart rate rises to an abnormally high level and it won't slow down or if the faint feeling persists, call 911. If water jets are available, instruct the client to let the pulses hit the most painful points on his or her body. For overall relaxation have clients vary the position of their body so the jets spray on the tender spots on their feet, ankles, calves, hamstrings, sacrum, gluteals, back, shoulders, and neck. A handheld shower massage using the same principles also works well for relaxing stiff musculature.

Dry Heat vs. Moist Heat

Other types of heat applications within the scope of massage therapy practice are dry and moist heat. Electric heating pads are a form of dry heat. Dry heat does not penetrate the soft tissues as deeply as moist heat and therefore is less effective at reducing pain. It also has a tendency to dry out the skin. Turning the temperature up to get deeper pain relief increases the risk of burns. Do not apply dry heat for more than a half hour at a time to allow the hyperemia (increased blood flow) to disperse, giving the tissue a chance to normalize. Remind your clients never to fall asleep while using a heating pad.

Moist heat is the deepest form of heat application in the scope of practice for massage therapists. Moist heat packs applied to the neck, shoulders, gluteals, back, and legs are a great way to start a stress reduction treatment. However, it is easier to burn a client using moist heat, so follow the following guidelines to avoid red skin, burns, and blisters.

Moist Heat Applications

Hot Packs **(hydrocollators)**: These are canvas packs filled with silica gel that release steam to provide soothing, moist, deep-penetrating heat to painful muscles and joints. Moist heat penetrates 2–4 cm into the soft tissues, unless blocked by the insulating effect of the subcutaneous fat. This type of heat is far more effective at reducing pain than dry heat heating pads that heat only near the surface of the body without penetrating into deeper tissue layers. Hot packs are available at pharmacies and medical supply stores. The standard-size packs are perfect for the back, hips, and legs; special cervical packs fit the neck and shoulder areas.

Soak new hydrocollator packs in water overnight before using (store them in sealed plastic bags in the refrigerator when not in use to prolong their effective life). Heat a pack for 20–30 minutes in clean, hot (160–175° F) water. Wrap the pack in some thick towels or commercially available—but expensive—pack covers and then place the pack on the painful area. Allow a few minutes for the heat to seep through and then adjust the towel layers for maximum comfort and safety. Check for burns; it just takes a small, uncovered corner of a pack to create some nasty blisters on your client's back.

Tips and Caution for Using Hot Packs:

- Be careful that you don't burn your hands when lifting the hot packs from the water. Use tongs or a chopstick to pull the pack from the water by one of its loops.
- Allow the excess water to drop off and then quickly place the pack in a commercially manufactured hot pack cover or in a towel. Always use a table or countertop to prepare the pack.

- Never place a towel on the client's back and then carry the dripping pack over the client's body because the potential for a hot drop of water burning them is too great.
- Experiment with different layers of towel until you find the right amount of comfortable heat. Six to eight layers of thin cotton towel or two to three layers of thick towels or commercial pack covers between the pack and the skin are usually sufficient.
- Place the packs on top of the area to be treated. Lying on a hot pack increases the potential for burns because the heat has no avenue to escape, which intensifies it. Use extra caution and extra layers of towels if you feel you must have a client lie on a pack.
- Keep the pack on the painful areas for 20–30 minutes or until it cools.

For stress reduction treatments place the packs on the client's neck, shoulders, back, and sacrum, while playing some relaxing music in the background and talking the client into a state of alert relaxation. Start the massage on the prone feet and legs and after about 10 minutes remove the sacral pack, take off a layer of cover, and place it on the soles of the client's feet over the draping. When you have completed the hip and gluteal work, remove the packs from the back, discard a layer of covering, and place it over tense leg areas. When you have completed the back work, remove the cervical pack and, if it still is warm, you can remove the layers of cover and place it over the back area. After the cervical region has been treated remove all the packs and turn the client over for the supine phase of the treatment. If the top sheet is wet from the steam packs, replace it with a dry sheet so the client does not get cold.

Microwavable Moist Heat Packs

Different manufacturers have marketed products that release soothing moist heat after being heated for 2–3 minutes in a microwave oven. These packs, which acquire ambient moisture from the air when heated, are filled with rice, beans, or some other pellets that are sewn into cases shaped like hydrocollator packs. These easy-to-use, convenient packs stay warm for 15–20 minutes. Some brands of these packs have safety indicators on them to prevent overheating and burning the client. Heating time depends on the strength of the microwave. Always follow the manufacturer's directions for heating and the rest time required before reheating these packs. Also cover the pack with a pillowcase before applying it to the client's skin. These packs don't put off as much steam as hydrocollators and don't stay warm as long but still are capable substitutes to use for treatments and are easy and safe for clients to use at home.

Cryotherapy

The term **cryotherapy** can be defined as the application of external sources of cold to the body for therapeutic purposes or, literally, "cold therapy" (Knight, 1995). Ice is an extremely effective tool to use to reduce the pain and swelling that occurs after a fresh injury. It is also a valuable aid to interrupt the pain-spasm-pain cycle and for relief of chronic pain. When ice is applied to a fresh injury, blood flow is reduced so less swelling occurs, reducing secondary tissue damage and decreasing the time it takes to heal. Cold applications also decrease muscle metabolism, so less oxygen is burned and fewer nociceptive chemicals and waste products, such as lactic acid, build up in the injured area, lessening the pain experienced. In addition, cold decreases nerve-conduction velocity, raising a person's pain threshold, and reduces muscle spasm and muscle tone by inhibiting the muscle spindles. Cold helps break the pain-spasm-pain cycle and relieves chronic pain by acting as a counterirritant that overrides pain impulses going to the spinal cord and brain.

When cold is applied to the body the client will experience cold for 1–3 minutes, which is followed by a burning sensation (this may occur between 2 and 7 minutes). After 5–7 minutes the area being treated turns numb. There is much confusion in the literature regarding what occurs next during an ice treatment. Some sources say never use ice on a fresh injury for more than 15–20 minutes because after that time the reverse vasodilation that occurs, called the "hunting response," will increase the circulation and lead to more damage to the effected area. This information is erroneous because, although cold-induced vasodilation does occur in some areas of the body, such as the fingers, the circulation to the area being treated is still far less than the original volume of blood that flows through the arteries. Knight wrote, "Vasodilation probably does occur during or following therapeutic applications of cold. If it does, it is only at the end of long-term applications. And its magnitude is minimal enough that average blood flow is much less than no application at all" (Knight, 1995: 125). Therefore, just because a blood vessel may dilate after long-term ice application, that does not mean that it is carrying more blood than it usually would.

Precautions for Using Ice

The massage therapist should adhere to the following precautions for using ice treatments.

- Keep ice treatments to less than 30 minutes.
- Avoid cold if the client does not like it.
- Avoid cold treatments if the client gets hives, pain, muscle spasms, excessive redness, or purpura (hemorrhage into the skin and mucous membranes).
- Cryotherapy can be used with individuals with a cardiac disorder or hypertension, but their condition must be monitored carefully during application.
- Avoid applying cold to a body area with diminished sensation and compromised local circulation because damage may occur without them realizing it.
- Individuals with Raynaud's disease and other vasospastic diseases, in which the arteries do not dilate normally, should never be treated with cryotherapy.
- Some commercially available gel ice packs are colder than ice so be careful when using them. In particular, avoid using them under a compression wrap.
- Many people with fibromyalgia are hypersensitive to cold, so avoid using cryotherapy with them.
- If the client demonstrates blisters and shivering, stop the treatment immediately.
- Individuals with anorexia nervosa are usually cold, so avoid using ice treatments with them.
- Avoid ice combined with compression over bony areas, such as the elbow and the head of the fibula, because the nerves near the surface may become damaged.

- Cold treatments increase tissue stiffness; therefore deep icing should not be used immediately before strenuous exercise because the tissue needs adequate time to warm up to prevent injury.

Cryotherapy and Stress Reduction?

For many ice is not very relaxing and may even increase the tension experienced by some overstressed clients. Before using cryotherapy it's always a good idea to ask the client whether he or she prefers heat or ice. If the client does not like ice, he or she will let you know very quickly. For those clients who have no restrictions and can tolerate the application of cold, ice is a valuable tool to help relieve pain. Combining cold application with some sort of movement is an even more valuable tool in the quest to relax tense musculature, reduce restrictions of normal movement, rebalance the posture, and relieve pain. Combining ice treatments with gentle, active, passive, and assisted movements; proprioceptive neuromuscular facilitation (PNF); and the skilled hands of a massage therapist is an effective way to help rebalance the body and eliminate pain at its source.

Before applying ice therapy to a client for the first time, describe to them the typical feelings they should expect during the course of a treatment. After ice is applied, talk the client through the stages, trying to distract his or her mind with thoughts of the beach or mention of some event of recent importance. The small talk is intended as a counterirritant or distraction, a way to occupy the client's mind so that he or she does not dwell on the physical sensations. You can also ask the client to imagine that the body part being iced feels numb and insensitive or that the feeling of ice next to the skin feels different but not painful.

Types of Cold Modalities

The following discussion outlines different ways to apply cold treatments.

- Crushed ice: A crushed ice pack can be applied to a fresh injury, edema, or area of chronic pain for up to 30 minutes. Place crushed ice in a plastic produce bag, but don't add too much ice because you want to try to keep the bag flat enough so that it can conform to the body. Remove the air from the bag, then twist the end and secure it with a twist tie. If you don't have crushed ice, use cubes or improvise with a bag of frozen peas. For most people it can be applied directly to the skin, with no danger of frostbite. For a fresh injury use the **RICE** principle (*r*est, *i*ce, *c*ompression, and *e*levation) for the first 48–72 hours. When injured rest the injured body part and apply compression with an elastic pressure wrap or even plastic cling food wrap. Wrap the area from distal to proximal, being careful not to wrap it so tight that you cut off the circulation. After the area is wrapped elevate the body part above the heart. To reduce swelling, crushed ice treatments can be repeated safely every hour during the acute phase of an injury.

- Ice massage: Ice massage is a valuable tool that uses an ice cup applied to the skin to help relieve pain and swelling. Ice cups can be used for a quick numbing or desensitization of a specific area of tissue so that active, assisted, and passive movements can be performed to help reduce myofascial restrictions. Icing a specific muscle with an ice cup will numb the area and increase the client's pain threshold, allowing the client to move actively with less pain. Ice massage can also be followed with PNF to help reduce myofascial restrictions. Fill paper cups (the 6–8-ounce variety) with water and put them in the freezer. When you want to use an ice cup, take it out of the freezer, peel some of the paper off, and rub your palm over the surface of the ice to remove any sharp points.

- There are two different ways to use an ice cup. You can place the flat, smooth surface of the cup on the target muscle and move it slowly along the treatment area. Keep the melted ice water mopped up. Don't push the cup down hard, particularly over bones; just let the weight of it touch the skin. Continue this procedure until the area becomes numb, but do not do it for more than 10 minutes. This type of icing is used to reduce localized pain and inflammation. The second method uses strokes applied using the side edge of the ice cup moved quickly along the entire length of a muscle, or group of muscles involved in a pattern of referred pain, to help reduce muscle spasm, relieve pain, and improve flexibility. The intent of this type of quick icing is to try to distract or trick a muscle (or group) that is in spasm into relaxing, which is then followed by stretching it through its comfortable range of motion. Apply the edge of the ice cup from tendon attachment to tendon attachment in line with the direction that the muscle fibers run. After one stroke is performed ensuing strokes are applied parallel to the first by moving a half-inch wide of the previous stroke. Usually one group of strokes consists of four to six nonoverlapping strokes covering the entire muscle or group involved. Remember to mop up all the melted ice after each stroke. After only one stroke is applied to each part of the entire muscle or group of muscles, the client actively moves, or is passively moved, through his or her comfortable range of motion. This procedure of quick icing and active or passive movements through the restricted range is then repeated four to six times. Brisk massage or the application of 4–5 minutes of heat is then used to rewarm the area after treatment.

- Gel packs: Soft, reusable chemical ice packs that are stored in the freezer can be used in place of crushed ice. Some of these packs are colder than ice, so don't use them directly on the skin, and to avoid frostbite don't use a compression wrap with them. These are easy to use and there is no mess, but they don't stay cold as long as ice so keep a few extras stored in the freezer.

- Ice bucket: A bucket or whirlpool full of icy, slushy water is an effective way to decrease swelling from an injury to the ankle, hand, or elbow. Although you can safely put the swollen area in the bucket for 15–30 minutes, treatments generally last from 7 to 10 minutes. To reduce the pain of submersion, use the toe and forefoot section of a diving bootie over the toes or fingers. Instruct the client to move the body part while in the bucket so the muscles act as pumps to assist venous return. If the ice bucket is too cold for the client, you can try building the client up to longer bouts of ice immersion by performing a series of 3–5-second quick dips in the bucket while moving the body part being soaked. The ice bucket is not something that is used frequently in a stress reduction treatment, but it is very effective for reducing edema.

- **Cryokinetics:** Cryokinetics literally means ice and movement. Cryokinetics can be performed with an ice cup. Massage an area with an ice cup for 10 minutes and then follow the icing with active or PNF stretching movements. This type of icing combined with movement can be applied to stress reduction treatments when trying to help the client rebalance the musculature and regain the full range of movement. Cryokinetics also can be performed with an ice bucket. After the acute phase of an injury place an injured area, such as the ankle, in an ice bucket for up to 10 minutes, constantly moving the foot around in all directions. After 10 minutes remove the foot from the ice and perform a series of strengthening exercises out of the bucket for 10 minutes. If the client had an inversion sprain, then have him or her perform heel raises, toe raises, and exercises to strengthen the peroneals, the everters of the foot. Balance activities on a Bosu ball and therapeutic elastic band strengthening exercises for the musculature also can be performed. After the 10 minutes of exercising, it is back in the ice bucket for 10 more minutes, once again constantly moving the foot and ankle. The movement contracts the muscles, which act like pumps to flush out the area being treated, which speeds healing. This technique is most effective for rehabilitating injured ankles and is generally not used in stress reduction treatments.

- **Contrast baths:** After the acute phase of an injury, alternating baths of ice and heat, combined with movement, is another technique used to reduce tissue inflammation. Contrast baths are not generally used in stress reduction treatments, but it is a useful technique to know because it helps improve the circulation of the blood and lymph to an injured area, flushing out the waste products and delivering more oxygen and nutrients. Place the ankle in an ice bucket for 2 minutes, moving the foot and ankle constantly. After 2 minutes place the foot in a hot tub for 2 minutes, once again moving the foot and ankle constantly. Repeat 4–5 cycles of alternate ice and heat soaks. Always start with ice and end with ice.

MASSAGE TO RELIEVE PAIN

Massage has been used for centuries as a natural way to relieve and control pain. Many different massage systems and techniques for pain control have been developed throughout the years. These systems of massage have charted the locations of painful points on the human body and labeled them with a variety of names, which include acupuncture points, pressure points, **neurolymphatic** points, tender points, **myalgic** spots, trigger points, and Ah Shi points. Regardless of what an author or massage system calls them, tender, painful points in the body are small palpable areas of hypertonic tissue located in the muscular and fascial tissues. The difference between tender points and trigger points is that when tender points are pressed localized pain is produced in the myofascial unit that is being touched, whereas when trigger points are stimulated pain refers in predictable patterns to locations outside of the myofascial unit being pressed. Trigger points can be active or latent. When stimulated active trigger points refer pain outside the muscle where it originates, whereas latent trigger points may exist in a muscle for years after an injury, with no indication of their existence except that they may limit the active range of motion of the client. Then suddenly overuse, overstretching, or even chilling of the muscle may suddenly revert latent trigger points to their active referred pain-invoking status (Travel, 1999).

In the Personal Stress Inventory you mapped and documented clients' painful points. To develop an effective treatment program the therapist must take into account whether they are treating trigger points or tender points and design the treatment plan accordingly. Did any of the points that you stimulated while palpating your client refer pain to another area of their body? If they did refer pain, study a chart of myofascial trigger points to help make sure that you have uncovered precisely where it originated. If you treat and eliminate the source of the pain, other areas of referred tenderness will disappear. However, you must realize that charts and books do have limitations because they only list the most commonly found trigger points; trigger points vary amongst people, and sometimes muscles develop multiple trigger points (Travel, 1999). Therapists should use the charts as a point of reference only and trust their palpation skills to determine the precise location of their clients' points to treat. Therapists should treat the active trigger points uncovered first, after which they should help the client achieve normal pain-free range of motion. After the first two goals have been achieved, release the client's tender points.

After a thorough review of clients' pain profiles the therapist must develop a multifaceted strategy to help them reduce the physical manifestations of their stress and reduce their pain. This strategy could include diaphragmatic breathing, relaxation and posture awareness training, active exercise, passive stretching, and the use of heat or ice and massage (of course). To reduce the client's pain the therapist should consider using both direct and indirect treatment techniques. Direct approaches are those techniques that apply force to remold and reposition the body and break down barriers that prevent normal pain-free range of movement. Examples of direct techniques are passive stretching, which can be combined with ice massage; gross and specific myofascial release; and PNF. PNF combines active motion with resistance and the use of reflex neurological activity to get through restrictive barriers. Indirect approaches are those techniques such as strain-counterstrain, also called PRT (positional release therapy) and the fold and hold method, which involves placing a person in a position of comfort or greatest ease for at least 90 seconds or until the tissues spontaneously release. Indirect approaches are not intended to force the client's body to change to a predetermined optimum; instead they place the body in a position of comfort, which helps the tissues relax, unwind, and readjust until they release their tightness and restrictions and return to their normal state of balance.

Direct pressure applied to painful points on the body is a pain-control technique that has been used for centuries. For stress reduction treatments another useful gentle technique for relieving sore, tender points on the body involves a combination of light pressure to the pain points and the client's conscious relaxation of those points. Most clients lack the ability to isolate and relax their tender points on their own. With this technique the relaxed but aware client uses the pressure and temperature feedback from the therapist's fingers to tune into the precise location of his or her hypertonic musculature, and then the client can use his or her mind to consciously let tension and pain melt away. For this type of work the client and the therapist must enter a state of focused relaxation.

The well-trained therapist should have a diversified collection of techniques at his or her disposal and should try different methods with clients until the right combination is found to relieve their pain. Clients react differently to different treatments. Some feel that indirect techniques are a waste of their time and money and are not willing to give them a chance, whereas other clients get relief from their pain through strain–counterstrain in a matter of a few minutes and really appreciate an indirect approach. The therapist must be willing to adjust, revise, and adapt his or her treatments according to the needs and response of the client.

DEVELOPING A PAIN-CONTROL PLAN

The following suggestions will help you develop an effective pain-control program for your client.

- Conduct a thorough assessment: Use results of the client's posture, flexibility, breathing, and painful point assessment from the Personal Stress Inventory and any other pertinent information gained from the subjective information that the client provides during the interview process to determine the location of problems and factors that could be contributing to them.
- Set up a pain scale: Before the first treatment session, ascertain where the client's pain from his or her major problems registers on a pain scale, such as 0 (no pain) through 10 (excruciating pain). Of course, this may vary for different areas of the body if the client has multiple problems.
- Determine goals for treatment: Taking all factors into consideration, realistically where do you expect the client's overall level of pain to register after a series of treatments, on a scale of 0 (no pain) through 10 (excruciating pain).
- Determine number of treatments: Estimate the number of treatments you will need to bring the client to the goal range (1–10).
- Plan and implement a treatment program: Don't begin without a plan. Use heat or ice as indicated, use direct and indirect techniques, and give the client homework assignments as an adjunct to the treatments. Keep revising the treatment program according to the evolving condition of the client.
- Treat the active trigger points uncovered first, then help the client achieve normal pain-free range of motion. After the first two goals have been achieved, release the client's tender points.
- Chart progress: Record which techniques you have used, those that the client liked, and those that produce the most effective results. Also record strategies that you want to use in the client's next treatment.
- Reassess: After the designated number of treatments, reevaluate the client's posture, flexibility, breathing, and painful points

using the pain scale to determine the effectiveness of your plan. Ask yourself the question, "What could I have done differently that would have produced better results?"

MASSAGE TECHNIQUES FOR PAIN CONTROL

Experiment with the following techniques to learn how to properly apply them and determine their effectiveness with relieving muscle spasm and pain.

Strain–counterstrain requires that the therapist have an understanding of muscle attachments and all the planes of joint movement for each muscle being treated. When a painful point is isolated, the therapist should press it hard enough to elicit a mild pain response or, as some say, a good hurt. While maintaining contact with the painful point, shorten the muscles being treated by approximating the origin and insertion. Adjust the position of the joint by internally or externally rotating, flexing or extending, adducting or abducting, or whatever motion is needed until a position is found that eliminates the pain. If the muscle crosses two joints, positional adjustments may have to be made involving that joint as well. Use all the planes of movement to help find the optimal position of ease, the part of the muscle range where the pain is alleviated. Hold the pain-free position until the area releases or for a minimum of 90 seconds; then very slowly return it to its normal resting position. Some believe that applying mild longitudinal force into the area being treated speeds up this process. For example, when releasing a neck muscle, position the neck in the optimal position and then press gently on the top of the head to mildly compress the area being released. This gentle force may help the musculature relax and unwind more quickly, so experiment with it and formulate your own opinion. This technique can be applied to any muscle. The creative use of bolsters and pillows can help the client maintain the ideal position, easing the burden on the therapist.

Applying direct pressure to clients' painful spots is an effective pain-control technique. Press clients' painful points with the pads of the fingers, reinforced thumbs, knuckles, or the elbow hard enough so they know exactly where they are but not so hard that they jump, cringe, or tighten up. It is important to instruct clients to take long, slow, deep, nourishing breaths as you press on these areas. Try to breathe with your clients as you tune into their muscles and try to help them relax. You can go deeper as their body allows you to, but you must work at the pace that the body dictates. Going too deep too fast will make for less beneficial treatments. A therapist can stimulate these points for 10–30 seconds or until he or she feels the client relax.

Instruct the client to use his or her mind to tune into the exact spot that you are touching and to breathe through that spot. Tell them to mentally picture the muscle fibers lengthening; unwinding; and growing long, loose, limp, heavy, and deeply relaxed. Tell the client to focus his or her entire awareness on the spot and to feel the muscle tension dissolving and pain subsiding. As you go deeper instruct the client to exhale; when the client exhales, you exhale with them. Breathing awareness and coordination with the client helps the therapist get more in synch with the client and helps improve intuition. Intuition and visualization are extremely important for this type of work. Intuition helps the therapist find the client's areas of tension and helps the therapist tune more effectively into the client's body. It is as if the pads of the fingers develop eyes that can see areas of hypertonicity. Therapists should try to put their mind into the muscle that they are working on and think about what they can do to soothe this muscle to make it relax and feel good.

The therapist can visualize the direction of the muscle fibers being contacted and then picture them releasing and relaxing. The therapist projects warmth and compassionate touch from his or her hands, and the client uses this pressure and warmth to tune into this area of the body and let tension and spasm melt away. The therapist can apply pressure on the point(s) until he or she feels a pulse, which indicates that the client has tuned into the feedback from the therapist's contact and that the relaxation process of the muscle has begun. As the muscle releases the therapist can adjust the angle of the pressure applied or move along the length of the muscle fibers searching for other points because sometimes multiple points must be found and treated, or the therapist can move on to another area. Don't work in an area too long; after the pulse is balanced and the texture of the tissue feels more relaxed it is time to move to another area. Some passive range of motion and a few cleansing effleurage strokes are a great way to bid farewell to one area and move on to the next area that needs to be addressed. This technique is more effective when combined with therapist-guided relaxation suggestions for the client. Points can be addressed bilaterally and unilaterally, and even different muscles involved in a pattern of referred pain can be worked on simultaneously. It also helps to start with the more proximal tender and trigger points and then work on the distal points.

An ice cup massage combined with active range of motion or PNF can be used to break the pain-spasm-pain cycle. Quick icing with the corner edge, not the flat, smooth part of an ice cup, can be applied along the entire length of the fibers of any muscle or group of muscles. The muscles are then stretched actively, or the neurological reflexes can be used to help improve flexibility. For example, you have a client who has a 10-degree limitation of active neck rotation in a counterclockwise direction. You have determined that the right sternocleidomastoid (SCM) is hypertonic and is the cause of the restricted movement. If they have no contraindications for using ice, apply one stroke to each part of the right SCM with the ice cup, mopping up all melted ice. After the SCM has been iced, have the client actively rotate his or her head counterclockwise as far as is comfortable. Then place your hand on the left side of the client's head and instruct the client to try to rotate his or her head counterclockwise against your force for 6 seconds. After the 6 seconds, pause for 2 seconds and then have the client actively rotate the head counterclockwise once again. Repeat the quick icing, resistance, and active movement 4–6 times. Always start the resistance from the new end of the client's range of motion.

DESIGNING A PAIN-REDUCING, STRESS REDUCTION MASSAGE

The therapist should think about which strokes he or she should use for a pain-reducing, stress reduction massage. A useful exercise for students is to record on paper a generalized stress reduction massage sequence of strokes. They can adapt the basic plan for different clients and incorporate the pain-control techniques into this sequence when indicated. When designing this sequence it is important to remember not to overstimulate the stressed client by working too hard and too deeply. For the highly stressed client avoid deep-tissue work unless the client is used to it and craves it. Slow your work down and use more effleurage, rocking, and gentle pétrissage, and combine the friction strokes you use with the relaxed focus of the client. Instead of trying to reshape their muscles with your force and strength, have the clients melt away their tension with their own minds.

It's a good idea to use the modalities at the beginning of the treatment. The heat will help relax clients, improve their circulation, and reduce their spasm, and the ice will reduce their spasm and pain and allow you to help them get back their restricted range of motion. Remember that cryotherapy is not for everyone. Try to add the positional release and focused relaxation techniques into your routine because these are very effective for highly stressed clients. Before using the focused relaxation techniques, the therapist must be relaxed and well-grounded. Figure 10.1 provides a sample grounding exercise that is useful preparation for this sort of treatment. The therapist also must be able to talk the client into a state of focused relaxation, so refer to Chapter 8 for techniques to help your client relax.

THE TREATMENT

After the therapist is relaxed and grounded, position the client on the table using as many bolsters and pillows and whatever configuration is needed to get him or her as comfortable as possible. Apply moist heat to the client's painful points or substitute ice if desired. Then talk the client into a state of relaxation. Instruct the client to take some slow, deep, diaphragmatic breaths and to let the tension flow out with each exhalation. Use muscular relaxation, autogenic training, visual imagery techniques, and suggestions to induce the proper state of alert relaxation. In the course of your massage routine address the client's painful points using any of the aforementioned techniques. These points can be stimulated from 10 to 30 seconds or until you feel the client relaxing. Use your intuition and judgment on how long to work on your client. Eventually you will feel these points melting under your fingers.

Record the following script with some relaxing music playing in the background and then listen to it while seated in a quiet room. This exercise should take about 20 minutes.

To begin close your eyes and take a long, slow, deep, relaxing complete breath, in through your nose for six seconds, filling your lungs completely, and then exhale slowly for eight seconds through the nose. When you exhale let all the tension flow out of your mind and your body. Each breath relaxes you more and more. Now relax all the muscles of your forehead and scalp. Let this wave of relaxation spread down to the muscles of your eyebrows, eyelids, and eyes. Relax the muscles of your cheeks, jaw, mouth, lips, and tongue. Let all the muscles of your face and head deeply relax. Now let this peaceful wave of relaxation flow down to the muscles of your neck and shoulders. Relax the muscles of the front, the sides, and the back of your neck where so much tension accrues. Let gravity pull your shoulders and arms down towards the floor. Give in to the pull of gravity; don't fight it. Let all of your tension flow out of you. Let this relaxed feeling now spread to the muscles of your arms. Relax the biceps and triceps of the upper arm, the flexors and extensors of the fore-arms, the hands, and all the way to the tips of your fingers. (Pause) Now repeat the following phrases silently to yourself.

My right arm and hand is growing warm and heavy; warmth is flowing into my fingers.
My left arm and hand is growing warm and heavy; warmth is flowing into my fingers.
My arms and hands are warm, heavy, and completely relaxed.

Now let this wave of relaxation and warmth spread down your back, relaxing all the muscles along the vertebrae and between the scapulae, all the way down to your gluteals and hips. Relax all the muscles of your chest and abdomen. Allow this wonderful feeling of relaxation to continue its path down to the thighs, relaxing the front, side, and back of the thighs. Now let this relaxed, heavy feeling flow down to the calves, feet, and all the way to the tips of the toes. Repeat the following phrases silently to yourself.

My right leg and foot is growing warm and heavy; warmth is flowing into my toes.
My left leg and foot is growing warm and heavy; warmth is flowing into my toes.
My legs and feet are warm, heavy, and completely relaxed.
My mind and body are completely relaxed.
Warmth is flowing into my toes.

Enjoy this relaxed feeling for a few minutes, then continue. Now picture in your mind that your feet have sprung roots like a tree. These roots extend from the bottom of your feet deep down into the center of the earth. Let all of your negativity, all of your anxiety, all of your problems, trials, and tribulations flow out of your body through these roots, right into the center of the earth. You feel totally relaxed, cleansed, and peaceful. You feel totally confident, yet still relaxed.

Now that you are deeply, deeply relaxed, picture in your mind a beam of light entering your forehead between your eyebrows. This light fills you with inspiration, peace, happiness, and tranquility. Let this light now flow down into your heart and solar plexus and then out to your hands. Picture this healing light flowing through your body and into your hands. Picture this energy flowing right through the palms of your hands and your fingertips. Now realize that whenever you are touching a client with compassion you can picture a flow of energy emanating from your hands and fingers tips to help them relieve their pain and tension. (Pause briefly.)

Now place the tip of your thumb against the tips of your ring and middle fingers. Placing these finger tips together puts you into your quick grounding elevator. You start on the third floor. Picture the number three in your mind three times, then as you descend to the second floor picture the number two three times, and as you descend to the bottom floor picture the number one three times. You have instantly transferred your mind to a deeply relaxed state. This is a way to quickly ground yourself before and between treatments. Realize from this moment forward whenever you want to ground yourself all you have to do is touch your fingertips together in this fashion, take some deep breaths, descend in your elevator, and relax. Your thoughts will instantly grow calm and peaceful; the light will flow into your body and you will project positive healing energy from your hands and fingers. Now, it's time to slowly come back and gently regain your conscious awareness. When I count to three open your eyes feeling much, much better than before. You will feel totally relaxed and refreshed. One: coming up slowly; two: still relaxed and feeling wonderful, but more awake; and three: eyes open, relaxed but awake and alert, ready to perform a truly effective treatment.

Figure 10.1

Grounding skills training exercise

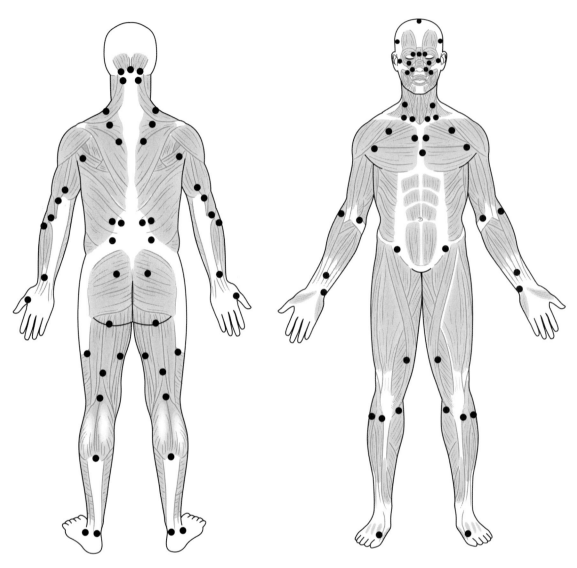

Figure 10.2

Back stress points

Figure 10.3

Front of the body stress points

FREQUENTLY PAINFUL STRESS POINTS

Figures 10.2, 10.3, and 10.4 present a collection of points that are frequently tense on stressed people. Check out these points on your client and treat them when indicated. They also can be shared with the client to use in his or her self-massage homework.

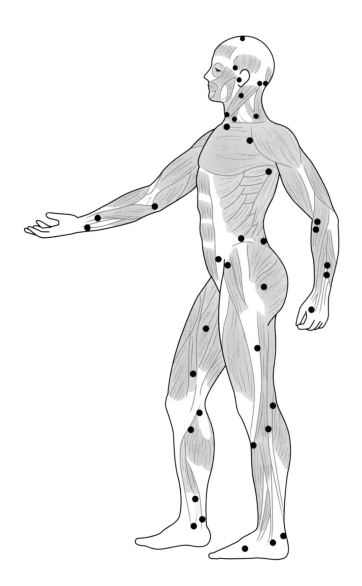

Figure 10.4

Stress points on the medial and lateral body

SELF-MASSAGE

The following self-massage techniques can be shared with the client for use as homework to relieve pain and relax muscles. If they can reach them, clients can massage the painful points on their own body. They can use a cane or two tennis balls tied in a sock to help apply pressure to their painful muscles. The use of balms or a warming and lubricating medium such as Prossage Heat™ may be used to add some glide and soothing penetrating heat to help relax tight musculature.

Self-Foot Massage

Our poor feet are often neglected and abused. We suffocate them in socks, cram them in shoes, pound them on hard pavement, and probably spend little time caring for them. Foot massage can improve circulation, reduce pain, and produce an overall feeling of relaxation in the body. Following is a technique for self-foot massage that works well. Wash the feet in warm water and soap, and after a 10-minute soak dry them well. Dry between the toes and then give each toe a gentle pull using the towel for a better grip. Have a seat in a chair and place a very small amount of lotion, balm, or oil on the hands. Squeeze one foot between the hands, starting at the toes and working toward the ankles. Next glide the hands over the sole and top of the foot, around the malleoli (ankle bones) and along the sides of the big tendon (calcaneal or Achilles tendon) on the back of the ankle. Next glide the knuckles three times firmly along the sole of the foot, starting at the base of the toes and working toward the heels. Press the knuckles in firmly, as if you were pushing a tack into wood, but go lighter along the arch. If you find a particularly tender area while gliding, come back to it and press a knuckle into it. You can move the knuckle around in small circles or you can curl the foot around the point of contact until it relaxes. Work each of the tender points at the bottom of the foot in this fashion. Next bend the toes forward (flexion) and back (extension) and then rub the space between each toe with the little finger. Now squeeze the tip of each toe and then use the fingers to corkscrew around each toe, moving toward the heart. Then run the thumbs in between the tendons and bones on the top of the foot. Next place one hand on each side of the foot and run both thumbs between each tendon while pushing up with the fingers in between the same bones on the sole of the foot. Follow this by grasping the metatarsals two at a time and then gently separating and stretching them by moving them up and down. Figure 10.5 demonstrates a technique for separating the metatarsals. Start at the groove separating the big toe from the second toe and work each pair of metatarsals progressing toward the little toe, separating all of the metatarsals.

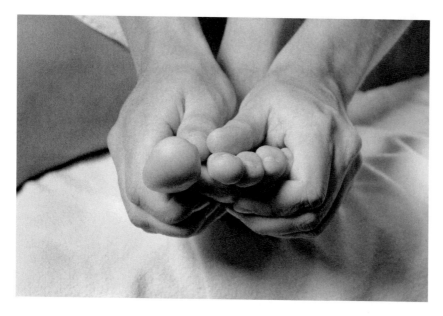

Figure 10.5

Separating the metatarsals

When you have completed stretching the gaps between all the metatarsals, grasp the calcaneal tendon and roll it between the thumb and index finger, searching for tender areas. Next massage the top of the ankle around each malleoli (ankle bone), and then press along the sides of the foot, searching for tender points. Finally, put one hand on top of your foot and the other on the bottom. Think about heat, warmth, and relaxation for 10–15 seconds. Now, feel the difference between your feet. Repeat the massage on the other foot.

Self-Massage to the Lower Legs

Sit down and flex one knee and hip and then place this leg over the other so you can easily touch the medial malleolus. Apply some lotion, balm, or a warming medium to your hands and warm up the entire calf and lower leg with some effleurage or compressions. Start lightly and progress to deeper strokes. If you are flexible enough you can even use your forearms. Next use your thumbs or reinforced fingers to slide up the musculature on the medial side edge of the tibia from just above the medial malleolus up toward the knee. Figure 10.6 demonstrates a technique for gliding along the medial tibia.

Glide as far as you can, tracing along the edge of the bone. If you find any tender spots on your glides, come back to them

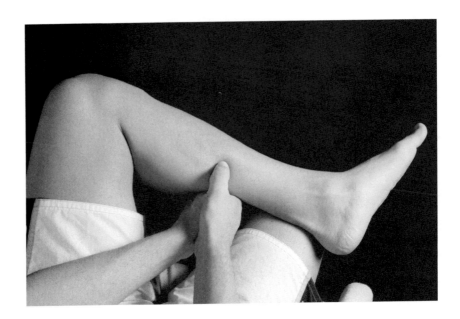

Figure 10.6

Gliding along the medial tibia

and press them for 10–30 seconds, or do some friction circles or cross-fiber friction to try to release them. You can continue by rubbing all over and around the entire medial aspect of the knee, searching for and trying to relieve any tender spots.

Next use the knuckles and slide up the lateral side of the tibia over the tibialis anterior muscle. Figure 10.7 shows a reinforced-wrist, knuckle-gliding technique for performing this stroke.

After warming the area up with a few strokes you can dig in deeper and slide up this anterior compartment of the lower leg while slowly plantar flexing and dorsiflexing the ankle. If you find a very tender spot, work it out with some circular or cross-fiber friction. Figure 10.8 demonstrates a cross-fiber friction technique to the tibialis anterior.

Now move to the lateral aspect of the lower leg and slide the knuckles all the way up the ankle everters to just below the head of the fibula; once again try to work out any tender points with some friction. After the peroneals have been worked, turn your attention to the calf. The hip and knee can be flexed or extended to give easier access to the part of the calf being worked. Now slide the pads of the fingers along the sides of the calcaneus tendon up the calf until just below the popliteal fossa; after gliding back to the start, work your way laterally with the same techniques covering the entire calf. Next slide on top of the calcaneus tendon and work

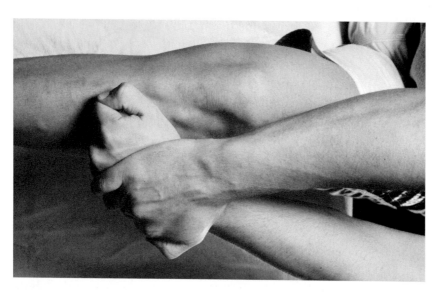

Figure 10.7

Knuckle gliding along the tibialis anterior with a reinforced wrist

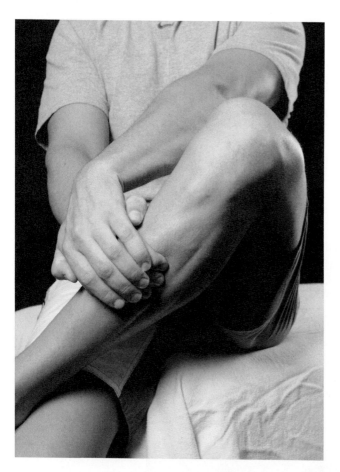

Figure 10.8

Cross-fiber friction to the tibialis anterior

along the entire posterior side of the tibia up to the popliteal area. Continue by covering the entire calf with some deeper pressure using the knuckles, working the soleus and then the two heads of the gastrocnemius as they cross the back of the knee. Start lightly and work progressively deeper. Take as many knuckle glides as you need to thoroughly cover the entire **triceps surae.** After the gliding strokes, perform a series of 10 deep thumb presses up the backside of the tibia by flexing the hip and knee, then pressing deeply with one or both reinforced thumbs into muscle and then flicking across the fibers. Work from the distal to the proximal, moving a half an inch superior on each successive stroke along the backside of the tibia. Add or reduce the number of presses according to the size of your legs. Thumb presses to the calf are featured in Figure 10.9.

This can be followed by some friction circles or cross-fiber work to any hypertonic spots uncovered on the soleus and both heads of the gastrocnemius. Finish the work to the lower leg with a cleansing effleurage to all the musculature, or if you prefer you can use some rolling, vibration, or tapotement. Another easy way to perform a calf massage is to long sit on the floor and place a tennis ball or a massage ball with some firm spikes on it

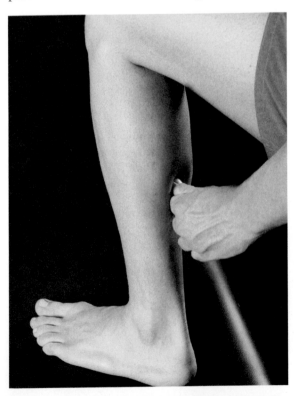

Figure 10.9

Reinforced thumb presses to the calf

underneath the calf. Use the force of gravity to apply pressure as you move the ball underneath the calf to work out the tense and painful areas. When using a spiked massage ball, work on the sides of the calcaneal tendon and by the musculotendinous junction, but avoid digging into the tendon just above the calcaneus.

Self-Massage to the Upper Legs

Once again sit down and apply some warming lubrication to your hands and forearms. Begin this upper-leg massage by gliding with the forearms or hands along the quadriceps, adductors, and hamstrings and following the iliotibial band (ITB) from the lateral knee up and around the greater trochanter of the femur. If you desire to address the hip abductors, perform some gliding or compressions to the gluteus medius and minimus, working from the crest of the ilium down to the greater trochanter. Figure 10.10 depicts the

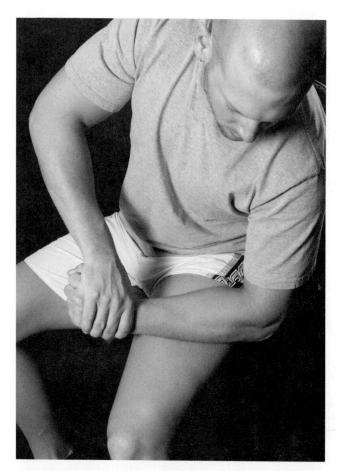

Figure 10.10

Forearm gliding to the quadriceps

application of a gliding forearm stroke to the quadriceps. Continue with some palmar or forearm compressions to the anterior, medial, and lateral musculature.

Next scoot to the edge of the chair and use the forearm like a rolling pin on the hamstrings, working from the back of the knee up to the ischial tuberosity, engaging the tissue by using a forward and backward rolling motion (not gliding). Figure 10.11 demonstrates the rolling pin action of the forearm to the hamstrings. Follow the rolling pin by pressing the triceps firmly into the adductors.

Figure 10.12 demonstrates working the adductors with the triceps. After the upper leg has been thoroughly warmed up, apply some friction with the elbow, knuckles, or reinforced fingers to any areas of hypertonicity that have been uncovered in the quadriceps,

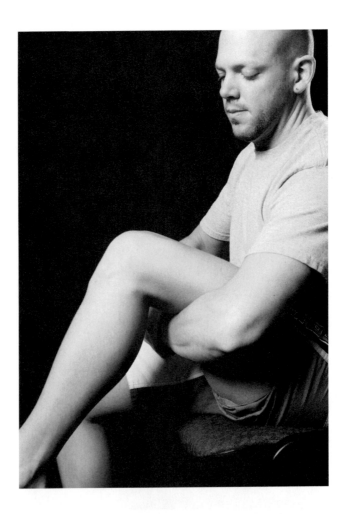

Figure 10.11

Rolling pin forearm to the hamstrings

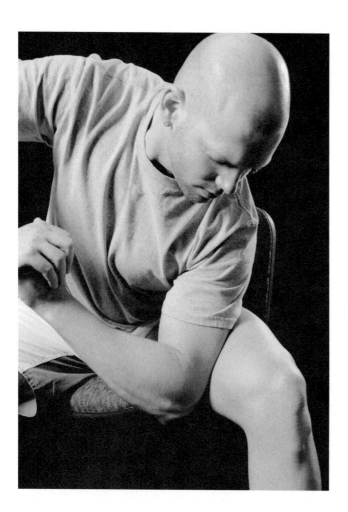

Figure 10.12

Triceps press to the adductors

adductors, and hamstrings. Also apply some friction to ITB and all the musculature around the greater trochanter and to the hip abductors if desired. Figure 10.13 demonstrates the application of friction with reinforced fingers to the ITB.

Finish this self-massage to the upper leg with a cleansing effleurage and if you desire some vibration or tapotement.

Self-Massage to the Hands and Arms

To perform a self-massage to the hands and arms, sit with the legs under a massage table, or, if you don't have one, you can use a kitchen table or a desk with a pillow on it. Use some lotion, balm, or warming oil on the hand or forearm to warm up all of your other hand and arm

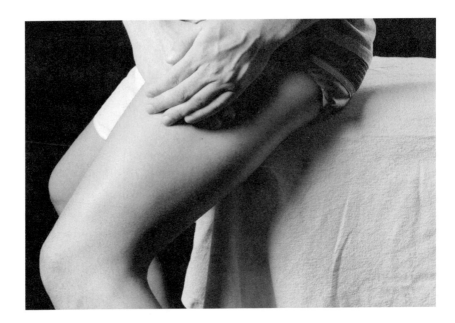

Figure 10.13

Reinforced finger friction to the iliotibial band

with some effleurage. Effleurage all the way up to the axilla, and if your flexibility is adequate, also work the anterior, middle, and posterior deltoids. Work both sides of the hand and forearm while resting on the pillow and elevate the arm to work the upper arm and deltoids, progressing from light to deep strokes. Figure 10.14 demonstrates an elevated arm gliding warmup stroke to the triceps.

After the warmup glide back to the hands and gently envelop and squeeze each finger between the thumb and fingers of the other hand, moving distally to proximally. After the finger compressions stretch, flex, and extend each finger and then give it a gentle pull. Next rub the web area between each finger, spending extra time at the junction between the thumb and index finger. Search the web area between the thumb and index finger for tension and pain, and if discomfort exists, apply pressure or circular friction for 10–30 seconds toward the index finger with the thumb or a finger of the other hand. Next separate all the metacarpal bones by placing the fingertips on the top of the hand and the thumb on the palm side and then gliding from distal to proximal between the bones. After separating the metacarpals, work the entire palm with the knuckles of the other hand. Be sure to thoroughly work both the thenar and hypothenar eminences. Apply friction to any tender spots found on the base of the palmar surface of the hand, particularly in the area

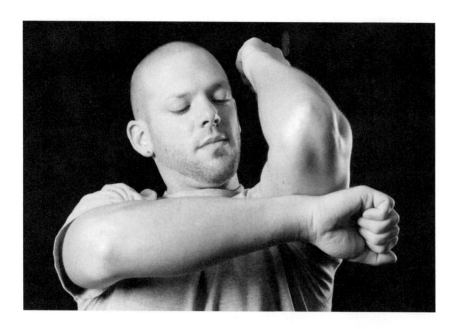

Figure 10.14

Warming up the triceps

over and near the transverse carpal ligament. After completing the base of the hand friction, let's move our attention to the forearm.

Perform some deep gliding to the supinated forearm with the other forearm or the knuckles. The forearm can be used as a rolling pin, with small back-and-forth movements moving from distal to proximal, or the knuckles can be used to deeply glide from distal to proximal. Of course, avoid putting hard pressure over the cubital fossa, the anterior fold of the elbow. Next use the reinforced thumb to glide along the edge of the radius, the ulna, and then between these bones. Perform some sustained friction to any areas of hypertonicity uncovered. Pay particular attention to tension in any of the wrist and hand flexors or pronators that attach to the common flexor tendon that originates at the medial epicondyle of the humerus. If the common flexor tendon area on the medial epicondyle is very tender, you can try some friction or even a positional release technique for relief. Figure 10.15 demonstrates a positional release technique applied to the common flexor tendon. Press the tender area and then bend the joints involved, adjusting in all planes of movement until you find the client's position of greatest ease. Hold that position for 90 seconds and then slowly move back to the anatomical position. After the forearm flexor work has been completed, pronate the forearm and let's concentrate on the extensor side.

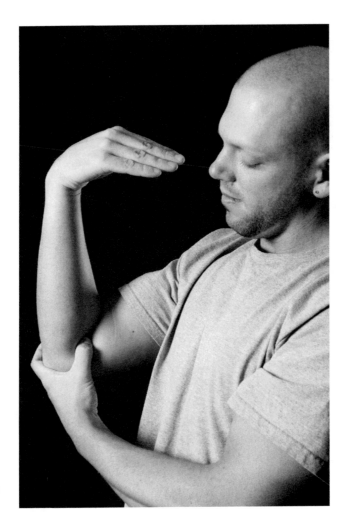

Figure 10.15

Positional release to the common flexor tendon

Place the pronated forearm on the table and perform a deep glide with the forearm or knuckles over the brachioradialis and all of the wrist and forearm extensor musculature. Follow this with a reinforced thumb glide along the inside edge of the radius, the ulna, and then over the extensor muscles in between, gliding all the way to the lateral epicondyle of the humerus. Continue by applying some friction to any areas of hypertonicity uncovered. A useful way to apply friction to the posterior forearm musculature is by placing the forearm being worked on in mid position (thumb up). Then place the thumb or fingertips of the free hand on the brachioradialis or extensor muscle being worked on. Sink slowly but deeply into the muscle mass and then slowly supinate and pronate the forearm. Work along

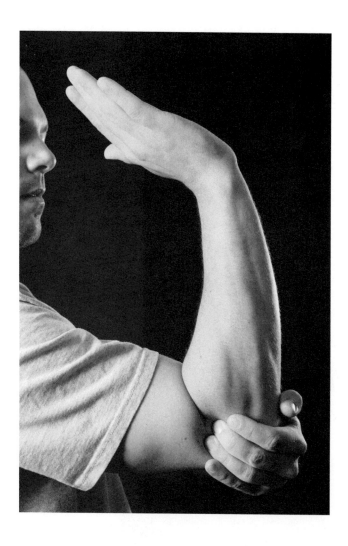

Figure 10.16

Positional release to the common extensor tendon

the length of the muscle, working out all the tender areas. This technique is also effective on the muscles attaching to the common extensor tendon, which originates from the lateral epicondyle of the humerus. Use mild force applied to a painful spot combined with the supination and pronation motion to help you apply effective friction. The positional release technique also can be applied to reduce tension and pain experienced in the musculature attaching to the common extensor tendon. Figure 10.16 demonstrates a positional release technique applied to the common extensor tendon.

After the forearm extensor work has been completed it is a good idea to stretch out all of the forearm, wrist flexor, and extensor muscles. To stretch the flexors extend the elbow of the arm being stretched and then extend the wrist by grasping the metacarpals of that hand with the other hand. Apply force to the metacarpals to gently stretch the wrist to its full range of motion. To stretch the forearm extensors, flex the shoulders to 90 degrees, extend the elbows, turn the thumbs down, and interlace the hands. Keeping the fingers interlaced, simply extend the opposite wrist to stretch the wrist and finger extensors. You can shake the hands and wrists out after stretching.

Now move up to the upper arm and begin with some deep knuckling or rolling-pin action to the biceps and triceps. Next perform some circular or cross-fiber friction applied with the knuckles or fingertips to any areas of excess pain, tension, or hypertonicity uncovered. Continue by performing some deep gliding, followed by some friction

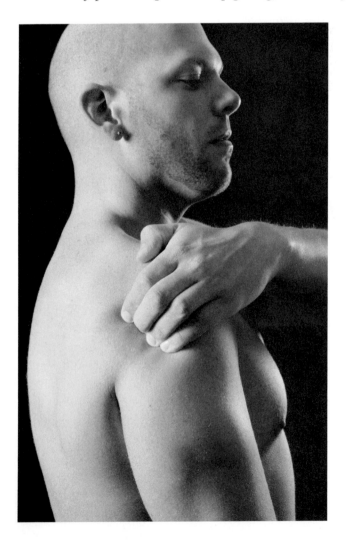

Figure 10.17

Friction to the posterior deltoid

to the anterior, middle, and posterior heads of the deltoids. Figure 10.17 demonstrates a technique to apply friction to the posterior deltoid.

After completing hand and arm work on both sides, briefly shake out the shoulders, arms, and hands, allowing them to feel long and loose, limp and relaxed. You can also interlace the hands, turn the thumbs down, extend both elbows, take a deep breath while raising both arms over the head, and then exhale while lowering the relaxed arms and shoulders.

Self-Massage to the Neck and Shoulders

The following techniques to the neck and shoulders can be performed supine or seated; try it both ways and determine which you prefer. Cut and file your fingernails before starting this procedure. Use a very small amount of lotion, balm, or warming oil when performing these techniques because overslippery fingers will reduce the ability to perform effective friction. Try working both sides simultaneously; however, if having both hands in the designated positions is uncomfortable, just do one side at a time. Start with some gentle effleurage to the muscles on the back of the neck, gliding with the fingertips placed just lateral to the spinous processes and working from the first thoracic vertebrae up along the spinous processes traveling past the base of the skull to the occipital ridge. Continue successive passes by moving laterally and gliding up and over the mastoid processes. Next glide from the spinous processes of the cervical vertebrae out laterally across the neck musculature to the anterior edge of the SCMs, working from C7 or T1 up to the base of the skull. While performing this lateral gliding activity be careful to avoid pressing firmly behind the angle of the jaw, just inferior to the ear lobe. After the area has been warmed up with effleurage, sink the fingertips firmly into the posterior neck paraspinal muscles right next to the spinous processes of C7 and flick the muscles laterally. Work your way up, flicking the paraspinals away from the spinous process from C7 to the base of the skull. Do another pass over the same muscles, except during the second pass apply small friction circles to the same area. Continue this pattern by performing one pass of flicking and one pass of friction circles by moving a half an inch laterally after each set of passes. Work the back and sides of the neck in this fashion, avoiding the area behind the angle of the jaw and below the ear lobe. Next move up to the mastoid processes and perform some friction circles around these bony prominences. Then, while tilting the chin up slightly, apply some friction circles to the base of the skull, working in from the mastoid processes toward the foramen magnum. Next place the knuckles or the tips of the fingers on each side of the foramen magnum and on the base of the skull. (This technique is easier to perform while lying supine.) Just tilt the chin up slightly and hang out there for a minute, letting the suboccipital muscles relax and unwind. Figure 10.18a and b demonstrate techniques for relaxing the suboccipital muscles.

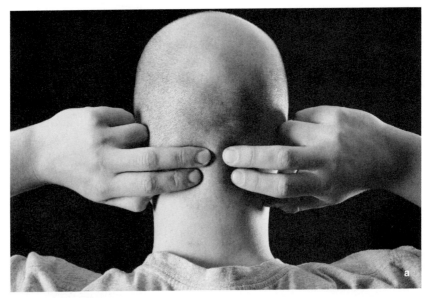

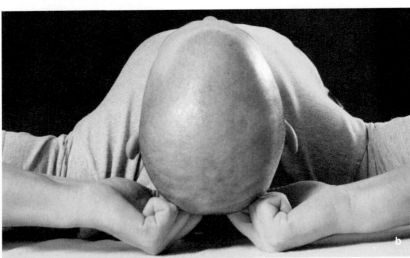

**Figure 10.18
a and b**

Relaxing the
suboccipital muscles

Next do a few soothing circular palm strokes to complete the work to the back and sides of the neck. To continue, perform some one-handed effleurage to the opposite side's upper trapezius, SCM, and scalene muscles. After warming up these muscles, follow up with some circular or cross-fiber friction. Apply friction down the upper trapezius all the way out to the acromion process, lingering for 10–30 seconds at each major point of hypertonicity discovered, trying to breathe and consciously relax these points of tension. Then follow the SCM down from the mastoid process, applying friction circles or working across the fibers to areas of pain and tension along the whole muscle. Continue the friction strokes down to and over the clavicular and sternal attachment of the SCM. For a really tight SCM you can also try combining a stripping stroke with active movement. If you have a tight left SCM, laterally flex and rotate the neck to the left. Then use firm reinforced thumb pressure to strip down the left SCM from the mastoid process to the clavicle or sternum while actively rotating the neck to the right. Perform four to six stripping strokes to the SCM, covering the whole muscle, while actively contracting it to rotate the neck to the opposite side. Figure 10.19a and b demonstrate this active stripping technique to the SCM. After working both sides of the neck, perform some cleansing effleurage and gently stretch the relaxed musculature into lateral flexion and then rotation to each side.

Self-Massage to the Face and Head

Because we will be working around the eyes, don't use any oil, balm, or lotion while performing this work. This work can be performed seated or lying supine. Start at the forehead and perform some gentle circles with the fingers, working from the center of the forehead laterally over the frontalis muscles out to the temples. Spend extra time at any area where pain, tension, or discomfort is felt. After the temples are relaxed continue the circles, moving up to the hairline and then back along the hairline to the top center of the forehead. From this point work down toward the nose, performing gentle circles to the area located midway between the center of the eyebrows. Project some warmth and relaxation to this point for 10–30 seconds, then continue by gently massaging over the eyebrows and then around the entire ridge of the eye sockets. If tenderness is present, spend extra time pressing on the indentation located on the inner ridge of the eye sockets by the medial edge of the eyebrows. Proceed by applying

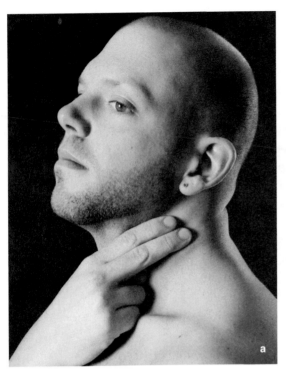
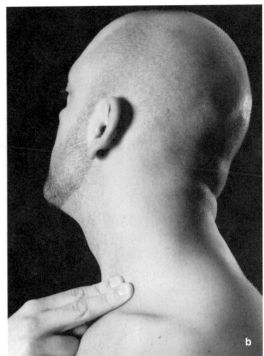

Figure 10.19 a and b

Active stripping to the sternocleidomastoid

small gentle circles from the bridge of the nose along the top of the zygomatic bone around the cheeks and then back over the bottom edge of the zygomatic bone to the nose. Press on the sides of the base of the nose, then move down to press on the center of the maxilla and work with small circles laterally along the maxilla and then up to the temporal mandibular joint (TMJ). If you desire, you can use a drop of warming oil to rub into the muscles around the TMJ. Spend some time rubbing all over and around the TMJ. Then slide the fingers down to the mandible. Glide along the mandible and then perform thumb or finger circles, working the muscles of mastication, and then continue toward the center of the jaw. Next move to the bottom edge of the mandible and glide over the musculature with the thumbs. Perform some friction to these muscles that attach to the underside of the jaw. If you find a really tender spot, you can press it while depressing the jaw or you can try actively moving the jaw to the side while applying pressure. Figure 10.20 demonstrates applying friction to the

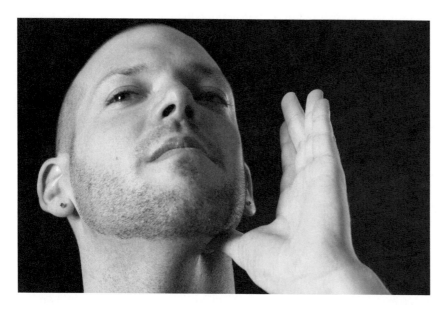

Figure 10.20

Friction to the muscles under the mandible

muscles under the mandible. Next continue by sliding the hands up the side of the face to the ears. If you are inclined you can massage all over and around the ears and even give them a little lateral pull and a waggle forward and back while pulling them gently. Next move the hands above the ears, and with the hands flat perform whole palm circles moving slowly up the side of the head. Work the palm circles all over and around the temporalis muscle. Figure 10.21 demonstrates the technique for performing palm circles to the temporalis muscles.

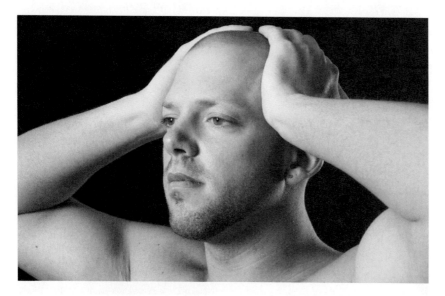

Figure 10.21

Palm circles to the temporalis muscle

You can also apply upward pressure to the temporalis with the fingers or palms while depressing the jaw. Hold this stretch for 10–20 seconds. Next perform a scalp massage with the fingertips. Move the scalp forward, back, and side to side and press along the entire top and center of the skull, trying to relax any tender areas. Finish with some gentle stroking of the hair or, if you prefer, a gentle hair pull.

Self-Massage to the Clavicles and Chest

It is best to perform the self-massage of the clavicles and chest lying supine. Apply some lotion, balm, or warming oil to the hands and begin by sliding the fingertips or thumbs along the inside top edge of the clavicle. Do not press down into the brachial plexus; just work along the entire inside edge of the bone. Take three or four gliding passes and then apply some cross-fiber friction to the tender spots uncovered. If this is too painful, try elevating the shoulder while applying pressure to these tender spots. Figure 10.22 demonstrates the elevated shoulder technique for working the inside edge of the clavicle.

After clearing out all the tender spots on the inside edge of the clavicle, we next move to the chest. Perform some effleurage to the chest musculature. Start at the sternal notch and glide under the clavicle to the shoulder. Overlap the first stroke with the next stroke, which should glide from the sternum to the serratus anterior or if

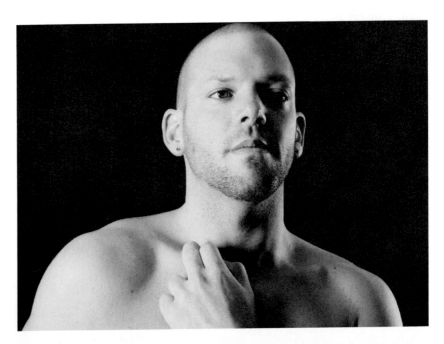

Figure 10.22

Elevated shoulder clavicular clearing technique

flexible enough the latissimus dorsi (move the nonmassaging arm out of the way to provide more access). The next stroke should start at the sternum and then sculpt the lower fibers of the pectoralis major and then run laterally over the rib cage. We continue by applying some more gliding strokes but reversing their direction. Start where you finished the last stroke but move from lateral to medial (from the side to the sternum). This time dig in more deeply, raking the muscles with the fingertips. Figure 10.23 demonstrates this raking stroke to the chest.

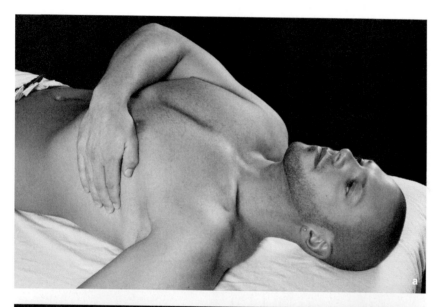

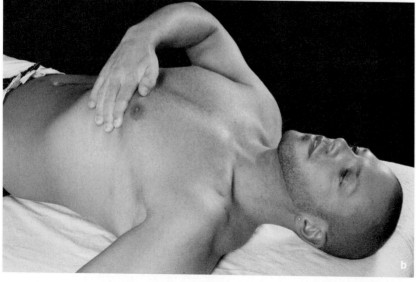

Figure 10.23 a and b

Raking the chest

Once again overlap each successive stroke as you progress from inferior to superior. Once this series of deeper gliding strokes is completed, we now perform some friction. Starting at the sternal notch apply some friction circles to this area and then move laterally to the underside of the clavicle. Continue with this circular friction for the entire underside of the clavicle. Make sure that you release around the coracoid process. Continue by coming back to the sternum but moving inferior to the space between the sternum and the next rib. Apply some friction to the space at the junction of the rib and the sternum and then follow the intercostal muscles laterally, applying friction as you progress. Apply friction to the spaces between the sternum and ribs 1–7 or the costal cartilage and rib 8–10 in this fashion. Figure 10.24 demonstrates how to apply friction to the intercostals.

If they are tender, spend some extra time releasing the fibers of the pectoralis minor, which runs from the coracoid process inferiorly and slightly medially to the third, fourth, and fifth ribs. Next move down to the tips of the ribs and apply some gentle friction to all of them. Finish with cleansing effleurages to the whole chest and rib cage, directing the force of these strokes to the axilla.

Now that we have completed our discussion of self-massage techniques, let's turn our attention to relieving a great source of pain for many clients—headaches.

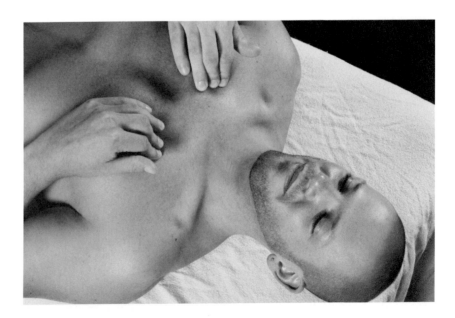

Figure 10.24

Friction to the intercostals

RELIEF FROM HEADACHES

Headaches are another source of pain that virtually everyone experiences at one time or another. Although many different types of headaches have been identified in the literature, only tension headaches and migraine headaches will be discussed here. The stress reduction principles discussed in this book including exercise, diet, and deep relaxation and some specific massage work can help individuals plagued by headaches. However, if any of your clients are suffering from very severe headaches, have them see their doctor before treating them to eliminate the possibility that they have a disease such as encephalitis or meningitis or even a brain tumor.

Tension headaches usually are caused by poor posture; a cervical vertebrae being out of alignment; or excessive muscle tension resulting in painful points in the muscles of the neck, shoulders, face, or scalp. The forehead, the temples, the jaw muscles around the TMJ, and the eye muscles can also contribute to tension headaches.

The following acupressure points for headache relief can be pressed by the therapist or can be taught to the client for self-treatment to provide relief from symptoms. If headaches persist, clients should consult their doctor. Figures 10.25 and 10.26 depict some commonly used headache relief points. Press these points for 10–30 seconds or until they relax. Try practicing focused breathing and relaxation while pressing them. Please note: If your client is pregnant never press LI4 because it may induce labor. Also, GB21 should be pressed only lightly on pregnant women (Gach, 1990).

Migraine headaches are a debilitating, referred pain type of headache that produces throbbing pain generally on one side of the head that may last for a few days. They are frequently felt in the face around the eye socket, in the sinus, or by the jaw or the neck area. The factors that may contribute to a migraine are diet, unchecked stress, nicotine use, exposure to bright lights and fluorescent lights, and missing a meal or a sleep cycle. The dietary factors that may trigger migraines include ingesting nuts, pickled foods, chocolate, cheese, excessive alcohol, monosodium glutamate (MSG), and caffeine, There appears to be a strong familial link for those who suffer from migraines. Many people who have migraine headaches experience an aura or warning sign that one is on the

GV16

GB20

B10

GB21

Back of the head
and shoulders

GV24.5

B2

S3

Front of the head

Ex2

SI19

Side of the head

Figure 10.25

Acupressure points for
headache relief

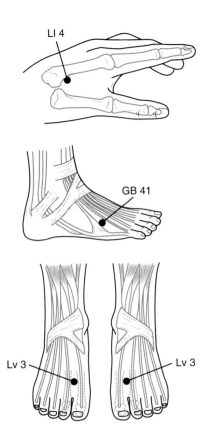

LI 4

GB 41

Lv 3

Lv 3

Figure 10.26

Acupressure points for
headache relief

way 20 minutes to 1 hour before an attack. Flashing lights, spots, wavy lines, and blind spots are some of the auras.

The pain from migraines is caused by swollen blood vessels of the brain. For this reason migraines also are referred to as vascular (blood-vessel) headaches. The excess blood causes pressure against the meninges (membranes that cover the brain), which produces migraine pain. Autogenic training, a relaxation technique that uses passive suggestions of warmth and heaviness to increase the blood flow to the distal extremities and the fingers and toes, has proved useful in combating migraines. When the client experiences an aura of a migraine he or she should use autogenic training before the headache becomes debilitating. Learning to bring more blood to the hands and feet may reduce the engorgement of the arteries in the brain and help the client to naturally eliminate headaches. If any of your clients do not receive any sign that a migraine is on the way, ask them to check the temperature of their hands and feet the next time they have one. If they are cold, tell them to try the following approach the next time they experience a migraine. They should sit or lie down in a quiet comfortable place; take some long, slow, deep breaths; relax; and use the autogenic suggestions to passively will their hands and feet to warm up.

A misaligned TMJ may also contribute to pain and headaches. To check the TMJ place the index fingertips in the notches right in front of the ear canals. Then have the client slowly open and close the jaw. If the client experiences pain or muscle spasms or perceives a clicking in the joint, it may be out of alignment and contributing to the headaches. Dentists specializing in TMJ problems can tell if the client needs a MORA (*m*andibular *o*rthopedic *r*epositioning *a*ppliance), which realigns the jaw, positioning it properly with the rest of the skull bones. The MORA is worn on the bottom teeth and does not interfere with eating or talking. Ice and massage to the surrounding musculature also can help relieve pain.

EXERCISES TO RELIEVE EYESTRAIN

Working long hours in front of a computer, watching lots of television, reading, and other close-up activities can lead to eyestrain and fatigue, which can contribute to headaches. The muscles responsible for eye movement are similar to other muscles in the body—they need exercise. The following set of eye exercises can provide the necessary movements to reduce eye-related stress and strain. While performing these exercises only move the eyes, not the head.

1. Look straight ahead and then roll just the eyes upward as far as they will go. Hold for 5 seconds and then roll the eyes downward toward the floor as far as they will go. Hold for 5 seconds.
2. Roll the eyes to the right and hold for 5 seconds. Then roll the eyes to the left for a 5 count.
3. Roll the eyes in the largest clockwise circles possible. Repeat three times. Next perform three circles in the counterclockwise direction.
4. Try the 20/20 rule. For every 20 minutes of close-up work, stand up and focus the eyes on an object as far away as you can for 20 seconds.
5. Close the eyes and gently massage the eyelids for a few seconds. If you wear contact lenses, please take them out before doing this activity. Also make sure that you don't have soap or any other irritant on the fingers before trying this technique.
6. Massage all around the outside edge of the eye sockets. Spend extra time on any painful points you find.

Try any of the natural pain-control strategies that have been outlined in this chapter deemed appropriate for your clients. Relieving their pain can add quality to their lives and help free them to concentrate on eliminating other factors in their lives that are contributing to their stress.

SUMMARY

Before we move forward to discuss dietary recommendations that reduce food-induced stress, some key pain-control concepts to review follow:

- Finding the cause of a painful condition and then trying to eliminate it at its source with safe, natural techniques is a wiser choice than taking drugs that merely mask the symptoms of the condition.
- Heat, ice, and massage can interrupt the pain-spasm-pain cycle.

- Modify activities of daily living and avoid hobbies that contribute to pain and discomfort.
- Postural awareness and realignment training can help reduce pain and muscle tension.
- Taking the mind off of pain by occupying it with other stimulation reduces the amount of pain perceived.
- Heat application increases circulation; reduces muscle spasm, pain, and stiffness; and produces an overall feeling of relaxation. Never apply heat to a fresh injury.
- Combining cold application with movement can relax tense musculature and help reduce restrictions in movement.
- Use the RICE principle for the first 48–72 hours after an injury.
- Direct approaches for relieving pain are those techniques that apply force to try to break down the barriers to normal movement. These include passive stretching, PNF, and gross and specific myofascial release.
- Indirect approaches for pain control such as positional release therapy place the body in a position of greatest ease until the tissues spontaneously unwind and release.
- An effective pain-control technique for stress reduction treatments combines light pressure to pain points combined with the client's conscious relaxation of those points.
- Teach clients self-massage techniques to practice as homework to help them relieve their pain and tension.

Diet and Stress

Dietary changes are the next component to consider adding to a client's personal stress reduction plan because unhealthy eating habits can greatly contribute to stress and pain. Although it is unethical for a massage therapist to give nutritional counseling unless he or she has been properly trained and certified, sharing common-sense dietary tips with clients to help reduce their stress is not. This chapter discusses suggestions to help your client reduce eating-related stress. A healthy eating plan, the dangers of fad diets, general tips for reducing food-induced stress, and information about eating disorders also are detailed.

Most people don't think twice about how diet affects their health. This is unfortunate because a poor diet can lead to obesity, cardiovascular disease, high blood pressure, diabetes, insomnia, cancer, allergies, muscle tension, osteoporosis, depression, a poor self-image, digestive and bowel problems, headaches, and stress. Nutritional inadequacies are also considered a crucial perpetuating factor for keeping trigger points activated (Travel, 1999:178). Although no single diet is adequate for everyone, following certain dietary principles will improve health, will eliminate some stress, and may improve the effectiveness of your massage treatments.

IDEAL BODY COMPOSITION

A good nutritional program is one that helps a person maintain or achieve ideal body composition while providing all of the nutrients essential for good health. **Ideal body composition** refers to more than just a good height-to-weight ratio; it also includes a person's percentage of body fat. The optimal percentage of body fat for men is 15–20 percent; for women it is 18–24 percent. The population average for American men is 25 percent fat and for women it is 28–30 percent fat. Finding out percentage of body fat can be calculated with skin-fold calipers, with electrical impedance machines, and by comparing a person's land weight with their underwater weight. **Body mass index (BMI)** is another common health measurement tool.

Body Mass Index

BMI is used to classify the health risks of having a body weight and waistline too great for one's height. BMI is calculated by multiplying the weight in pounds by 703 and then dividing the product by the height in inches squared

$$BMI = \frac{Weight\ (pounds) \times 703}{Height^2\ (inches)}$$

The metric formula is calculated by dividing the body weight in kilograms by the height in meters squared.

$$BMI = \frac{Weight\ (kg)}{Height^2\ (Meters)}$$

This BMI number and a person's waist size are then compared to a disease risk chart. Refer to Figure 11.1 to compare your client's results to the BMI disease risk chart. A BMI score over 25, combined

Figure 11.1

Classification of overweight and obesity by body mass index (BMI), waist circumference, and associated disease risk* (From National Heart, Lung, and Blood Institute. 1998. *Clinical Guidelines on the Identification, Evaluation, and Treatment of Overweight and Obesity in Adults: The Evidence Report.* Bethesda, MD: National Institutes of Health. http://www.nh1bi.nih .gov/guidelines/obesity/ e_txtbk/intro/12.htm retrieved 2/8/06)

Disease Risk* Relative to Normal Weight and Waist Circumference				
	BMI (kg/m^2)	Obesity Class	Men ≤102 cm (≤40 in.) Women ≤88 cm (≤35 in.)	Men >102 cm (>40 in.) Women >88 cm (>35 in.)
Underweight	18.5		-----	-----
Normal†	18.5–24.9		-----	-----
Overweight	25.0–29.9		Increased	High
Obesity	30.0–34.9	I	High	Very High
	35.0–39.9	II	Very High	Very High
Extreme Obesity	≥40	III	Extremely High	Extremely High

*Disease risk for type 2 diabetes, hypertension, and CVD.
†Increased waist circumference can also be a marker for increased risk even in persons of normal weight.

with a waist size of 40 inches or greater for a man and 35 inches or greater for a woman, may suggest a greater risk of diseases such as high blood pressure, heart attack, stroke, diabetes, gall bladder disease, liver disease, sleep apnea, irregular menstrual periods, and some types of cancer. Please note that the BMI does not always accurately predict when weight could lead to health problems, particularly in individuals with a great deal of muscle mass, African-Americans, Latinos, older people, and very short individuals.

BLOOD CHEMISTRY

A proper nutritional program will help a person maintain or achieve ideal blood chemistry. Of particular interest is **cholesterol,** a type of fat produced by the body and found in meat, dairy, fish, and poultry. Although a certain amount of cholesterol is needed for normal body functions, too much in the bloodstream can occlude the arteries and cause them to lose their flexibility and may increase a person's chance of experiencing a heart attack or stroke. It is recommended that a person maintain a cholesterol level of less than 200 mg/dL to reduce the risk of heart disease.

Cholesterol travels through the bloodstream attached to a protein molecule; the combination of these compounds is called a lipoprotein. There are two major categories of lipoproteins found in the body that are commonly measured in blood tests: **high density lipoproteins (HDLs)** and **low density lipoproteins (LDLs).** HDLs are referred to as "good cholesterol" because they capture and remove excess cholesterol from the blood and bring it back to the liver for elimination. Aerobic exercise can increase blood HDL levels, and a higher HDL level actually may decrease a person's risk of coronary artery disease, heart attack, and stroke. An HDL level higher than 60 is most desirable, as is a ratio of 4 or less when cholesterol is divided by HDL.

Ideal cholesterol and HDL ratio

$$4 \text{ or less} = \frac{\text{Cholesterol}}{\text{HDL}} = \frac{200}{60} = 3.3$$

LDLs are referred to as "bad cholesterol" because they carry cholesterol from the liver through the bloodstream and may adhere to the artery walls, making them sticky and more susceptible to the buildup of plaque. A high LDL level can increase the risk of heart disease and stroke. It is recommended that a person maintain an LDL level of less than 100 mg/dL. Triglycerides are another form of fat that is found in food and floating in the bloodstream that may also increase a person's risk of cardiovascular-related diseases. Triglycerides are the way that the body transports and stores fat. It is recommended that fasting triglyceride levels be maintained at less than 150 mg/dL.

Ideal Blood Chemistry Recommendations

Cholesterol level: < 200 mg/dL

HDL cholesterol level: 40–60 mg/dL (the higher the better)

LDL cholesterol: < 130 mg/dL (the lower the better)

Triglycerides: < 150 mg/dL (the lower the better)

CALORIC INTAKE

The big problem with the way most people eat is that they take in more calories than they burn and they select the wrong foods. If a person does not balance his or her caloric intake with his or her energy expenditure, the excess food ingested will be stored as fat and the person will put on weight. Beginning around age 25 years, the body needs less and less food—about 10,000 calories less per year, or about 25 less calories per day each year. Of course, a person may increase his or her activity level to burn more calories or try to develop more muscle mass by lifting weights. Muscle mass acts like a furnace—the more muscle mass a person has, the more calories he or she burns at rest. The body burns 25–50 kilocalories per day per pound of muscle. Therefore the first principle to abide by when changing one's eating habits to maintain weight is calories in = calories burned.

A healthy eating program is made up of 15 percent protein, 10 percent sugar, 30 percent fat, and 45 percent complex carbohydrates. In this country the average person eats more than enough protein and way too much simple sugar. In fact, in 1900 the average person ate 4 pounds of sugar a year, which is a paltry sum compared to the 120 pounds or more per year that the average person eats today. The average American of today has way too much fat in his or her diet. The area where our modern diet falls short is that most do not eat enough complex carbohydrates.

A HEALTHY WAY TO EAT

For optimal health a person should eat the rainbow diet, which essentially is eating foods representing all the different colors of the rainbow every day. Different-colored foods provide different nutrients, which includes vitamins, minerals, and antioxidants. If a person eats a little bit of each color and type of food every day, he or she will not overindulge in one of the food group areas, which decreases the possibility that he or she will develop a deficiency (or excess) of one nutrient. The six food groups areas are as follows: (1) breads, cereal, rice, and pasta; (2) vegetables; (3) fruit; (4) milk, yogurt, and cheese; (5) meat, poultry, fish, dry beans, eggs, and nuts; and (6) fats, oils, and sweets. The following guidelines, developed by the United States Department of Agriculture, designate the recommended daily serving for each of the major food groups.

Breads and Cereals

Eat 6–11 servings of the breads and cereals food group each day. Select breads, cereals, and pasta products made from whole grains. These and other complex carbohydrates, such as potatoes and brown rice, provide fiber, which helps prevent constipation and other more serious bowel disorders. Avoid white rice and white bread. A serving of bread is usually 1 slice, whereas a serving of cereal is 1 ounce (although the typical cereal bowl is 6 ounces).

Vegetables

Eat 3–5 servings of vegetables every day because they provide a person with fiber, vitamins, carbohydrates to burn, and other nutrients. Vary the colors and types and don't worry too much about the serving size unless there is butter, cream, or cheese sauce on it. Select fresh products whenever possible because canned products are full of salt and may contain fewer nutrients. Eat vegetables raw or steam them only briefly to keep them crisp (overcooking removes the nutrients). Also try to avoid frozen products that have sauces because those calories add up. Beans and tofu have been shifted to this category, although they are also good sources of protein and can be used as alternatives to meat.

Fruit

Consume 2–4 servings of fresh fruits each day, varying the types and colors. These provide a person with fiber and carbohydrates and are a rich source of vitamins. A serving is the size of an apple or a handful of grapes.

Dairy

Consume 2–3 servings of dairy products each day. Dairy is high in protein, carbohydrates, and calcium. Drinking nonfat milk or eating nonfat yogurt and low-fat cheese reduces the fat intake. The size of a serving is a cup of milk or yogurt and 1.5–2.0 ounces of cheese, depending on the type of cheese.

Meat, Poultry, Fish, Dry Beans, Eggs, and Nuts

Eat 2–3 servings of meat, poultry, fish, dry beans, eggs, and nuts each day. These foods provide a person with proteins, B vitamins, and iron. Increase consumption of white fish; skinned poultry; and vegetable sources of protein such as nuts, tofu, legumes, grains, and seeds. These less fatty sources of protein are healthier because they reduce the risk of getting heart disease. Reduce beef and pork consumption to two to three times a week. A serving is about the size of a deck of cards.

Fats, Oils, and Sweets

Sweets and products with fats and oils are high in calories and have little nutritional value so a person should limit their intake of them. Butter, margarine, oil, mayonnaise, sweets, and salad dressing should all be used in moderation.

GENERAL TIPS FOR REDUCING FOOD-INDUCED STRESS

Try the following suggestions to see if they help reduce your symptoms of stress.

Eliminate Caffeine

Typical caffeine-rich foods are coffee, tea, chocolate, and soda. If you are highly stressed, caffeine, very powerful in its own right, will arouse your already-overactive nervous system and, in essence, will compound your problems. Try drinking herbal teas or beverages that have no caffeine.

Eliminate or Drastically Cut Back on Sugar

Eating foods having a high percentage of sugar produces dramatic blood sugar–level fluctuations that may lead to between-meal hunger, sluggishness, and irritability. White and brown sugar, honey, syrups, candy bars, doughnuts, pastries, cookies, and ice cream all produce a sugar rush of energy that quickly brings you up, lasts for a brief time, and then drops you down in the dumps. When you come down off your "sugar high" there is also a greater tendency to snack on more sugary foods to quickly bring yourself back up once again. Think of it this way: one piece of chocolate is too many and a million aren't enough. Overconsumption of sugar products can also lead to tooth decay, increased body fat, and diabetes. Fruit is a much better way to take in sugar. Fruit gradually releases sugars into your system. Your increased energy level remains high longer, and then it gently dissipates without any withdrawal symptoms. Fruit also is a good source of fiber, vitamins, and other nutrients. To illustrate your daily intake of sugar, take 21 teaspoons of sugar out of your sugar jar and put them on a plate. If you eat the average American diet, that's how much sugar you eat each and every day! Now, think again about cutting down on sugar.

Reduce Consumption of Salt and Foods High in Salt

Too much salt (sodium, sodium nitrate, sodium benzoate, and monosodium glutamate [MSG]) in your diet, and hence too much sodium in your body, may lead to high blood pressure, which in turn increases the risk of stroke, heart attack, and kidney damage. Although many foods don't taste salty, they are. For example, seafood, dairy products (including cheese), canned vegetables and soup, baked goods, and cereals are all loaded with salt or salt additives. In fact, one fast food meal alone may account for more than half your daily salt needs. As an alternative to salt, experiment with lemon juice, lime juice, garlic, fresh ginger, dill, tarragon, and other spices to enhance the flavor of food without endangering your health.

Avoid Fatty and Greasy Foods

Fatty and greasy foods tremendously increase the risk of cardiovascular disease. No more than 30 percent of total calories should come from fat, and at least half of total fat intake should come from unsaturated fat sources such as corn, olive, sunflower, soybean, and canola oils. Unsaturated fats are generally liquid at room temperature, whereas saturated fats are generally solid at room temperature. Lowering your cholesterol level 10–15 percent by cutting down on fat and cholesterol can reduce your chance of having a fatal heart attack by 20–30 percent. A low-fat diet is even more important if you're under stress because blood cholesterol levels increase during peak periods of stress.

Cholesterol Adjustments

If you have a cholesterol level higher than 200 mg/dL on a blood test or are overweight, restructure your diet away from animal fats and the "invisible" fat found in products such as mayonnaise, snack crackers, butter, cheese, eggs, potato chips, olives, nuts, and chocolate. Avoid foods that contain hydrogenated oil and trans fats because they raise the LDL cholesterol level that can increase the risk of heart disease. (Food manufacturers use trans fats, which are made by adding hydrogen to healthy oil, to extend the shelf life of products.) When preparing your meals, broil or bake foods instead of frying them. Also, eat more high-fiber foods such as oats, dried beans and peas, and fruits. These foods can actually lower cholesterol levels by increasing the speed that food moves through the intestine. In addition to eating less fat, aerobic exercising increases your level of cleansing HDLs.

Reduce Alcohol Consumption

Alcoholic beverages are high in calories and low in nutrients. Excessive indulgence can alter the way your body absorbs and uses food; too much alcohol can also impair sleep quality and lead to serious health problems. Try plain or flavored mineral waters, spring water, iced green tea, or natural fruit juices as healthier alternatives.

Learn to Say No to Food When You Aren't Hungry

The next time you sneak to the refrigerator, ask yourself the following questions: "Am I really hungry?" "Do I need to eat?" "Is the food nutritious?" "How will I feel after I've eaten?"

Eat Foods That Make You Feel Good and Avoid Foods That Upset Your System

You may be allergic to some foods or cannot digest them properly. Avoid artificial ingredients such as food coloring, preservatives, and flavor enhancers; stick to the real thing. The next time you feel sick, think about what you ate recently.

Chew Your Food Well

Many people under heavy stress bolt their food down and do not take the time to chew it adequately. Savor each bite. This helps you stop rushing for a few moments, and it will make your digestive tract's job much easier.

Record Caloric Intake

If weight control is a problem, it is important to chart the number of calories eaten on a typical day and week to get a firm grip on where adjustments should be made. Reading food labels and controlling the size of the portions eaten are also important habits to acquire. The older and less active a person becomes, the less the person should eat.

Take Appropriate Vitamin Supplements

Do you need vitamin supplements? It depends. If you're healthy and you eat well, the answer is no. If you don't eat a balanced diet and are subject to a high degree of stress, absolutely yes. Vitamins help your body perform functions essential to health and life. Without them you can suffer all sorts of maladies ranging from scurvy (lack of vitamin C) to a general malaise and feeling of discomfort. Smoking, air pollution, drug and alcohol use, infections, and burns all increase the body's demand for vitamins. Treat vitamins as you would any other drug and do not exceed the recommended daily doses. The old philosophy that if some is good then more is better is not true for vitamins. Excessive vitamin intake can disrupt your metabolism, affect your hormone levels, cause sensory damage (blindness), and in some cases can even be fatal.

FAD DIETS ARE DANGEROUS

Be wary of fad diets because they do not work and they can leave a person in a weaker, fatter state than when he or she started because most quick weight loss comes from the loss of muscle and water, not fat. Avoid any diet plan that recommends that you cut out essential food groups. For instance, the popular Atkins diet vilifies carbohydrates and instructs abstinence from them. Carbohydrates supply the brain with glucose, and eliminating them from the diet leads to fatigue, irritability, and memory loss and will require the body to convert the protein from muscle tissue to glucose so that the brain isn't starved for energy. So after an initial loss of fat the weight loss achieved comes from the loss of water and muscle mass. The low-carbohydrate diet also puts the body in an unhealthy state called ketosis, which can result in kidney damage if the condition exists for a long period.

PERSONAL STRESS INVENTORY DIET RESULTS

Now let's refer back to your client's Personal Stress Inventory results regarding the question about diet. Which diet most closely resembled the client's diet?

> Diet A: A healthy, balanced diet that follows the guidelines outlined by the United States Department of Agriculture. If the client's BMI numbers and cholesterol numbers are in the healthy range, then the client should continue with this program.

> Diet B: The fast food/junk food diet. Clients in this category need to explore healthy modifications to their diet to help them reduce their stress. If they don't change their eating habits, they should keep their life insurance up to date.

That way their diet-induced abuse to their body will have some benefit to their next of kin. They should strive to eat a healthy diet at least 80 percent of the time and minimize their junk food to 20 percent.

Diet C: The meat and potatoes diet. If they don't change, these individuals should prepare themselves for a life of bowel problems, hardened arteries, and increased risk of heart attack. They need nutrition from all of the food groups and must adapt their diet to help reduce their food-related stress. Vegetables are not just for rabbits; humans need them too.

Diet D: Vegetarian. If any of your clients are vegetarian, they must learn to balance their meals to get the right combination of amino acids. For the body to obtain the right balance of protein from foods, we need to ingest all nine essential amino acids. However, three of the amino acids, known as limiting acids, are particularly important because without them the other six are useless, even if available in the right quantities. Very few vegetarian foods contain all nine of the amino acids; thus it's crucial to balance meals appropriately. Vitamin balance in a vegetarian diet is also important. Vitamin B_{12} deficiency is a common flaw in many vegetarian diets because it is found primarily in animal sources, although certain cereals are fortified with it. Overall, vegetarian diets can be healthy and life prolonging. They just take a little more planning than a burger and fries does.

EATING DISORDERS

Eating disorders are a serious worldwide problem affecting all segments of society, regardless of ethnicity, financial status, or age. Research reported by Anorexia Nervosa and Related Eating Disorders, Inc. has shown that in the United States roughly 1 percent of the population has **anorexia nervosa** and about 4 percent of the population of college-age women experience **bulimia nervosa.** Up to 4 percent of the adults in the United States experience binge-eating disorder. Anorexia nervosa and bulimia primarily center on women; only 10 percent of those suffering from the disorders are male. Both sexes, however, are well-represented with those prone to periods of uncontrollable bouts of eating. Many sources blame the media for the unrealistic ultra-thin look that is in style. Particularly affected are teenage girls, who are all too frequently dieting in an unrealistic attempt to look like cover girl models. They don't realize that cover girls are born with their physiques and the average person will never look like one, no matter how much dieting they do. It is unfortunate that many girls do not get adequate nutrition during the time when they need to store bone density for later years. It's tragic that sometimes this obsession with being thin takes innocent lives.

Anorexia nervosa is essentially self-starvation brought on by the obsession with not becoming fat. Because of a poor body image or the fear of being fat, sufferers limit their intake of adequate sustenance or seriously reduce the nourishing effects of what they do ingest by compulsively exercising; vomiting; or using laxatives, enemas, or diuretics. They become unhealthily thin. A BMI score of 17.5 and being < 85 percent of normal body weight are indicators used to distinguish cases of it. Anxiety, absence of normal menstrual periods, not eating in front of others, tooth damage, erosion of the esophagus, weak, brittle skin and nails, lowered pulse rate, and obsession about calorie intake are all signs and symptoms of this disorder. Anemia, osteoporosis, depression, and heart disorders are also associated conditions. One in 10 of those afflicted with anorexia dies. A relaxing massage may help this client feel better about his or her body. Avoid deep work in the later stages of this disorder.

Bulimia nervosa is a condition in which a person takes in the proper amount of food, or more than they need, but then vomits or purges from the system what they have ingested by using laxatives, enemas, or diuretics. Many are able to hide the disease for years, and many become reclusive so no one will find out their secret. The vomiting erodes the enamel of the teeth, damages salivary glands, and at times ulcerates the esophagus. Individuals with bulimia have a higher predisposition toward heart attacks. Many people with anorexia develop bulimia. As with anorexia, gentle massage techniques work best with clients with bulimia.

Binge eating or compulsive overeating occurs when a person has repeated episodes of eating constantly, unable to stop although they are full. It is estimated that this disorder affects up to 12 million people in the United States. Many have a long history of diet failure and are subjected to feelings of helplessness and guilt. Depression and obesity are frequent companions with this disorder. Massage can help relax them and help them get more in tune with their bodies.

RISK FACTORS APPRAISAL TEST

Factors in diet, lifestyle, and heredity may contribute to the risk of having a heart attack or stroke. Here is a quick test that can be shared with clients to assess their risk and help them realize that they need to modify their eating habits and lifestyle. Appendix 10 is a clean copy of this test that you can reproduce and share with your client.

Heart Attack and Stroke Risk Self-Appraisal

1. Male   Female
2. Age
3. If you are overweight, estimate how many pounds over your ideal weight you are at this moment.
   0–5 pounds   5–10 pounds   10–20 pounds
   20–30 pounds   More than 30 pounds.
4. Do you smoke? Yes   No
   If yes, estimate how many cigarettes do you smoke each day: _____.
5. Has any member of your immediate family died of a heart attack or stroke?
   Before the age of 65? Yes   No
6. Do you eat red meat 3 or more times a week? Yes   No
7. Do you eat organ meats (liver, kidneys, etc.) more than once a month? Yes   No
8. Do you eat 5 or more eggs a week? Yes   No
9. Do you eat hot dogs, cold cuts, or luncheon meats 3 to 5 times a week? Yes   No
10. Do you consume whole milk, cheese, or ice cream 3 to 5 times a week? Yes   No
11. Do you eat deep-fried foods about 3 to 5 times a week?
    Yes   No
12. Do you use mayonnaise and butter 3 to 5 times a week?
    Yes   No
13. Do you frequently enjoy sweets every day (sugar or honey in your hot drinks, soda, candy, jelly, cake, cookies, etc.)?
    Yes   No

14. How often do you perform aerobic exercise in your target range each week?
    A. 20 nonstop minutes 3 times a week   B. Sometimes
    C. Never
15. Do you always add salt to your food? Yes   No
16. Do you practice some form of deep relaxation at least 3 times a week? Yes   No
17. Is your life full of deadline and time pressures? Yes   No
18. Select the category that your most recent blood pressure measurement falls into:
    A. 119/79 or less   B. Between 120/80 and 139/89
    C. Between 140 and 159/99   D. 160/100 or higher
19. Men, is your waist circumference 40 inches or larger?
    Yes   No

    Women, is your waist size 35 inches or larger? Yes   No

What to do with the results?

1. Score 1 point if you are a man; 0 points if you are a woman.
2. Add 1 point if you are older than age 35.
3. Add 1 point for every 10 pounds that you are overweight.
   10 pounds = 1 point; 10–20 pounds = 2 points; 20–30 pounds = 3 points; More than 30 pounds = 4 points (Even someone 50 pounds overweight will just get 4 points.)
4. Add 0 points if you don't smoke; add 1 point for each half pack you smoke each day.
5. Add 1 point for each member of your immediate family who died of a heart attack or stroke before the age of 65 years.
6. Add 1 point if you eat red meat 3 or more times a week.
7. Add 1 point if you eat organ meats once a month.
8. Add 1 point if you eat 5 or more eggs a week.
9–13. For these questions, add 1 point for up to 2 yes answers and 2 points for 3 or more yes responses.
14. Subtract 1 point if you exercise 20 minutes 3 times a week; add 1 point if you get some exercise; add 2 points if you do not exercise.
15. Add 1 point if you always add salt to your food.
16. Subtract 1 point if you practice deep relaxation 3 times a week. Add 0 points if you don't.

17. Add 1 point if your life is full of deadline and time pressures.

18. Subtract 1 point for 119 or less; add 0 points for between 120 and 139; add 1 point for between 140 and 159; and add 2 points for 160 or higher.

19. Men, add 1 point if your waist size is 40 inches or larger; women add 1 point if your waist size is 35 inches or larger.

Total

Now, total the points up and compare your results to the corresponding statement that follows.

0–4: Congratulations! A score of 4 or less indicates that for your age and sex you have a very low risk of experiencing a heart attack or stroke.

5–7: Your score in this range indicates that you demonstrate a below-average risk of having a heart attack or stroke. However, you may want to modify certain aspects of your life to either decrease or maintain your risk at this level.

8–10: Your score in this range indicates that you have an average risk of experiencing a heart attack or stroke. Have your physician give you a stress test. Ask about changes in diet, exercise, and lifestyle that can reduce the risk. Become serious about sticking to your personal stress reduction plan so you don't slip into the high-risk category.

11–13: You have a high risk of experiencing a heart attack or stroke. Have a complete medical checkup including a stress test; a percent of body fat test; and blood analysis to assess cholesterol, triglyceride, and lipoprotein levels. Adhere to your physician's recommendations and stick with your personal stress reduction program.

Higher than 14: Danger! You have an extremely high risk of having a heart attack or stroke. Have a complete medical checkup immediately! Make sure the checkup includes a stress test; a percent of body fat test; and blood analysis to assess your cholesterol, triglyceride, and lipoprotein levels. Your doctor will advise you of essential changes to your diet, exercise, and lifestyle that you must make. Your personal stress reduction program is more important than ever.

SUMMARY

People experiencing stress-related physical and psychosocial problems should consider modifying their diet to reduce the impact that the quantity and quality of foods and beverages that they ingest has on their lives. Before we proceed to the next chapter to discuss relieving psychosocial stress, let's review some key concepts a person should adhere to so as to reduce the negative effects that their diet has on their stress level.

- A good nutritional program helps a person maintain or achieve an ideal body composition while providing all the nutrients essential for good health.

- BMI is used to classify the health risks of having a body weight and waistline too great for one's height. Try to keep the BMI less than 25.

- A person should strive to achieve an ideal blood chemistry, which includes cholesterol at < 200 mg/dL, HDL cholesterol at 40–60 (the higher the better), LDL cholesterol at < 130mg/dL (the lower the better), and triglycerides at 150 mg/dL (the lower the better).

- To maintain weight, ensure calories in = calories burned.

- For optimal health eat the rainbow diet—eat foods representing all the different colors of the rainbow every day.

- Eat whole grains and avoid processed foods.

- Cut down on caffeine, sugar, salt, saturated fat, fried foods, lunch meats, mayonnaise, artificial flavors and colors, and fast food.

- Reduce alcohol consumption.

- Avoid fad diets.

- Eating disorders such as anorexia nervosa, bulimia, and compulsive overeating are a worldwide problem. Individuals with these problems should seek help from professional counseling services and support groups.

More Tips for Managing Stress

In the preceding chapters we have reviewed many strategies for relieving the physical manifestations of stress. However, a comprehensive stress reduction program is not complete if it doesn't help a person develop strategies to successfully cope with the psychosocial aspects of his or her stress. The problem is that most massage therapists are not professional psychologists and therefore are not trained to help clients eradicate or at least reduce the intensity of their fear, anxiety, panic attacks, anger, hostility, depression, and phobias. Psychological counseling is not within the scope of practice of massage therapy. However, massage therapists should have a basic understanding of these conditions so they can be sensitive to the needs of these clients while treating them and should know when to refer them out for professional help. Massage therapists should also understand techniques for improving organizational and time-management skills so that they can share these with their clients. This chapter discusses common psychosocial manifestations of stress and their implications for massage. The chapter also offers suggestions on developing and maintaining ethical relationships with clients suffering from stress, using a balance sheet to make major decisions, improving organizational skills, dealing with timelessness, setting goals, and modifying behavior. A summary of stress reduction tips that can be shared with clients also is discussed.

The mind and the body are inseparable. Our thoughts, feelings, and emotional responses to stressful situations and events can have a tremendous impact on our physical health. Conversely, physical problems and pain associated with stress and trauma affect how we think, feel, and react to different stressors. It is important that the massage therapist have a basic understanding about emotions, anxiety, depression, and panic disorders and the potential effects that they may have on the psyche of clients. The therapist must be prepared to handle different situations as they arise during the course of treatments. For example, how would you react when a client has a panic attack on your table? Or what would you say to a client who experiences an emotional release and starts crying uncontrollably during a treatment? The massage therapist should understand some basic self-help strategies for coping with emotional and psychological stress. If appropriate, these strategies can be shared with clients to try to help them cope with these forces so they don't reverse the positive gains that have been achieved in the course of a treatment program.

COPING WITH PSYCHOLOGICAL AND SOCIAL STRESS

The psychological, emotional, and social manifestations of stress are often the most debilitating. Inability to cope with this aspect of stress may interfere with mental health and happiness, impair the ability to raise a family and to work, erode social relationships, reduce job performance, and damage physical health. If clients respond on their Personal Stress Inventory (PSI) that they often or always experience anxiety because of reasons that they could not pinpoint, irritability, strained relationships, easily aroused hostility, anger, depression, procrastination, panic attacks, trouble turning off the mind at night, stressful dreams, low motivation, pessimism, worrying, lack of control over their life, a short-fused temper, or drug and alcohol abuse, it is absolutely essential that they try to unearth the factors contributing to these problems and then take action to try to eliminate them.

Pinpointing the causes of chronic psychosocial stress symptoms is the first step toward relieving them. This, however, is much easier said than done. Uncovering this information demands that clients thoroughly analyze their behavior and life with an open mind. They must take an in-depth look at each of their problems and try to figure out why they're reacting to their stressors the way they are. There's no magical way to do this. A person must simply sit quietly and think about his or her problems and their causes. They must be honest, thorough, and above all patient with themselves. This self-appraisal should first look at emotions.

Emotions are a combination of our thoughts, feelings, perceptions, and the physical responses and actions that they produce. Anger, fear, rage, guilt, sadness, love, and hate all produce physical responses in the body. Emotions excite us and can lead us to take action. Our morals, values, and belief systems and the way we interpret events can influence our emotions and the intensity of those emotions. Unfortunately, if we allow our emotions to rule our lives we may end up doing and saying things that we may later regret. Here is an example. Joe was on the highway driving home after a stress-filled day at work. A driver talking on a cell phone and not paying attention to the driving conditions cuts in front of Joe and slams on the brakes to avoid the traffic stopped up ahead. Joe in turn has to slam on his brakes to avoid hitting him. Joe immediately experienced fear and anxiety because his life was in danger. Then Joe started thinking that the no-good, idiot, reckless driver is going to kill someone someday. The driver needs to be set straight about driving. The fear and anxiety Joe initially experienced quickly gave way to anger, rage, and aggression. So Joe honked his horn, held up the finger of scorn, and offered a few choice words that aren't generally part of his vocabulary. The driver in front saluted Joe back and this further enraged him. Joe became so angry he followed the car, honking his horn until the driver pulled off the road at a rest area. At the rest stop the two started fighting until the police came by and arrested them for road rage.

We can't afford to be like Joe and allow our emotions to dictate our behavior. We must learn that different emotions bring about different intensities of reactions and these reactions do not last forever—they come and go like the ocean's tides. If we learn to count to 10 or even 20 before reacting to our emotions, we may be able to avoid saying or doing something that we will regret. In the heat of the moment, instead of acting impulsively, say to yourself "This emotion will soon pass." Stay strong and resist the temptation to quickly fly off the handle. Take some long, slow, deep breaths to help you calm down, and bite your tongue if you have to. Try to become more aware of your emotional outbursts and overreactions. Ask yourself the question, "Why do I behave and react emotionally to situations the way I do?" An increased awareness of one's emotions is the first step toward controlling them.

People who are quick to anger and frequently experience hostility and strained relationships must learn to pick their battles. Not every disagreement in life should result in a major confrontation that produces ill will and negativity. We must recognize that at times many of us blow minor incidents way out of proportion. When we look at the whole scheme of things the cause of many disagreements is really not that important. Before you overreact to a situation and a major confrontation erupts, it is a good idea to try to change your perspective and look through the eyes of the other person for a moment. Try to understand their point of view. It is important to learn not to be so headstrong and to cooperate with others. Try to be flexible without losing your integrity, of course. Ultimately, don't sweat the small stuff; worry about major problems.

A massage treatment combined with moist heat, diaphragmatic breathing, and relaxation can offer clients a positive experience that can help calm them, break their stress response, and release pent-up emotional distress. Many individuals internalize their stress and never adequately release it. In their soft tissues they store traumatic events, suppressed feelings and memories, and unreleased emotional reactions to situations that have occurred in their past. If the client feels safe and secure with you and in your environment, he or she may experience an emotional release on your table. When you release an area of built-up muscle tension that a client has been carrying for years, the client may start sobbing uncontrollably and may not even understand or realize why he or she is crying. The client may become embarrassed and upset and feel as if he or she has lost control. If this happens on your table, tell the client that releasing this tension is natural and a normal part of the healing process. Let the client know that it's healthy and good to let go and release these suppressed feelings. Not releasing these armored points of tension may contribute to depression, anxiety, and panic attacks.

Depression is a temporary or sometimes chronic mental state that is characterized by low energy and lack of initiative and feelings of sadness, isolation, despair, guilt, dread, loneliness, and low self-esteem. Individuals with depression frequently have low motivation, lack self-confidence, and have a negative outlook on life. Changes in sleep cycles and eating habits frequently coincide with depression. We have all felt the blues at times, but individuals suffering from depression seem to be stuck in a rut and they always dwell on the negative. Many stop caring about their physical appearance and lose interest in sex and healthy pursuits, whereas some stop bathing and suspend personal hygiene. They frequently have aches and pains, and some entertain thoughts of suicide. Massage therapy can help an individual who is depressed to get moving once again. A nurturing touch by a caring individual who is concerned with the individual's health and well-being can help relieve aches and pains and add to feelings of self-worth. Massage treatments will help them break out of their isolation and help them take a more positive view of themselves and their life. They must be reassured that they are important, they are unique, and they deserve good times and happiness in their lives. Anxiety and panic disorders are frequently interrelated with depression.

An **anxiety disorder** refers to the chronic psychological state that occurs when a person excessively worries and irrationally anticipates that events will lead to doom and calamity. Even innocuous situations may be interpreted as dangerous and a threat to their safety. Muscle aches and pains, fear, irritability, reduced decision-making skill, memory, and concentration are frequent symptoms of anxiety. A panic attack is the manifestation of this response, in which a person feels terror from an event or fear of something, which results in a state of sympathetic nervous system arousal in the body (i.e., a racing heart, labored breathing, gastrointestinal disturbances, sweaty palms, dry mouth, and excess muscle tension). Even the apprehension of experiencing another episode of what a person fears can set a person off into an attack of anxiety or panic. For example, if a person with insomnia dwells on the fear that they won't be able to sleep that night, he or she will have an anxiety attack, which arouses the sympathetic nervous system, which will interfere with sleeping. Panic attacks don't occur frequently during massage sessions; in fact, the author has only seen one during his many years in the profession. Here is a description of that one instance. Fifteen minutes into some prone bodywork the client reared up out of the face cradle gasping for air through his mouth; his heart was pounding, and his stress response was fully activated. Because of the danger of hyperventilating, he was instructed to try to exhale, to relax his shoulders, and to try to calm his mind and relax. Hands were placed on the client's shoulders to try to get him to relax and to breath more diaphragmatically. He started to relax in a few moments, and when his breathing returned to normal he was offered a glass of water, which he gratefully accepted. He was questioned as to what happened. He said that with his face in the face cradle his nose got all plugged up and he couldn't breathe through his nose. So he was breathing through his mouth and his mouth and throat got dry; after a while he said he just panicked. He said that his heart started racing and he had to move because he feared that he would suffocate. When the client rose up he was truly terrified, as if a lion were chasing him. If a client has a panic attack on your table, get him or her in a comfortable position. Try to get his or her mind off the pattern of thought that set him or her off. Use a calming voice and instruct the client to breathe and relax; try to help them get to a better place mentally. Also, if the client gets claustrophobic when putting his or her face in the face cradle, avoid prone position work. To help the client relax more, use the sidelying, supine, and seated positions instead.

REFERRING A CLIENT FOR COUNSELING OR PSYCHIATRIC SERVICES

Referring a client for professional counseling or psychiatric services is a delicate matter that should be handled carefully because many people have the misconception that they'll be labeled as "crazy" if they seek help for an emotional or psychological problem. Let the client know that the reverse is true because it takes a more "together" person to realize that he or she needs professional help and then seek it out. Some people are just not able to ameliorate their problems by making behavioral changes; instead they need medication, professional guidance, or both to help control their emotions and suppress their fear, nightmares, anxiety, depression, and phobias. A client should be referred to counseling if they have recurring nightmares; show signs of severe depression such as no energy, lack of motivation, procrastination, deteriorating hygiene, self-depreciation, constant negativity, and weight fluctuations; or mention suicide. Take a client seriously if they make a comment such as "Things would be easier if I were dead." This could be the client crying out for help, so confront him or her about this sort of statement and follow up. The therapist should also consider referring the client to professional help if they demonstrate dramatic mood swings, if they are a threat to themselves or another person, and if their anxiety appears to be growing so bad that it is interfering with their ability to function normally in their daily lives. The massage therapist should try to develop professional relationships with psychologists and, if possible, psychiatrists in their community to ask questions when the need arises and to have names and phone numbers available for clients who are interested in pursuing help. These professionals may also become great sources of referral because research has shown that many individuals with psychological and emotional problems benefit greatly from massage therapy.

DEVELOPING AND MAINTAINING ETHICAL RELATIONSHIPS WITH HIGHLY STRESSED CLIENTS

The following recommendations will help you establish the proper framework for treating highly stressed clients in your practice. You have the opportunity to add quality to their lives, so make the most of your time spent with them. Creating the proper environment for your treatments will help you positively influence the clients' spirits as you calm their minds and bodies.

- Be punctual and prepared for these treatments. Don't add to your client's stress by wasting his or her valuable time. Sloppy business practices will cost you clients.
- Try to create a safe, nonthreatening atmosphere in your treatment room and during your treatments. This is particularly important for those who have suffered from abuse and trauma.
- Be a good listener, but don't bring your life into the conversation. Try to let the client rest and relax during stress reduction treatments. If the client wants to vent, let him or her but don't get involved in barbershop conversation. If the client tries to keep involving you in a conversation, instruct him or her to take some deep breaths and to relax the mind and body. Encourage the client to let go and unwind.
- Don't be judgmental.
- Always keep within the legal scope of practice for massage therapy in your community. Remember that unless you have the degree and training, you are not a psychological counselor, nutritionist, or personal trainer, so refrain from stepping beyond the limitations of your credentials.
- Know when to refer a client. If a client's pain is exacerbating, if he or she is extremely depressed or suicidal, or if the challenges presented are beyond your experience and expertise, refer the client to the appropriate professionals.

- Try to nurture and boost the spirits and self-image of highly stressed clients. Positively reinforce their behavioral changes and the progress they have made on achieving their goals.
- If any of your clients experience an emotional release on your table, reassure them that it is normal and natural and part of the healing process. Inform them that it is healthy for them to release this repressed stress from their minds and their tissues.

SLOW DOWN OR SPEED UP

It is important to find the proper balance of work and play in our lives. Different people are on different ends of the pendulum of stress. Some need to pick up the pace and achieve more because they are suffering from the effects of too little stress and too few challenges. Most people fall into the other category. They are over-loaded and need to slow their lives down because they don't have enough time in the day to do everything they want and need to do.

NOT ENOUGH TIME IN THE DAY

Timelessness is not having enough time in the day to do everything you need to do or want to accomplish. Timelessness is a major cause of stress in our frantic world. People constantly run from one project to the next without ever taking time to rest, to think their own thoughts, enjoy the beauty of a sunset, marvel at a flower, or spend time with family and loved ones. Unlike a simple hamster that jumps off its treadwheel when it's tired, many human beings obsessed with work, money, fame, prestige, and power cast aside logic and reason and literally work themselves to death. People can avoid this "hurry sickness syndrome," reduce stress, and add qual-ity to their life by learning how to get the most out of their time.

USING TIME MORE EFFECTIVELY

Get organized. Use a weekly calendar schedule organizer or an elec-tronic organizing device such as a personal digital assistant (PDA). Set up a weekly schedule that allows time for work, aerobic exercise and muscle toning, deep relaxation, breathing and postural realign-ment training, massage treatments, preparing and eating healthy meals, social events, and community responsibilities. If at all possible don't neglect your health and family for work. If the schedule is too hectic, then readjust it so that it is more realistic. To reduce stress it is important to have a plan, and organizing how you use your time is an important part of that plan.

Every day record a list of what you want and need to accomplish. When you complete a job on the list, give yourself a pat on the back and take a few moments for yourself. Tasks impossible to finish should be carried over to the next day's list. Don't put matters off too long because unfinished business can be stressful and take its toll on your mind and body. Even if the list seems overwhelming, chip away at it and you will eventually get through it. Procrastination causes more stress, whereas closure reduces it.

Handle each piece of paper as little as possible. When you receive a piece of paper with information about an appointment, a meeting, or an event that you plan on attending, enter the information immediately into your schedule book or PDA and then file any maps and directions included into a future-events folder or recycle the paper. You will save time because you will not have to shuffle the paper again. This also will reduce clutter and anxiety about forgetting about something you wanted or needed to do. I can't think of anyone who has never said, "There is something that I wanted to do today but I just can't remember what it was." Separate your paperwork into three groups: (1) urgent and top priority; (2) tasks that need to be done soon; and (3) trivial pursuits (for when you have nothing else to do). Don't procrastinate with your paperwork—get it done and get it off your mind—and then proceed to your next task.

Use your time wisely. Study your behavior to determine the time of day that you work most effectively. For instance, if you write your best in the morning, schedule your writing then and leave the rest of the day for other jobs. Schedule your time according to your personality.

Learn to say "no." Some people accept too much responsibility. Learn your limitations and capabilities. If you spread yourself too thin, your work performance and health will suffer. Assert yourself; take care of yourself, and if you really don't want to do something or don't have the time to do it, don't do it—and don't feel guilty about your decision.

Take time out. When you feel your stress level getting out of control, call a time out. Rearrange your schedule to take time for relaxing and recharging your energy. If you can't spare the time to have some fun and relax, deep relaxation is your only healthy alternative. Wake up a few minutes early and do some deep relaxation first thing in the morning, or listen to a relaxation recording during your coffee break or at lunch. Regardless of when you practice deep relaxation, it will help break the stresses of constantly rushing through life. Believe it or not, taking time for yourself improves your productivity and reduces the amount of time it takes you to get a job done.

Uncloud your thoughts. If you are having difficulty thinking clearly, step back from your daily routine, look at your life, and objectively (and honestly) determine the cause of your fuzzy thoughts. Is it a work overload, the medication you're taking to reduce your blood pressure or muscle tension, lack of sleep, drug or alcohol abuse, or the inability to cope with your stress? Once you isolate the cause of your problem, you can eliminate it. Then, with clear eyes and sharp thoughts you can get your jobs done in a fraction of the time it might have taken you. Generally, you should avoid caffeine and if possible daily dependence on sleeping pills and muscle relaxants. Follow the suggestions in Chapter 9 for improving your sleep, practice focused breathing and deep relaxation, exercise more, seek professional help for a drug or alcohol problem, consider changing jobs if necessary, and follow your personal stress reduction plan.

JOB, LIFESTYLE, AND BEHAVIORAL CHANGES

For many people, reducing stress may require a change of jobs, lifestyle, relationships, habits, or behaviors. Before change is attempted a person must first determine what changes he or she needs to make to reduce stress. Sometimes taking a long, hard look at one's life is the best way to determine the most beneficial course of action. Clients must ask themselves the following questions: "What do I want to do with my life, and how am I going to get there?" Frequently, an honest answer requires job, lifestyle, and behavioral changes. For instance, if a client is a workaholic (and can't stop working or thinking about work), although the hard work pays the bills, is it worth jeopardizing his or her health and relationship with the family? Sometimes people set their goals unrealistically high and put too much pressure on themselves, whereas others experience stress as a result of the guilt caused by having too much fun and not working hard enough to realize their full potential. Sometimes stress is caused by parents forcing their expectations for life on their children—for example, forcing a career path on their child instead of allowing him or her to seek his or her own. Our habits and behaviors can also become major contributors to our stress.

We all have our own unique eccentricities, fears, quirks, habits, behaviors, and rituals that are part of our lives. Some we have learned, and others we have developed on our own. The human mind is an amazing computer that records an incredible amount of diverse data over the course of our lives. Our parents, close relatives, and environment are major influences in the development of our interpersonal skills and behaviors. Without realizing it we learn from and subconsciously assimilate many of our behavioral responses to different situations from them—some of them good and some not so good. We learn eating habits, emotional reactions, how to love and nurture, or how to lash out physically or verbally in anger or to withdraw and isolate ourselves when upset. Few people can honestly say that they have never thought to themselves after chastising a child, "Oh no, I sound just like my parents." The first step to changing learned behavioral responses requires taking a close look at our reactions to different situations and asking ourselves, "Is this how I want to act in these situations?" When the behavioral areas you want to change are uncovered, you then must ask, "How can I change my behavior to become the person I want to become?"

The survey presented in Appendix 11 will help your clients think about their job, lifestyle, and behavior to help them determine if changes are needed in these areas to reduce their stress. This survey will also have clients think about their long-term lifelong goals and short-term goals. The job lifestyle survey will also help clients formulate some ideas on how to institute the changes they want to make in their lives. Appendix 11 is a clean copy of this survey that you can reproduce and share with your clients.

Have your clients complete this survey as homework, and when they return it to you go over their responses with them. Explain to the client that the purpose of this assignment was to evaluate their current state of happiness with their job and lifestyle and to think about their goals for the future. To reduce stress clients must first do a good job setting lifelong goals and then develop some short-term goals to help achieve their long-range plans.

Goal Setting

In the job lifestyle survey (Appendix 11) the client was asked to record lifelong goals and some short-term goals. The client must think about where he or she wants to be in 20–30 years. The client also may want to think about where he or she wants to be in 5 years, in 1 year, in 6 months, and even in 1 month. It greatly reduces a person's stress to have a plan or a direction in place, instead of just wandering through life without a vision. After the long-term goals have been set it is essential that the client set sharp, clearly defined, short-term goals that can be measured and that he or she can take pride in achieving. Short-term goals must be small, realistic, attainable steps that help the client on the path to achieving a long-range plan. If goals are set properly, the client can see forward progress, which will boost self-confidence and chances for success, whereas short-term goals that are too ambitious can lead to frustration and failure.

After the goals have been set, review the other questions in the job lifestyle survey with the client. If the survey indicated that changes in job, lifestyle, or behavior are in order, it is important that the client thinks about how these changes will affect his or her quality of life. It's up to the client to decide if action is the answer. Ask the client, "Do you think some changes are needed in your life or are you willing to continue with your current situation?" The next section on effective decision-making will help the client reduce stress while making major decisions.

EFFECTIVE DECISION-MAKING

When making critical decisions about one's lifestyle, job, or future (e.g., managing money, changing jobs, getting married, buying a home, making investments, moving, going back to school) a decision balance sheet can help clearly indicate the optimal choice. Using the balance sheet method, one can make a side-by-side comparison of the positive and negative aspects of each alternative choice of action. This way major decisions are not based on gut feelings alone because many other factors are weighed into the equation. Figure 12.1 provides an example of how to complete a balance sheet. Appendix 12 provides a blank balance sheet that you can reproduce and share with your clients.

Lifestyle Items	Choice I Stay the same	Choice II Move	Choice III School/retraining
I. Family and Significant Others			
a. Spouse or lover	−2	−2	2
b. Parents	0	−2	0
c. Children	−2	−2	2
d. Friends	−2	−2	2
e. Colleagues	2	−2	−2
f. The community	0	0	2
g. Other (Volunteer work)	2	−2	2
II. Career			
a. Financial situation	2	−2	−2
b. Your interest in the work	−2	0	2
c. Chances for promotion	0	0	2
d. Creative challenge	−2	0	2
e. Security	2	−2	−2
f. Free time	−2	2	−2
g. Status	−2	0	2
h. Other (list them)	0	0	0
III. Self Considerations			
a. Your personal values	0	2	2
b. Your moral standards	0	2	2
c. Contribution to community or society	−2	1	2
d. Control over your life	−2	2	2
e. Self-image	−2	2	2
f. Prestige	0	0	1
g. Gut feelings	−2	1	2
h. Environment	0	2	0
i. Stress level	−2	1	1
j. Health	−2	1	2
k. Other (knowledge)	0	0	2
IV. Life Goals			
a. Achievement of long-range objectives	2	1	2
b. Pursuit of happiness	−2	1	2
c. Retirement	2	0	2
d. Other			
Total	**−16**	**2**	**34**

Figure 12.1

Sample decision
balance sheet

Balance Sheet Directions

Clients first must select the three possible courses of action or direction for their life. They can use the ideas that they mentioned in their PSI or those they generated in their job lifestyle survey. They may have more than three choices, but let's start with three to demonstrate how to use the balance sheet.

For example, the client's three choices are the following:

Choice 1 = Stay the same.

Choice 2 = Move to the country.

Choice 3 = Go back to school to retrain for a new career.

The next step is for the client to rate these potential alternative pathways for his or her life on the balance sheet using the following evaluation scale:

Very Negative	Negative	Neutral (NA)	Positive	Very Positive
−2	−1	0	1	2

For each choice the client should rate how the variety of components of his or her life, which are listed in left column of the survey, will be affected by this decision by writing down the number from the evaluation scale corresponding to the element in question. Then the client totals the score for each vertical column; the highest score is the best possible course of action for them.

Analyzing the Balance Sheet Results

For our sample client's balance sheet the choice to go back to school to retrain was the obvious winner over the two other options, which were moving to the country with no secure job or career prospects and staying in the same uninspiring, dead-end job. After your client completes the balance sheet and adds all the columns for each of the potential courses of action, instruct the client to look back over his or her answers to see if he or she skewed any of them to influence the results. Once clients have made any adjustments, recalculated the results, and know for sure that all the answers were true and correct, they must then ask themselves the following questions, "Is this really the direction I want my life to take?" and "Am I willing to take the next step to change my life?" The choice to change is up to the client and the client only. The massage therapist should not offer advice or any pressure for the client to change. Remember we are using the balance sheet to help the client reduce stress, so don't add more. When the client feels that change is needed, he or she should design a plan, institute the plan, reinforce the proper behavior, and stick with the plan while keeping the future in mind.

Converting a Plan into Action

Now that the client has set lifelong goals and the short-term goals to help achieve his or her long-range plan, the next step requires that the client institute that plan. This plan includes a daily to-do list, weekly goals, monthly goals, and yearly goals. Clients can even include a 5-year plan if they so desire. If any of your clients do decide to change, one way to help them put their plan into action and succeed is to for them to write a formal contract on a piece of paper. Clients should place this paper in a prominent place so that they frequently see it. This contract should include rewards for completing the contract and a penalty for failing. For instance, a contract may read:

> Within six months from the date of this contract I will have found a job that gets me out of the dead-end job that I am in. The new job will be interesting and will give me an opportunity for advancement. On finding this job I will join the health club and use it 3–5 hours a week. If I do not find the job within 6 months, I will stop watching my favorite TV program and will no longer eat desserts with my meals.

The client should sign the contract, date it, put it in on display, and then begin the next phase of his or her life.

It is important that the client not try to change too many behaviors at once. For instance, quitting smoking and no longer drinking alcohol are two tough propositions that are more difficult to accomplish than trying not to snack on a candy bar in the afternoon or not yelling so much at one's children. Clients should concentrate on simple behaviors to change first and then, after they gain confidence and they are ready, progress to the major changes on their list. The progress that they achieve in changing and then maintaining their new behaviors will intrinsically reward them and hopefully spur them on to greater successes. Clients also must realize that setbacks may occur in this process. If clients do transgress into old behaviors, they must recognize them and try to get back on track as soon as possible. Remind the client that to err is human and all is not lost with a setback—it's just a speed bump in the road that slows a person down but does not stop their progress.

REDUCING JOB AND SCHOOL STRESS

If left unchecked, job- and school-related stresses and strain might take a severe toll on a person's health and productivity. Follow these recommendations to help you survive in the workplace or to help you cope with the never-ending deadlines that plague a student's life.

Be prepared. Go to work or school every day ready to do the best job that you possibly can. When you're given a task to do, always produce your highest-quality work and try to finish on time. Don't wait until the last minute to complete assignments. Deadline pressures add to your stress, inhibit your creativity, and can reduce the overall quality of your work. As a rule, try to complete major projects a few days before they are due so you have adequate time to review them and make any necessary corrections.

Be punctual. Make it a habit to arrive at appointments or classes a few minutes early. Punctuality will add to your credibility and reduce your stress by eliminating the anxiety and physical stress responses that occur when you are constantly late.

Know what is expected of you. It is essential that you know and understand the scope and responsibilities of your job or the assignments that are due for school. Stress occurs when you don't have a clear picture of who you report to and who reports to you, what your specific duties are, the limits of your authority, and the criteria used to evaluate your performance. If your job has recently changed or has never been clearly defined, ask your supervisor or manager to provide you with a written, up-to-date job description. Students, if you are not clear on the due date or the directions for an assignment, talk to your instructor and get clarification, but don't wait until the last minute.

Be a team member. If possible, treat your work colleagues or fellow students working on a group project as teammates whose major goal is the same as yours: to win for your organization. Pull your part of the load. Don't rely on others to carry the burden for you. Unfortunately, many negative things occur in the workplace (such as jealousy, deceit, backstabbing, lying, personality clashes, idea stealing, and power coalitions) that prevent feelings of team camaraderie. If you're experiencing these problems at work, some suggestions to help you improve your work relationships follow:

- Be sensitive to the feelings and needs of your colleagues; they may return the courtesy. Never talk derisively about your fellow workers. If you do, they'll probably do the same to you. Essentially, treat others as you want to be treated.

- Try to be courteous and friendly but always maintain a professional approach toward work. Keep your private life out of the workplace. Think twice before dating or getting involved with someone at the office. In addition, never trust anyone at work with a secret. Even best friends have been known to break confidences if they can personally gain. Secrets are ammunition your enemies can use against you.

- Confront negativity and hostility and determine its cause. If you perceive that a serious communication barrier exists between yourself and a co-worker, family member, or fellow student and you don't know what is causing it, confront the individual directly. Come right out and ask the person questions such as: "What have I done to you? I sense negativity and hostility from you. What can we do to eliminate this problem?" Getting personality conflicts out in the open as soon as possible keeps the work, home, and school environment from becoming an unfriendly battleground. Although some people may never be able to work together comfortably, an uneasy coexistence is better than a high degree of work-related stress.

- Stand up for your rights. When you are unfairly blamed for a problem, don't sit back and take the abuse passively. If someone slanders you for no apparent reason, first get to the root of the problem. Gather all the facts of the situation, then tactfully and unemotionally present your side of the story to your supervisor. Dealing with this sort of problem as soon as possible will minimize its impact on your mind, body, and overall stress level.

- Maintain your integrity. At times, some employers ask you to do things that go against your values and better judgment. If you refuse an assignment on moral grounds, you risk losing your job, but you can maintain your self-esteem; if you neglect your true feelings, you risk losing your self-respect. You do have a choice. If your job frequently compromises your values, morals, and ethical standards, change jobs.

- Relax during breaks. If you're having a very trying day, go for a brisk walk during a break or between classes, or do some stretching, eye exercises, self-massage, focused breathing, or deep relaxation. These activities will help take your mind off your problems, uncloud your thoughts, and help you relax. You can also try sitting in your car or in a private, quiet room at the office and listen to a relaxation or self-improvement recording.

ASSIGNING CLIENTS HOMEWORK AND FOLLOWING UP

After each treatment it is important that you assign clients some self-help homework. Use the stress reduction reference chart in Appendix 13 for ideas of homework assignments to give clients for their particular problems. Try not to overwhelm them and add more stress to their busy lives by giving them too many things to do. Write down their assignments and activities on paper, copy pictures of the exercises that they need to practice, and give them clear instructions on how often or how many times they need to perform the activities. Assignments might include aerobic and postural realignment exercises, deep relaxation and deep breathing practice, and using modalities and self-massage techniques. You may also recommend basic dietary changes, such as cutting out caffeine; organizational and time management skills; and lifestyle changes. The job lifestyle survey, balance sheet, and heart attack and stroke risk test are other good assignments for clients in need of stress reduction. Pick a new area or two to add to the client's self-help program after each treatment. Record the assignments that you have doled out on the client's SOAP note form. The next time that you treat the client, ask how the homework went, how well the techniques worked, and if he or she has any questions or problems. This information can also be ascertained by using the reproducible pre-treatment status form located in Appendix 5.

REASSESS AFTER 10 WEEKS

Over the course of 10 weeks (try to get in at least 10 treatments over this period) you have experimented with different techniques to reduce your client's physical and psychosocial manifestations of stress. You have recorded each treatment using the SOAP note format. Now, it's time to readminister the original battery of tests to determine if any measurable progress was made in reducing the client's overall stress. You will once again use the PSI to check for physical and psychosocial stress symptoms, posture, flexibility, painful points, breathing mechanics, lung capacity, and diet. Use Appendix 6, the stress profile summary chart, to compare the new results with the results of the original PSI and document all the areas of progress that were achieved. Use the new data in your hands to try to interpret the results by answering the following questions:

- Which techniques worked and which did not?
- What could you have done differently that would have produced better results?
- How well did the client cooperate with homework assignments, and did the client stick to the stress reduction program?
- What kind of progress has the client achieved and in which areas?

Stress Reduction Massage Treatments

Massage therapy can be a tremendously effective way to help reduce the negative impact that the stresses and strain of our fast-paced world place on the human spirit, mind, and body. A practice specializing in performing stress reduction treatments demands more than just performing relaxing massage. To achieve the greatest results and have objective data to verify client success, a systematic comprehensive stress reduction program is needed, such as the process outlined in this book, which includes the following:

- Pretreatment assessment
- Anti-stress program design and implementation
- Trial and continuous revision of the treatments using both direct and indirect techniques
- Homework and follow-up
- Post-treatment reassessment
- Program success evaluation

Each client's status must be measured at the beginning of the process. Use the results of the assessments to help the client understand his or her stress and its effect on the mind and body. This will help clients get to the root of their problems. Use the assessment information to help clients develop a comprehensive plan to combat their stress and then institute that strategy. This program may require that clients add the routine practice of aerobic and postural realignment exercises, deep relaxation, and deep breathing practice to their busy schedule and incorporate dietary, lifestyle, and behavioral changes into their lives. Encourage clients to stick to their plan and positively reinforce their successes. The treatments must evolve as the client's status changes, and the therapist should try direct and indirect techniques to determine which are most effective for the client. The treatments should include the use of focused relaxation and, if indicated, the use of moist heat. Clients must be given homework, and the therapist must follow up on the homework to help clients achieve their goals. Then after a series of treatments each client's condition must be reevaluated to determine the effectiveness of their stress reduction program and the treatments used. The objective data gained by documenting the techniques used and the outcomes achieved can help provide valuable research as to the efficacy of a comprehensive stress reduction massage treatment program in combating stress-related physical, psychological, and emotional problems.

The most difficult task for the massage therapist performing stress reduction treatments is to find a way to persuade clients to institute and stick to the positive health and lifestyle changes that they need. For a treatment program to be most effective, clients must be ready to change. With the client working together with the therapist, the causes of stress, pain, and tension can be reduced and the negative effects of overall stress can be minimized.

SUMMARY

Share the following list of stress reduction tips with your clients, and if you desire use them to help relieve the stresses and strains in your own life.

- The best way to reduce your stress is to enjoy your life.

- Take control and responsibility for yourself. Direct your energies on the path that best fulfills your needs, wants, aspirations, and goals while allowing for your pursuit of happiness.

- Don't live to fulfill someone else's expectations.

- Your mind and the body are one, so incorporate activities in your life that tone the body and calm the mind.

- Pick your battles; not every disagreement should lead to a major confrontation.

- Love and pamper yourself; schedule special activities that bring you pleasure.

- Keep learning and growing intellectually your entire life.

- Keep a positive attitude, have confidence in your abilities, avoid negative thinking, and don't belittle yourself. If you keep saying negative things about yourself, you'll eventually begin to believe them.

- Take time to relax and think your own thoughts. It's unhealthy to be constantly preoccupied with work or your problems. Let your mind have a rest by giving it a chance to think about fun and beauty. Enjoy your time off and don't feel guilty about it. You deserve it. When you come home from work, take a shower, put on relaxing clothes, and separate yourself from the tension of the day.

- Participate each week in at least three aerobic exercise sessions that maintain your heart rate in your target range for at least 20–50 minutes. Exercise and deep relaxation are the cheapest, most effective health insurance available.

- Maintain your personal hygiene. Floss and brush your teeth and keep your toenails trimmed and your body clean because this helps a person feel good physically and mentally.

- Try to practice some techniques of deep relaxation for at least 20 minutes 3 times a week. Deep relaxation is productive time that will help you perform your job more effectively.

- Each day, perform a few quick exercises for improving your posture, breathing, and flexibility.

- Try to get 6–8 hours of sleep each night.

- Experience a relaxing massage at least once a week.

- Eat a well-balanced diet avoiding caffeine, salt, sugar, grease, too much fat and cholesterol, artificial flavoring and coloring, and junk food.

- If you have a drug or alcohol problem, get professional help. You may have to change your life (and your circle of "friends"), but it's in your best interest that you sober up.

- Participate in hobbies that keep you physically active. Move it, use it, or lose it.

- Don't try to relax when you have a lot to do. Get your work done first. When you finish, sit back and completely enjoy your relaxation. You've earned it.

- Be productive without killing yourself. Set attainable goals that help you achieve your long-range objectives. Reward yourself when you succeed.

- Modify your behavior or life by making the changes that reduce your stress.

- Don't exaggerate the importance of your problems. In the whole scheme of things many problems are actually inconsequential.

- Enjoy your life as you did when you were a child.

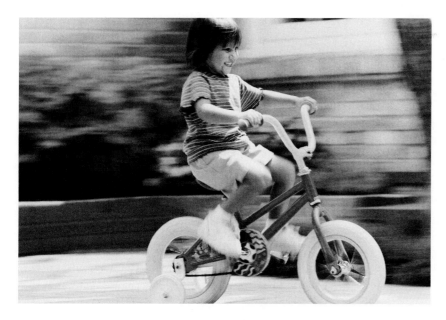

Figure 12.2

Remember how to play and laugh and enjoy special moments to their fullest

Massage Therapy Research Studies

MASSAGE THERAPY RESEARCH STUDIES

Authors/Year of Publication	Title	Benefits
Hart, S., Field, T., Hernandez-Reif, M., Nearing, G., Shaw, S., Schanberg, S., et al. (2001).	Anorexia symptoms are reduced by massage therapy. *Eating Disorders, 9,* 289–299.	• Reduced anxiety, depressed mood and salivary cortisol (stress hormone) levels and resulted in decreased body dissatisfaction associated with anorexia
Hernandez-Reif, M., Field, T., Krasnegor, J., & Theakston, T. (2001).	Low back pain is reduced and range of motion increased after massage therapy. *International Journal of Neuroscience, 106,* 131–145.	• Massage decreased low back pain • Depression and anxiety reduced • Improved sleep • Improved range of motion • Serotonin and dopamine levels were higher
Field, T., Shanberg, S., Kuhn, C., Fierro, K., Henteleff, T., Mueller, C., et al. (1997).	Bulimic adolescents benefit from massage therapy. *Adolescence, 33,* 555–563.	• Improved body image • Decreased depresion and anxiety symptoms • Decreased cortisol levels • Increased dopamine and serotonin
Cullen, C., Field, T., Hartshorn, K., Gruskin, A., Hernandez-Reif, M., Escalona, A., et al. (In review).	Carpal tunnel syndrome symptoms are lessened following massage therapy. *Journal of Bodywork and Movement Therapies, 8,* 9–14	• Daily self-massage for stretching tendons alleviated pain after 1 month

MASSAGE THERAPY RESEARCH STUDIES—continued

Authors/Year of Publication	Title	Benefits
Field, T., Sunshine, W., Hernandez-Reif, M., Quintino, O., Schanberg, S., Kuhn, C., et al. (1997).	Chronic fatigue syndrome: Massage therapy effects on depression and somatic symptoms in chronic fatigue syndrome. *Journal of Chronic Fatigue Syndrome, 3,* 43–51.	• Reduced depressed moods and anxiety • Decreased stress hormone (cortisol) • After 10 days of massage therapy, fatigue-related symptoms—anxiety and somatic symptoms—were reduced • Reduction in depression, difficulty sleeping
Field, T., Ironson, G., Scafidi, F., Nawrocki, T., Goncalves, A., Burman, I., et al. (1996).	Massage therapy reduces anxiety and enhances EEG pattern of alertness and math computations. *International Journal of Neuroscience, 86,* 197–205.	• Decreased frontal electroencephalogram (EEG) alpha and beta waves; increased delta activity consistent with enhanced alertness • Math problems were completed in significantly less time with significantly fewer errors after the massage • Anxiety, cortisol, and job stress levels were lower at the end of the 5-week period
Field, T., Hernandez-Reif, M., LaGreca, A., Shaw, K., Schanberg, S., & Kuhn, C. (1997).	Massage therapy lowers blood glucose levels in children with diabetes mellitus. *Diabetes Spectrum, 10,* 237–239.	After 1 month of parents massaging their children with diabetes: • Children's glucose levels decreased to the normal range and dietary compliance increased • Parents' and children's anxiety and depression levels decreased

(continued)

MASSAGE THERAPY RESEARCH STUDIES—continued

Authors/Year of Publication	Title	Benefits
Sunshine, W., Field, T., Schanberg, S., Quintino, O., Fierro, K., Kuhn, C., et al. (1996).	Fibromyalgia benefits from massage therapy and transcutaneous electrical stimulation. *Journal of Clinical Rheumatology, 2,* 18–22.	When compared to transcutaneous electrical stimulation, massage therapy resulted in the following: • Improved sleep patterns • Decreased pain, fatigue, anxiety, depression, and cortisol levels
Field, T., Cullen, C., Hartshorn, K., Hernandez-Reif, M., & Sunshine, W. (In press).	Fibromyalgia pain and substance p levels decrease and sleep improves after massage therapy. *Journal of Clinical Rheumatology, 8,* 72–76	• Patients with fibromyaglia sleep better (showed lower activity levels, suggesting more deep sleep) • Lower substance P levels and less pain following a month of biweekly massages
Field, T., Quintino, O., Henteleff, T., Wells-Keife, L., & Delvecchio-Feinberg, G. (1997).	Job stress reduction therapies. *Alternative Therapies in Health and Medicine, 3,* 54–56.	When hospital nursing and physician staff members were provided massage, relaxation, and music therapy, they experienced • Reduced anxiety, depression, and fatigue • Increased vigor
Hernandez-Reif, M., Field, T., Krasnegor, J., Theakston, H., Hossain, Z., & Burman, I. (2000).	High blood pressure and associated symptoms were reduced by massage therapy. *Journal of Bodywork and Movement Therapies, 4,* 31–38.	• Decreased diastolic blood pressure, anxiety, and cortisol (stress hormone) levels
Field, T. (1998).	Massage therapy effects. *American Psychologist, 53,* 1270–1281.	Infant, child, and adult massage therapy studies ranging across many conditions—including attention disorders, depression, addictions, pain syndromes, and immune and autoimmune disorders—are reviewed along with potential underlying mechanisms

MASSAGE THERAPY RESEARCH STUDIES—continued

Authors/Year of Publication	Title	Benefits
Hernandez-Reif, M., Field, T., Field, T., & Theakston, H. (1998).	Migraine headaches were reduced by massage therapy. *International Journal of Neuroscience, 96,* 1–11.	• Decreased the occurrence of headaches, sleep disturbances, and distress symptoms and increased serotonin levels
Hernandez-Reif, M., Martinez, A., Field T., Quintino, O., Hart, S., & Burman, I. (2000).	Premenstrual syndrome symptoms are relieved by massage therapy. *Journal of Psychosomatic Obstetrics & Gynecology, 21,* 9–15.	• Improved mood • Reduced anxiety, pain, and water retention
Field, T., Morrow, C., Valdeon, C., Larson, S., Kuhn, C., & Schanberg, S. (1992).	Massage therapy reduces anxiety in child and adolescent psychiatric patients. *Journal of the the American Academy of Child and Adolescent Psychiatry, 31,* 125–130.	After five 30-minute massages, child and adolescent patients: • Had better sleep patterns • Lowered depression and anxiety • Lowered cortisol and norepinephrine level
Hernandez-Reif, M., Field, T., & Hart, S. (1999).	Smoking cravings are reduced by self-massage. *Preventive Medicine, 28,* 28–32.	• Cravings, anxious behavior, and the number of cigarettes smoked reduced by self-massage (rubbing ear lobes or hands whenever subjects experienced a craving)
Diego, M., Hernandez-Reif, M., Field, T., Brucker, B., Hart, S., & Burman, I. (2004).	Spinal cord patients benefit from massage therapy. *International Journal of Neuroscience, 112,* 133–142.	• Improved functional abilities, range of motion, and muscle strength in patients with spinal cord injury

Personal Stress Inventory

Personal Stress Inventory, Section 1, Part A: Physical Symptoms of Stress

Instruct the client to use the following scale to answer the questions and circle those that apply.

1 = Never	2 = Rarely	3 = Sometimes
4 = Often	5 = Always	

To what extent do you experience the following?

    1 2 3 4 5   Sweaty palms

    1 2 3 4 5   Cold hands and feet

    1 2 3 4 5   Tension headaches

    1 2 3 4 5   Migraine headaches

    1 2 3 4 5   Teeth grinding

    1 2 3 4 5   Neck pains

    1 2 3 4 5   Uncontrollable muscle spasms

    1 2 3 4 5   Pains in the shoulder, upper back, or both

    1 2 3 4 5   Low back pain

    1 2 3 4 5   Pain down the back of your leg(s)

    1 2 3 4 5   Shortness of breath

1 2 3 4 5   Susceptibility to minor illness

1 2 3 4 5   Poor-quality sleep

1 2 3 4 5   Hair, eyelash, or beard pulling

1 2 3 4 5   Nail biting

1 2 3 4 5   Frequent trips to the toilet

1 2 3 4 5   Gastrointestinal pain or discomfort

1 2 3 4 5   Diarrhea

1 2 3 4 5   Constipation

1 2 3 4 5   Nausea

1 2 3 4 5   Chronic fatigue

1 2 3 4 5   Binge eating

1 2 3 4 5   Do not eat because you fear becoming fat

1 2 3 4 5   Bulimia

1 2 3 4 5   General malaise

1 2 3 4 5   Cold sores, hives

1 2 3 4 5   Restless legs or feet (toe or finger shaking)

1 2 3 4 5   Repetitive joint cracking (neck, knuckles, etc.)

Personal Stress Inventory, Section 1, Part B: Psychosocial Symptoms of Stress

Continue using the same scale:

1 = Never	2 = Rarely	3 = Sometimes
4 = Often	5 = Always	

How frequently do you experience the following? Circle the answers that apply.

1 2 3 4 5   Not enough time in the day

1 2 3 4 5   Trouble concentrating (difficulty thinking clearly)

1 2 3 4 5   Anxiety from causes that you cannot pinpoint

1 2 3 4 5   Irritability

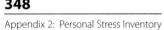

1 2 3 4 5	Strained relationships
1 2 3 4 5	Easily aroused to hostility or anger
1 2 3 4 5	Job dissatisfaction or prolonged unemployment
1 2 3 4 5	Depression
1 2 3 4 5	Taking work home with you
1 2 3 4 5	Thinking about work even when relaxing
1 2 3 4 5	Being a workaholic
1 2 3 4 5	Trouble turning off your mind at night
1 2 3 4 5	Decision-making anxiety
1 2 3 4 5	Stressful dreams
1 2 3 4 5	Nonstop rushing around
1 2 3 4 5	Low motivation
1 2 3 4 5	Pessimism
1 2 3 4 5	Worrying
1 2 3 4 5	Lack of control over your life
1 2 3 4 5	A short-fused temper
1 2 3 4 5	An unhappy home environment
1 2 3 4 5	Isolation or loneliness
1 2 3 4 5	Procrastination
1 2 3 4 5	Panic attacks
1 2 3 4 5	So impatient that you finish others' sentences
1 2 3 4 5	Functioning subnormally or missing work because of drug or alcohol abuse

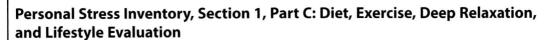

Personal Stress Inventory, Section 1, Part C: Diet, Exercise, Deep Relaxation, and Lifestyle Evaluation

Circle the diet that best describes your eating habits on a typical day.

a. Lots of fruit and vegetables (salads), whole grains, and legumes; less than 30% of all food consumed comes from fat; at least two glasses of dairy products (unless allergic) each day; low cholesterol; little sugar; more fish, turkey, and chicken than red meat.
b. Lots of fast food, junk food, soda, and grease.
c. Meat and potatoes.
d. Vegetarian.
e. A combination of _____ and _____.

How many cups of stimulants do you drink each day (include coffee, tea, hot chocolate, and soda)? _____

List the name and dose of any medications you are currently taking (including appetite suppressants and vitamin pills): _____

_____

How frequently do you practice a form of deep relaxation (such as meditation) each week?

Never _____ Days a week _____ Duration _____

How frequently do you participate in vigorous, nonstop aerobic activities that elevate your heart rate to your target range?

Never _____ Days a week _____ Duration _____

How often do you perform postural realignment or stretching exercises?

Never _____ Days a week _____ Duration _____

How frequently do you lift weights, perform calisthenics, or participate in any other activities that tone your muscles?

Never _____ Days a week _____ Duration _____

What time of the day do you feel most stressed? What happens at these times (i.e., commute in traffic, children fighting at the dinner table, the daily meeting with the boss)? Use more paper if necessary.

_____

_____

The following factors are common contributors to stress. Put them in the order that you think they contribute to your stress level. Put a 1 next to the element that causes the most stress, then a 2 next to your second biggest stressor, and so on down the list.

_____ Job or lack of a job

_____ Studies

_____ Family members

_____ Social relationships

_____ Sexual issues

_____ Financial issues

_____ Health

_____ Living situation

_____ Environmental pollution

_____ The world situation

_____ Other _____

List three lifestyle or behavioral changes that you think may improve the quality of your life.

_____

_____

_____

List some ideas for coping with, or eliminating, your stressors. Include even the most

bizarre alternatives that you can imagine. Don't inhibit your creativity.

_____

_____

_____

Personal Stress Inventory, Section 2, Part A: Posture Evaluation

Follow the directions outlined on page 28 of the text. To get a true evaluation, instruct your clients to stand in their relaxed habitual posture, and then compare what you see with the pictures in the PSI in Chapter 2. Record which picture most closely resembles the client's posture on this form.

Forward Head

Normal Posture   Mild   Moderate   Severe

Comments _____

Kyphosis

Normal Posture   Mild   Moderate   Severe

Comments _____

Elevated Shoulder

R or L   Normal   Mild   Moderate   Severe

Comments _____

Head Tilt

R or L   Normal   Mild   Moderate   Severe

Comments _____

_____

Elevated Hip

R or L   Right High _____ inches   Left High _____ inches

Comments _____

_____

_____

C or S Curve of the Spine

Normal   C right   C left   LTRL   RTLL

Rib Cage Rotation L R

Comments _____

Hyperlordosis (Exaggerated Lumbar Curve and Anterior Pelvic Tilt)

Normal Posture   Mild   Moderate   Severe

Comments _____

ASIS Rotation

Normal   Right low _____ inches   Left low _____ inches

Comments _____

Leg Length

To measure for imbalances in leg length in the supine position, follow the directions out-lined on page 34 of the text. Record your results on this form.

Equal length _____   Left short _____ inches   Right short _____ inches

Comments _____

Personal Stress Inventory, Section 2, Part B: Flexibility Evaluation

Evaluate the following muscle groups and check their lengths compared to the pictures beginning on page 36. Have the client try to assume the positions indicated without warming up first. Instruct them not to strain or cause any pain or injury. Record the appropriate positions they can comfortably attain on this form.

Hip Flexors

R Normal Length   Mild   Moderate   Severe

L Normal Length   Mild   Moderate   Severe

Comments _____

Quadriceps

R Normal Length   Mild   Moderate   Severe

L Normal Length   Mild   Moderate   Severe

Comments _____

Low Back Muscles

Normal Length   Mild   Moderate   Severe

Comments _____

Hamstrings

R Normal Length   Mild   Moderate   Severe

L Normal Length   Mild   Moderate   Severe

Comments _____

Hip Lateral Rotators

Measure the distance from the bottom of the patella perpendicular to the table.

Compare sides.

R _____ inches   L _____ inches

Comments _____

Hip Adductors

R Normal Length   Mild   Moderate   Severe

L Normal Length   Mild   Moderate   Severe

Comments _____

Tensor Fasciae Latae and Iliotibial Tract

Follow the directions for this test outlined on page 40 and refer to the pictures on page 41.

R Normal   Inches from table _____

L Normal   Inches from table _____

Comments _____

Gastrocnemius

Place the hands on the wall, extend one knee completely, and slide the foot flat on the

ground back as far as possible. The foot should be kept straight ahead, and the heel

should not rise up. Measure the distance from the toes to the wall. Compare sides.

R _____ inches   L _____ inches

Comments _____

Soleus

Place the hands and the sole of one foot on a wall, raising the toes as high as they can

comfortably go. Flex the knee and bring the patella toward the wall; then measure the

distance from the patella to the wall.

R _____ inches   L _____ inches

Comments _____

Longitudinal Arch, Calcaneal Tendon Angle, and Toe Deviations

Observe the client's feet while he or she is standing barefoot. Look for a flat or extra high arch, deviations of the calcaneal tendon angle, hammer toes, and big toe deviations.

R Longitudinal arch: Normal _____ Flat _____ High

L Longitudinal arch: Normal _____ Flat _____ High

R Calcaneus tendon angle: Straight   Medial deviation

L Calcaneus tendon angle: Straight   Medial deviation

R Toes: Normal deviation observed

L Toes: Normal deviation observed

R Big toe; Normal   Lateral deviation observed

L Big toe: Normal   Lateral deviation observed

Shoulder External Rotation

R Normal   Mild   Moderate   Severe

L Normal   Mild   Moderate   Severe

Comments _____

Shoulder Internal Rotation

R Normal   Mild   Moderate   Severe

L Normal   Mild   Moderate   Severe

Comments _____

Shoulder Flexion

R Normal   Mild   Moderate   Severe

L Normal   Mild   Moderate   Severe

Comments _____

Shoulder Extension

R Normal Length   Mild   Moderate   Severe

L Normal   Mild   Moderate   Severe

Comments _____

Over and Under

R over   Normal (Fingers touch) _____ inches between fingers

L over   Normal (Fingers touch) _____ inches between fingers

Comments _____

Personal Stress Inventory, Section 2, Part C: Muscle Tension Evaluation

Now let's evaluate and map areas of tension and pain in your client's body. Draw a dot on the points that are hypertonic. Draw an X on those that are painful; use wavy lines (≈) for points that the client reports radiate pain. Press all over the client's body from the top of the head to the bottom of the feet.

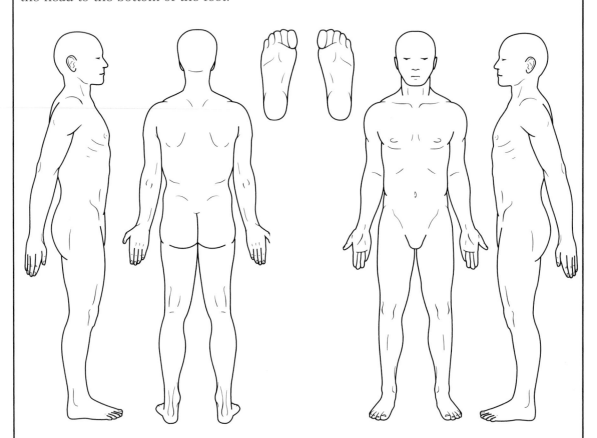

Personal Stress Inventory, Section 2, Part D: Breathing Evaluation

The way a person breathes can contribute to his or her level of stress. You will be evaluating five breathing factors that include the following: the length of inhalation, length of exhalation, shoulder elevation, action of the diaphragm, and overall control. Have clients sit in a chair and relax. Use your clock or stopwatch to measure the time it takes for them to fully inhale and exhale. Instruct them to take long, slow, deep, complete breaths in through the nose, breathing as slowly as possible. Then instruct them to release the breath, exhaling through their nose as slowly as possible. Record the time it takes for them to inhale and exhale. Perform two trials, and record them both.

Trial I

Inhalation _____

Exhalation _____

Trial 2

Inhalation _____

Exhalation _____

Now perform the following tests. Place your hands on their upper trapezius muscles and have them continue to take long slow breaths in and out.

1. Do the client's shoulders move when they breathe?   YES   NO

Next place your hands on the client's diaphragm just below the xiphoid process and check the action of the diaphragm. (If the person practices the principles of Pilates, place your hands on the sides of the rib cage in the same region.)

2. When the client begins to take air in, does the action of the diaphragm push your hands out away from the client's body? YES   NO
3. Next ask the client if it feels to him or her that the inhalation travels from the bottom to the top of the chest. YES   NO
4. Ask the client if his or her breathing feels deep, relaxed, and coordinated. YES   NO

One-Week Stress Log

Date or Day	Time of Day	Stressor	Physical Reaction	Psychological Reaction	Coping Techniques

APPENDIX 3   ONE-WEEK STRESS LOG

Date or Day	Time of Day	Stressor	Physical Reaction	Psychological Reaction	Coping Techniques

APPENDIX 3 ONE-WEEK STRESS LOG

Health History/Intake Form

Personal Information

Name: _____ Age: _____ Date: _____

Address: _____ Phone Numbers: _____

City/State/Zip: _____ Day: _____

Email Address: _____ Evening: _____

Employer/Occupation: _____

Hobbies/Physical Activities: _____

Primary Health Care Provider: Person to Contact in Case of an Emergency:

Name: _____   Name: _____

Phone: _____   Phone: _____

Contact Preferences

Would you be interested in receiving appointment reminders via phone or email?

☐ Y/ ☐ N

Would you like to receive information about holiday specials, coupons, and events?

☐ Y/ ☐ N

Massage History Information

Have you received a professional massage before?   ☐ Y/ ☐ N

If yes, do you receive massage regularly?   ☐ Y/ ☐ N

How often? _____

Depth of massage pressure preferred:

☐ Light   ☐ Moderate   ☐ Firm   ☐ Deep

Do you have any allergies or sensitivities to lotions, oils, or fragrances?

☐ Y/ ☐ N/ ☐ Don't Know

If yes, please describe: _____

Do you have any music preferences during your massage treatment?   ☐ Y/ ☐ N

Describe: _____

Are there any areas you want avoided during every massage?   ☐ Y/ ☐ N

Where: _____

Please let us know how you heard about our services: _____

Medical History

Mark current conditions with an "X"

Mark previous conditions by filling in the box "■"

Condition	Condition
☐ Acute infectious disease	☐ Indigestion
☐ Allergies: _____	☐ Insomnia
☐ Arthritis—osteoarthritis	☐ Irritability/nervousness/stress
☐ Arthritis—rheumatoid	☐ Memory loss
☐ Asthma/difficulty breathing	☐ Muscle cramps/spasms
☐ Back pain	☐ Neck pain
☐ Blood clots/phlebitis	☐ Numbness/tingling
☐ Bruise easily	☐ Osteoporosis
☐ Bursitis	☐ Panic attacks/anxiety
☐ Cancer/tumors	☐ PMS (premenstrual syndrome)
☐ Cold/flu	☐ Poor circulation
☐ Cold hands or feet	☐ Poor posture
☐ Chest pain	☐ Pregnancy
☐ Depression	☐ Rashes
☐ Diabetes	☐ Skin problems
☐ Diarrhea/constipation/bowel	☐ Stroke
☐ Disc problems	☐ Scoliosis
☐ Dizziness	☐ Sinus conditions
☐ Earache/ringing in ears	☐ Swollen ankles
☐ Fatigue	☐ Swollen joints
☐ Foot problems	☐ Tendonitis
☐ Headache	☐ Tremors
☐ Heart disease	☐ Varicose veins
☐ Hernia	☐ Other_____

Are you currently under the care of a health practitioner for any of the above conditions?

□ Y/ □ N

If yes, please explain:_____

By signing below, I understand and accept that:

- I am solely responsible for my physical condition and for seeking medical treatment when necessary.
- Massage is not intended to be used in place of medical care by a doctor.
- I further authorize my massage therapist to contact my primary health care provider for information pertaining to my health and safety regarding massage.
- The above information I have provided is complete and accurate to the best of my knowledge.
- Unless there is an emergency situation, all cancellations of treatment require 24-hour notice. If no notice or late notice is given, I agree to pay the full appointment fee.

Signature: _____ Date: _____

Pretreatment Status Form

5

Current Health Status

Please check:

Blood Pressure: ☐ Low ☐ Normal ☐ High

Have you had any recent injuries? ☐ Y/ ☐ N

Where: _____

Have you had any recent illnesses? ☐ Y/ ☐ N

Describe: _____

Are you wearing any of the following:

☐ hard contact lenses ☐ hearing aid ☐ pace maker

Current Symptoms

Please indicate on the diagrams the area(s) where you are experiencing discomfort

or pain:

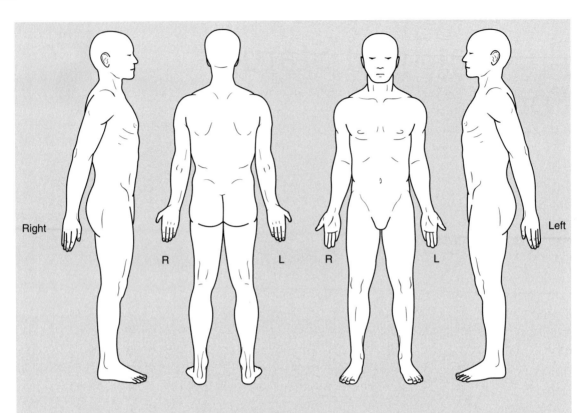

Right   Left

R   L   R   L

Which two areas would you like your therapist to focus on during this massage session?

Please be specific.

1.

2.

For each area, what is the symptom you are experiencing at these locations (example:

pain, tension, numbness, spasm)?

1.

2.

For each area, what is the symptom's intensity level you are experiencing? Use a 1–10 intensity level scale, where 1 is very mild, 5 is moderate, and 10 is severe.

1.

2.

For each area, how often does the symptom present itself—daily, weekly, monthly, once or twice a year?

1.

2.

For each area, how long does the symptom last once it has begun—minutes, hours, days, weeks, months?

1.

2.

For each area, do you know what causes the symptom to occur? Was there an original injury?

1.

2.

For each area, is there anything you can do to relieve the symptom once it has begun?

1.

2.

For each area, are there activities of daily living that make the symptom worse?

1.

2.

During your last treatment, were there any techniques that did not work well for you?

Explain.

During your last treatment, were there any techniques that worked extremely well?

Explain.

How often did you practice the homework/exercises given during your last session?

Stress Profile Summary Chart

6

Physical stress manifestations, Section 1, Part A: List all 4 and 5 responses.

Pscyhosocial stress manifestations, Section 1, Part B: List all 4 and 5 responses.

Section 1, Part C: Indicate if the client needs to add these components to his or her

weekly schedule.

Deep relaxation practice for 15-20 minutes three times a week	Y N
Aerobic exercise practice, elevating the heart rate to the client's target range for 20-50 minutes three times a week	Y N
Postural realignment exercises every day	Y N
Strength and toning exercises three times a week	Y N
Dietary changes	Y N
Stimulants: Does the client need to reduce the amount ingested?	Y N

Supplements and medications:

Time of day most stressed:

Top three stressors:

Lifestyle and behavioral changes listed by the client:

Ideas for coping:

Muscle tension evaluation: Summarize major areas of pain and tension noted on the body charts in Section 2, Part C of the PSI and any progress made in these areas.

Pertinent data from stress log: Look for patterns in the time of the day most stressed and physical symptoms.

POSTURE EVALUATION

	Pretest Date:_____	Posttest Date:_____	Comments
Forward head	Nor L M S	Nor L M S	
Kyphosis	Nor L M S	Nor L M S	
Elevated shoulder	Right: Nor L M S Left: Nor L M S	Left: Nor L M S Left: Nor L M S	
Head tilt	Nor L M S	Nor L M S	
Elevated hip	Right: Nor L M S Left: Nor L M S	Right: Nor L M S Left: Nor L M S	
C or S curve of spine	Nor C right C left LTRL RTLL Rib Cage RotationLR	Nor C right C left LTRL RTLL Rib Cage RotationLR	
Hyperlordosis	Nor L M S	Nor L M S	
ASIS rotation	Nor/Same Right: Low _____in Left: Low _____in	Nor/Same Right: Low _____in Left: Low _____in	
Leg length	Nor/Same Right: Short _____in Left: Short _____in	Nor/Same Right: Short _____in Left: Short _____in	

Nor, Normal; L, Mild; M, Moderate; S, Severe.

FLEXIBILITY EVALUATION

	Pretest	Posttest	Comments
Hip flexors	Right: Nor L M S Left: Nor L M S	Right: Nor L M S Left: Nor L M S	
Quadriceps	Right: Nor L M S Left: Nor L M S	Right: Nor L M S Left: Nor L M S	
Low back muscles (lumbar extensors)	Nor L M S	Nor L M S	
Hamstrings	Right: Nor L M S Left: Nor L M S	Right: Nor L M S Left: Nor L M S	

(continued)

FLEXIBILITY EVALUATION—continued

	Pretest	Posttest	Comments
Hip lateral rotators	Nor/Same Right: Short _____in Left: Short _____in	Nor/Same Right: Short _____in Left: Short _____in	
Hip adductors	Right: Nor L M S Left: Nor L M S	Right: Nor L M S Left: Nor L M S	
Iliotibial tract	Right: Nor L M S Left: Nor L M S	Right: Nor L M S Left: Nor L M S	
Gastrocnemius	Right _____in Left _____in	Right _____in Left _____in	
Soleus	Right _____in Left _____in	Right _____in Left _____in	
Longitudinal arch	Nor Flat High	Nor Flat High	
Calcaneus (Achilles) tendon angle	Straight Medial Deviation	Straight Medial Deviation	
Hammer toes	Nor___ deviated	Nor___ deviated	
Big toe	Nor_____ Lateral Deviation _____	Nor_____ Lateral Deviation_____	
Shoulder external rotation	Right: Nor L M S Left: Nor L M S	Right: Nor L M S Left: Nor L M S	
Shoulder internal rotation	Right: Nor L M S Left: Nor L M S	Right: Nor L M S Left: Nor L M S	
Shoulder flexion	Right: Nor L M S Left: Nor L M S	Right: Nor L M S Left: Nor L M S	
Shoulder extension	Right: Nor L M S Left: Nor L M S	Right: Nor L M S Left: Nor L M S	
Shoulder horizontal adduction	Right: Nor L M S Left: Nor L M S	Right: Nor L M S Left: Nor L M S	
Shoulder horizontal abduction	Right: Nor L M S Left: Nor L M S	Right: Nor L M S Left: Nor L M S	
Over and under	Right Over: Normal or Short _____in Left Over: Normal or Short _____in	Right Over: Normal or Short _____in Left Over: Normal or Short _____in	

Nor, Normal; L, Mild; M, Moderate; S, Severe.

BREATHING EVALUATION

Breathing Evaluation

	Pretest	Posttest
Trial 1	Inhalation Time:	Inhalation Time:
	Exhalation Time:	Exhalation Time:
Trial 2	Inhalation Time:	Inhalation Time:
	Exhalation Time:	Exhalation Time:
Do the client's shoulders move when he or she breathes?	YES or NO	YES or NO
Do the client's ribs and belly button push out when he or she begins to take air in?	YES or NO	YES or NO
Does the client's breath in travel from the bottom to the top of his or her chest?	YES or NO	YES or NO
Does the client report that his or her breathing feels deep, relaxed, and coordinated?	YES or NO	YES or NO

Additional comments:

_____

_____

_____

_____

_____

SOAP Note Review

GENERAL NOTES:

- Always use blue or black pen; never use pencil.
- If you make an error, simply put one line through the error and initial it. Never use white out, erase, or scratch out an entry.
- Always remember that SOAP notes are legal documents. Use professional language and avoid inappropriate side commentary.
- Use abbreviations throughout the body of the SOAP note text. Refer to standardized abbreviations to be consistent with other health professionals. An excellent reference is Diana Thompson's book, *Hands Heal*.
- Use symbols on the diagrams to denote client symptom locations. Do not use symbols in the text of SOAP notes. Symbols are visual cues, and abbreviations are shorthand for written words. Recognize this difference and their different applications. Use them appropriately.

S: (SUBJECTIVE)

This is the client's descriptions/perceptions of what is going on with his or her body. Use his or her terms and statements. If her or she give you a diagnosis of the condition, either use quotation marks or write Dx (diagnosis) by doctor. It is not in your scope of practice to diagnose client conditions.

- Goals: For first-time clients, determine what they want to get out of the massage.
- Update: For repeat clients, check in with the client to see if there is any information you should be aware of: new goal/focus, recent injury, illness. Also, check the previ-

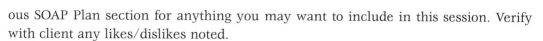

ous SOAP Plan section for anything you may want to include in this session. Verify with client any likes/dislikes noted.

- Symptom: What is the complaint: pain, numbness, swelling, limited ROM?
- Location: Where, specifically, is the symptom presented (e.g., right lateral knee pain)?
- Intensity: Use 1–10 pain scale or L, M, or S for low, moderate, or severe.
- Frequency: How often does this symptom present itself (seldom, intermittent, frequent, constant)?
- Duration: How long does the symptom last when it does occur (minutes, days, months)?
- Onset: When did symptom first appear? What was the client doing at this time? What does the client feel is the cause?
- Aggravating: Are there any activities of daily living that make the symptom worse?
- Relieving: Are there any activities that make the symptom better?

O: (OBJECTIVE)

This is the visual and palpable evidence presented. Use the diagrams to note all observations. This is also where you state all the treatments and modalities used to remedy the client's symptoms.

- Visual findings: Note imbalances with posture, muscle tone, gait (e.g., elevated right shoulder).
- Palpable findings: This is where you note any hypertonicities, ROM issues, spasm, tender points, trigger points, adhesions, scars, etc.
- Modalities/techniques used: State the stroke/technique used for each visual and palpable finding noted.

A: (ASSESSMENT)

This is the therapist's summary of the changes to the client's conditions directly resulting from the treatment provided. For every visual/palpable finding noted in "O," you must address the postmassage status. Any symptom and intensity level noted in the "S" section must also be addressed. Hopefully, your treatment will improve the client's status. If there is no change to certain symptoms or findings, please note.

- Symptom/intensity level: Any changes?
- Visual/palpable findings: Any changes?

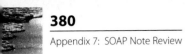

P: (PLAN)

Use this section to quickly communicate future treatment strategies to the next therapist working on this client—or as a reminder to yourself. Write down any home-care treatments you've suggested to the client so that you can follow up on their progress during the next session.

- Treatment plan
  - What techniques worked/did not work
  - Client preferences
  - Anything you didn't have enough time to address
  - Anything you want to check out next time
  - Anything you think the next massage therapist should know
- Massage frequency: How often should this client receive massage for adequate progress toward his or her goals?
- Homework: Any self stretches, recommendations, and assignments

SAMPLE
SOAP NOTES

APPENDIX 8

BLANK SOAP NOTES

Therapist Name: _____ SOAP Chart

Client Name: _____ Date: _____

Current Injuries and/or Medications: _____

S   (Subjective) Focus for Today

Symptoms/Location/Intensity/Frequency/Duration/Onset

Activities of Daily Living: Aggravating/Relieving

O   (Objective) Findings: Visual/Palpable

Modalities/Techniques Used:

A   (Assessment) Response to Treatment

P   (Plan) Future Treatment/Frequency/Techniques that worked
    /Techniques that did not work/Homework/Self-care

Therapist Signature_____ Date: _____

Legend:	℮ TrP	● TeP	○ Ⓟ	☀ Infl	≡ HT	≈ SP
	✕ Adh	≋ Numb	↻ rot	╱ elev	⤚ Short	↔ Long

Therapist Name: _____

Client Name: _____ Date: _____

Current Injuries and/or Medications: _____

S

O

A

P

Therapist Signature_____ Date: _____

Therapist Name: _____

Client Name: _____ Date: _____

Current Injuries and/or Medications: _____

S

O

A

P

Therapist Signature_____ Date: _____

Appendix 8
Example Soap Notes

Therapist Name: *John America*   SOAP Chart

Client Name: *Suzie Stone* _____ Date: *1-10-06*

Current Injuries and/or Medications: *NA* _____

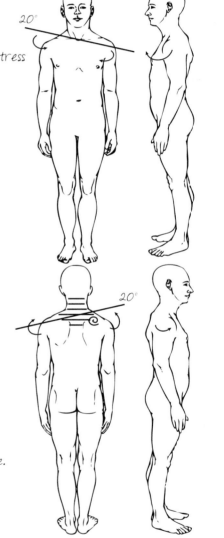

S   (Subjective) Focus for Today

↓ Neck/SH Ⓟ, ↑ Relaxation

Symptoms/Location/Intensity/Frequency/Duration/Onset

ⒷⓁ Neck/SH Ⓟ /⁸/10/cons./1+ mo/holiday & work stress

Panic attacks
& shortness / ⁷/10/interm./hrs/ thinking about
of breath   deadlines

Activities of Daily Living: Aggravating/Relieving
A: computer work; thinking about deadlines
R: massage, hot baths

O   (Objective) Findings: Visual/Palpable
V: ele Ⓡ Sh ~ 20°; L ⒷⓁ Sh rot;
    shallow, rapid breathing
P: HT ⒷⓁ lev scap, U-trap, pec min
    TrP Ⓡ lev scap ref. to head

Modalities/Techniques Used:
Heat pack to upper back & neck 10 min.
Full body eff, neck & Sh PROM, CRAC + TrP
release to Ⓡ lev scap, Pec pumping & DP

A   (Assessment) Response to Treatment
Client states "I feel so much more relaxed!"
↓ Ⓡ Sh ele ~ 20°∆ → 5°
TrP Ⓡ lev scap gone
↓ HT ⒷⓁ lev scap, U-trap
⊖∆ to pec min HT
Neck/Sh Ⓟ ∆ 8 → 3
RR: Exh > inhal, ⊖ sh ele c̄ breathing

P   (Plan) Future Treatment/Frequency/Techniques that worked

/Techniques that did not work/Homework/Self-care

• Pec pumping ineffective + Ⓟ-ful to ct. Try PR next time.
• Ct very responsive to CRAC @ lev scap
• Ct given diaphragmatic breathing exercises for H.W.
  Perform daily
• Ct encouraged to perform neck/Sh AROM + self massage
  during showers
• Request erg. @ work if poss.

Therapist Signature *John America* _____ Date: *1-10-06*

Legend:	☾ TrP	• TeP	○ Ⓟ	☀ Infl	≡ HT	≈ SP
	✕ Adh	≫ Numb	↻ rot	╱ elev	⤜ Short	↔ Long

Walking Endurance Improvement Plan

WALKING ENDURANCE IMPROVEMENT PLAN

Enter the number of steps that you take each day on the chart below. At the end of the week, tally the total number of steps taken and then divide by 7 to get the average steps taken per day.

	Monday	Tuesday	Wednesday	Thursday	Friday	Saturday	Sunday	Total number of steps per week	Average number of steps per day
Week 1									
Week 2									
Week 3									
Week 4									
Week 5									

Heart Attack and Stroke Risk Self-Appraisal

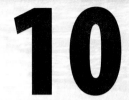

1. Male   Female

2. Age

3. If you are overweight, estimate how many pounds over your ideal weight you are

   at this moment.

   0–5 pounds   5–10 pounds   10–20 pounds

   20–30 pounds   More than 30 pounds.

4. Do you smoke?   Yes   No

   If yes, estimate how many cigarettes do you smoke each day: _____.

5. Has any member of your immediate family died of a heart attack or stroke? Before

   the age of 65?   Yes   No

6. Do you eat red meat 3 or more times a week?   Yes   No

7. Do you eat organ meats (liver, kidneys, etc.) more than once a month?   Yes   No

8. Do you eat 5 or more eggs a week?   Yes   No

9. Do you eat hot dogs, cold cuts, or luncheon meats 3 to 5 times a week?

   Yes   No

10. Do you consume whole milk, cheese, or ice cream 3 to 5 times a week?

   Yes   No

11. Do you eat deep-fried foods about 3 to 5 times a week?   Yes   No

12. Do you use mayonnaise and butter 3 to 5 times a week?   Yes   No

13. Do you frequently enjoy sweets every day (sugar or honey in your hot drinks, soda, candy, jelly, cake, cookies, etc.)?   Yes   No

14. How often do you perform aerobic exercise in your target range each week?

   A. 20 nonstop minutes 3 times a week

   B. Sometimes   C. Never

15. Do you always add salt to your food?   Yes   No

16. Do you practice some form of deep relaxation at least 3 times a week?

   Yes   No

17. Is your life full of deadline and time pressures?   Yes   No

18. Select the category that your most recent blood pressure measurement falls into:

   A. 119/79 or less   B. Between 120/80 and 139/89

   C. Between 140 and 159/99   D. 160/100 or higher

19. Men, is your waist circumference 40 inches or larger?   Yes   No

    Women, is your waist size 35 inches or larger?   Yes   No

What to do with the results?

1. Score 1 point if you are a man; 0 points if you are a woman.
2. Add 1 point if you are older than age 35.
3. Add 1 point for every 10 pounds that you are overweight. 10 pounds = 1 point; 10–20 pounds = 2 points; 20–30 pounds = 3 points; More than 30 pounds = 4 points (Even someone 50 pounds overweight will just get 4 points.)
4. Add 0 points if you don't smoke; add 1 point for each half pack you smoke each day.
5. Add 1 point for each member of your immediate family who died of a heart attack or stroke before the age of 65 years.
6. Add 1 point if you eat red meat 3 or more times a week.
7. Add 1 point if you eat organ meats once a month.
8. Add 1 point if you eat 5 or more eggs a week.
9–13. For these questions, add 1 point for up to 2 yes answers and 2 points for 3 or more yes responses.
14. Subtract 1 point if you exercise 20 minutes 3 times a week; add 1 point if you get some exercise; add 2 points if you do not exercise.
15. Add 1 point if you always add salt to your food.
16. Subtract 1 point if you practice deep relaxation 3 times a week. Add 0 points if you don't.
17. Add 1 point if your life is full of deadline and time pressures.
18. Subtract 1 point for 119 or less; add 0 points for between 120 and 139; add 1 point for between 140 and 159; and add 2 points for 160 or higher.
19. Men, add 1 point if your waist size is 40 inches or larger; women add 1 point if your waist size is 35 inches or larger.

Job and Lifestyle Survey

1. Are you satisfied with your job?   Yes   No   NA

2. Do you make enough money for what you do?   Yes   No   NA

3. Do you have a realistic chance for doing better?   Yes   No

4. Are you overloaded with work?   Yes   No   NA

5. Are you burned out (have lost enthusiasm for your job)?   Yes   No   NA

6. Do you feel part of the work team?   Yes   No   NA

7. Do you need new challenges?   Yes   No

8. Do you feel a change of jobs, career, or relationships would help?

   Yes   No   NA

9. Do you get along well with your colleagues, family, and friends?   Yes   No

10. Are you happy with your lifestyle?   Yes   No

11. Do you feel love at home?   Yes   No

12. Do you take time for your family?   Yes   No

13. What are the risks if you don't change?

_____

14. What are the risks if you do change?

_____

15. What are your possible courses of action?

_____

_____

16. List three long-term, lifelong goals for the future and discuss how you plan on

achieving them._____

_____

17. List three short-term, achievable goals and discuss how you plan to meet them.

_____

_____

18. List three or more behavioral changes that will help you become the person that

you want to be and then discuss strategies for instituting these changes.

_____

_____

Decision Balance Sheet

12

Select three possible courses of action or direction for your life and list them as the choices at the head of the columns below. Then use the following evaluation scale:

Very Negative	Negative	Neutral (NA)	Positive	Very Positive
-2	-1	0	1	2

Under each choice rate how each aspect of your life will be affected by your decision and write down the number corresponding to the element in question. Then total the score for each vertical column/choice; the highest score is the best possible course of action for your life.

	Choice I	Choice II	Choice III

I. Lifestyle Items

1. Family and
   significant others

   a. Spouse or lover

   b. Parents

   c. Children

   d. Friends

   e. Colleagues

   f. The community

   g. Other

II. Career

   a. Financial situation

   b. Your interest in the work

   c. Chances for promotion

   d. Creative challenge

   e. Security

   f. Free time

   g. Status

   h. Other (list them)

III. Self Considerations

   a. Your personal values

   b. Your moral standards

   c. Contribution to
      community or society

   d. Control over your life

   e. Self-image

   f. Prestige

   g. Gut feelings

   h. Environment

   i. Stress level

   j. Health

   k. Other (knowledge)

IV. Life Goals

   a. Achievement of
      long-range objectives

   b. Pursuit of happiness

   c. Retirement

   d. Other

Total

Stress Reduction Homework Reference Chart

13

Use the following quick-reference chart for ideas on assignments to give clients as homework to help relieve their stress-related problems.

Problems	Homework Recommendations
Sweaty palms	Reduce or eliminate caffeine intake and practice controlled diaphragmatic breathing and deep relaxation training for 15–20 minutes every day.
Cold hands and feet	Avoid caffeine and cigarettes and practice controlled breathing along with deep relaxation using passive suggestions of warmth and heaviness to the extremities on a daily basis. Daily practice of mild to moderate aerobic exercise and postural realignment exercises will be useful too.
Tension headaches	Practice neck and shoulder posture realignment exercises every day. Self-massage using the headache relief acupressure points. Use moist heat applications to tense neck and shoulder muscles. Muscle relaxation practice using the contract-relax or the diminishing tension techniques.
Migraine headaches	Avoid foods and activities that set off migraines. Practice deep relaxation on a daily basis using passive suggestions of warmth and heaviness to the hands and feet.
Teeth grinding	Practice self-massage techniques for the face, head, temporomandibular joint, and jaw on a daily basis. Also, perform the daily practice of deep relaxation with the client, focusing on having the jaw muscles growing loose and limp and deeply relaxed. Recommend that the client speak to the dentist about purchasing a custom-fit night mouth guard.

Problems	Homework Recommendations
Neck pains	Neck and shoulder posture realignment and kinesthetic awareness improvement practice on a daily basis. Self-massage techniques for the neck and shoulders. Use moist heat or ice applications to the painful areas. Perform deep relaxation training practice, focusing on relaxing all their tight neck musculature. Purchase a new neck contour pillow.
Uncontrollable muscle spasms	Daily posture improvement training and stretching exercises. Deep relaxation, muscle awareness, and tension reduction training. Use moist heat or ice applications. Self-massage to the area in spasm. Eating foods high in calcium, magnesium, and potassium.
Pains in the shoulders or upper back	Daily practice of posture realignment and stretching exercises. Using ice, heat, and self-massage techniques to the painful areas. Lie on a tennis ball (or two tied in a sock) and shift the body weight around to find and massage away the painful points. Deep relaxation training focusing on contracting and relaxing the client's hypertonic musculature. Also determine if the client's work station, hobbies, mattress, or pillow contribute to the problems and make recommendations accordingly.
Low back pain and pain down the back of the legs	Unless contraindicated, practice core strengthening exercises on a daily basis. Also the hip flexor, lumbar extensors, and hamstring muscles should be stretched gently every day. The client may also use heat, ice, and self-massage to the tight musculature. If the client has an old mattress, a new firm mattress may help. Clients should try to take breaks from sitting during the work day and spend a few minutes stretching.
Shortness of breath	Daily practice of controlled diaphragmatic breathing exercises emphasizing increasing lung capacity, exhaling for 2 seconds longer than they inhale, and not using unnecessary muscular activity. Abdominal and latissimus dorsi strengthening exercises. Chest and neck self-massage.
Susceptibility to minor illness	Eat a balanced diet and drink more water each day. Deep relaxation training practice. If sleep debt or quality is a problem, have the client keep a sleep log and then suggest some natural sleep improvement tips.
Poor-quality sleep	Keep a sleep log, make dietary changes, and perform deep relaxation practice. Self-massage using acupressure points for sleep. Get evaluated at a sleep clinic.

Problems	Homework Recommendations
Hair, eyelash, beard pulling, and nail biting	Deep relaxation training practice with passive suggestions of warmth, heaviness, relaxation, and visualization. While in a deeply relaxed state the client should visualize himself or herself free from the urge to perform these habits.
Frequent trips to the toilet	If the urge to urinate is to the result of stress and not a medical condition, such as an enlarged prostate, then deep relaxation practice is in order. The client should also cut down on caffeine products. Strengthening the abdominal and pelvic floor muscles will help the client void more completely.
Gastrointestinal pain or discomfort, diarrhea, constipation, nausea, and heartburn	If the client has these problems they should visit his or her primary care doctor for a thorough examination. If the doctor determines these symptoms are stress related, the client should practice deep relaxation on a daily basis. The client also should monitor what, when, and how he or she eats. He or she possibly should eat smaller and more frequent meals, avoid spicy foods, eat slowly, chew food thoroughly, and avoid eating heavy meals before going to bed. He or she may also need to restructure his or her diet so that it is more balanced. They must eat more fruit, vegetables, and fiber; reduce their saturated fat intake; and avoid foods that cause them distress.
Chronic fatigue	Keep a sleep log for a week and develop a sleep improvement plan. Practice deep relaxation every day and eat a well-balanced diet. Gradually increase the level of exercise practiced, progressively increasing strength and endurance.
Binge eating, not eating because of the fear of becoming fat, and bulimia	Seek out an eating disorders support group and attend a meeting and bring back educational information. Talk to a professional counselor, or a psychiatrist and follow their recommendations for coping with these problems.
General malaise	Have clients monitor their typical diet for a week and modify it as indicated. Make sure that they drink enough water each day. Have them routinely participate in deep relaxation and mild aerobic exercise. They should also assess their sleep quality and quantity experienced and if needed institute changes to help them sleep longer and deeper.
Cold sores and hives	There isn't much a person can do about these problems aside from eating a balanced diet with an adequate amount of calories, performing deep relaxation every day, and using natural sleep improving strategies when indicated.

Problems	Homework Recommendations
Restless legs and feet, toe and finger tapping, and repetitive joint cracking	Daily diaphragmatic breathing, deep relaxation, and total-body stretching practice. When clients have the urge to perform one of these actions, have them take a deep breath, realign their posture, and then relax the muscles involved.
Not enough time in the day	Have clients use a personal digital assistant (PDA) or a weekly schedule to organize their time and to record lists to accomplish each day.
Trouble concentrating and difficulty thinking clearly	Perform diaphragmatic breathing and deep relaxation practice. Have the client take a walk outdoors to smell some flowers or watch a sunset
Anxiety from causes you cannot pinpoint	Have the client think about and list potential reasons for their anxiety. They should practice diaphragmatic breathing, deep relaxation with visualization, and self-massage to their tense neck, shoulder, and chest muscles.
Irritability	Suggest that clients count to 10 before speaking when they are very irritable. Stretching, deep relaxation, and aerobic exercise are also great ways to positively alter a person's mood.
Strained relationships	Ask clients to reflect on the reasons that they often or always have strained relationships. Also have them try to view events from point of view of the other individual(s) involved. Ask them to list any changes that they can make to positively influence their interpersonal relationships and how they can actualize those changes. Have them practice deep relaxation and during the relaxation have them visualize themselves becoming the person that they want to be.
Easily aroused hostility or a short-fused temper	Have the client try to count to 10 and bite their tongue before speaking and lashing out. Have them practice deep relaxation on a regular basis. The client should to try to not blow minor problems out of proportion and should try to replace hostility with compassion.
Job dissatisfaction	Have them take the job and lifestyle survey and review their results with them. If they feel a change is indicated, have them complete the decision balance sheet for more accurate data on the best direction to proceed. Give them a copy of the list of tips for reducing job-related stress to read for homework.
Depression	If clients reported that they are often or always depressed, they should probably be under the care of a counselor or psychiatrist or should participate in a support group. Let clients know that

Problems	Homework Recommendations
Depression *(continued)*	they can get helpful information from on-line support groups that they can access from their personal computer. Deep relaxation training using visual imagery (trying to picture in their mind happy, positive experiences in their life) and aerobic exercise can help these individuals, if practiced on a routine basis. Also recommend that clients perform self-massage, maintain their personal hygiene, and avoid alcohol consumption.
Taking work home with you	If the client constantly takes work home, review with them the tips for using time more wisely, handling paperwork less and getting more organized. If their job is getting them down, have them complete the job lifestyle survey and balance sheet and read the tips for reducing job stress.
Thinking about work even when relaxing and being a workaholic	This client needs fun, active hobbies that can take his or her mind off of work and allow him or her to enjoy free time more. Share the list of general stress reduction tips with him. If the problem is an overwhelming job, then the client should complete the job lifestyle survey and balance sheet as homework and consider changes. The routine practice of deep relaxation training, using time more effectively, and improving organizational skills can also help clients that don't know how to turn off their job.
Trouble turning off the mind at night	Give this client a list of natural sleep improvement strategies to read and follow. Controlled breathing, aerobic exercise and deep relaxation training should be practiced on a routine basis. They should avoid exercising and doing intellectually stimulating activities close to bed time. Drinking a relaxing cup of herbal tea or a glass of warm milk might help calm their body and ease their minds.
Decision-making anxiety	Have the client complete the job lifestyle survey and decision balance sheet.
Stressful dreams	If the client repeatedly has stressful dreams or reoccurring nightmares, he or she should discuss this issue with a psychological counselor or psychiatrist. Share the natural tips for sleep improvement.
Nonstop running around	Deep relaxation training and using time more effectively are useful tools to relieve this problem. It will help the client to get more organized and to leave earlier for scheduled appointments.

Problems	Homework Recommendations
Low motivation, pessimism, worrying, lack of control over their life, or procrastination	Have the client take the job lifestyle survey to help him or her pinpoint the behaviors that he or she wants to change. Set goals and develop a plan to achieve those goals. The balance sheet and a behavior-change self-contract also are good assignments for clients with these sorts of issues.
An unhappy home environment, isolation/ loneliness, and panic attacks	Clients must explore why these are issues for them, then have them list what changes they can make to help relieve these problems. Counseling and support groups are excellent avenues for these clients to seek out. Daily practice of deep relaxation and aerobic exercise can help relieve some of this stress.
So impatient that you finish others thoughts	Have the client practice taking a deep breath and letting others speak their mind.
Missing work or functioning subnormally because of drug or alcohol abuse	Counseling and support groups can be important assets for a person trying to combat an addiction. A person must first recognize that he or she has a problem, and once clients make that realization they can develop a plan to change and if they desire seek help. Share the general stress reduction tips with them. Try to encourage them to participate in healthy activities and to eat a well-balanced diet. The regular practice of aerobic and stretching exercise and deep relaxation can be very beneficial.
Dietary problems	Have the client monitor their food and caffeine intake for 1 week. You can have them calculate the amount of calories ingested and compare it to the number of calories burned. They can also rate how balanced their diet is. The client can also be assigned the heart attack risk test for homework. They may also want to schedule an appointment with a nutritionist to help them develop a healthy eating plan.
Poor breathing mechanics and lung capacity	Have the client practice three diaphragmatic breathing exercises and using breathing as a relaxation tool at least three times a week. They should conduct self-massage to the neck, chest, and muscles of respiration.
Atypical posture and poor flexibility	Have the client practice postural realignment and flexibility-improving exercises at least three times a week. Build the client's homework exercise program according to the needs uncovered in his or her Personal Stress Inventory.

References

Aiello, D. (2004). The hot and the cold of it. *Rehab Management*, June.

Alter, M. (1996). *Science of flexibility.* Champaign, IL: Human Kinetics.

Anderson, D. L. (1995). *Muscle pain relief in 90 seconds.* New York: John Wiley and Sons.

Anorexia Nervosa and Related Eating Disorders, Inc. (2004). *Statistics: How many people have eating disorders?* [Online]. Available: http://www.anred .com/stats.html. [April 2006].

Beck, M. (2006). *Theory and practice of therapeutic massage* (4th ed.). Clifton Park, NY: Thomson Delmar Learning.

Benson, H. (2001). Mind body pioneer—Mind body medical institute, *Psychology Today*, May/June.

Bloomfield, H. H., Cain, M. P., & Jaffe, D. T. (1975). *TM: Discovering inner energy and overcoming stress.* New York: Delacorte Press.

Business & Health Bulletin. Richard Service, Editor. Denville, New Jersey; January 2000.

Cannon, W. B. (1939). *The wisdom of the body* (2nd ed.). New York: W. W. Norton.

Clarkson, H. M. (2000). *Musculoskeletal assessment: Joint range of motion and manual muscle strength,* (2nd ed.). Baltimore: Lippincott Williams & Wilkins.

D'Ambrogio, K. J., & Roth, G. B. (1996). *Positional release therapy: assessment and treatment of musculoskeletal dysfunction.* St. Louis: Mosby.

Dalton, E. (1998). *Myoskeletal alignment techniques.* Oklahoma City: Freedom From Pain Institute.

Daniels, L., & Worthingham, C. (1977). *Therapeutic exercise for body alignment and function,* (2nd ed.). Philadelphia: W. B. Saunders .

Daniels, L., & Worthingham, C. (1997). *Therapeutic exercise for body alignment and function,* (2nd ed.). Philadelphia: W. B. Saunders.

Dement, W. (1997). *Sleepless at Stanford: What all undergraduates should know about how their sleeping lives affect their waking lives.* Stanford, CA: Stanford University Center of Excellence for the Diagnosis and Treatment of Sleep Disorders, September.

Department of Health and Human Services. (1996). *Physical activity and health: A report of the Surgeon General.* Atlanta: DHHS.

Donatelle, R., Davis, L., & Hoover, C. (1988). *Access to health.* Upper Saddle Ridge, NJ: Prentice Hall.

Fahey, T. D., Insel, P. M., & Roth, W. T. (2005). *Fit and well: Core concepts and labs in physical fitness and wellness* (6th ed.). New York: McGraw Hill.

Forman, J., & Myers, D. (1987). *The personal stress reduction program.* Englewood Cliffs, NJ: Prentice Hall.

Gach, M. R. (1990). *Accupressure's potent points: A guide to self care for common ailments.* New York: Bantam Books.

Girando, D., Dusek, D., & Everly, G. (2005). *Controlling stress and tension* (7th ed.). San Francisco: Pearson Education, Inc./Benjamin Cummings.

Goldberg, P. (1978). *Executive health.* New York: McGraw Hill.

Greenberg, J. (1999). *Comprehensive stress management* (6th ed.). Boston: McGraw-Hill.

Health & Stress. (2001). The quandary of job stress compensation. *The Newsletter of The American Institute of Stress, 1*(3), 1–7.

Janda compendium, Volume II. Distributed by OPTP, Minneapolis, MN.

Janda, V. (1988). Muscles and cervicogenic pain syndromes. In R. Grant (Ed.), *physical therapy of the cervical and thoracic spine* (pp. 153–166). London: Churchill Livingstone.

Katon, W. J., & Walker, E. A. (1998). Medically unexplained symptoms in primary care. *Journal of Clinical Psychiatry, 59*, 15–21.

Kendal, F., McCreary, E., & Provance, P. (2005). *Muscles: Testing and function* (4th ed.) Philadelphia: Lippincott Williams & Wilkins.

Knight, K. (1995). *Cryotherapy in sports injury management*. Champaign, IL: Human Kinetics.

Magee, D. (1997). *Orthopedic physical assessment* (3rd ed.). Philadelphia: W. B. Saunders.

Marra, T. (2004). *Depressed and anxious: The dialectical behavior therapy workbook for overcoming depression and anxiety*. Oakland, CA: New Harbinger Publications.

Mattes, A. (2000). *Active isolated stretching*. Sarasota, FL: self–published.

McAtee, R., & Charland, J. (1999). *Facilitated stretching: Assisted and unassisted PNF stretching made easy*. Champaign, IL: Human Kinetics.

McCarberg, B., & O'Connor, A. I. (2004). A new look at heat treatment for pain disorders, Part 1. American Pain Society, November/December 2004 vol. 14, no. 6.

National Headache Foundation. Informational resources for headache sufferers. 2005.

National Institutes of Health. (2000). Restless leg syndrome. Detection and management in primary care. Washington, DC: NIH Publication No. 00-3788.

Neumann, D. (2002). *Kinesiology of the musculoskeletal system: Foundations for physical rehabilitation*. St. Louis: Mosby.

Norkin, C., & White, J. (2003). *Measurement of joint motion: A guide to goniometry* (3rd ed.). Philadelphia: F. A. Davis Company.

Rama, S., Ballentine, R., & Hymes, A. (2005). *Science of breath: A practical guide*. Honesdale, PA: Himalayan Institute Press.

Redline, S., Kirchner, H. L., Quan, S. F., Gottlieb, D. J., Kapur, V., & Newman, A. (2004). The effects of age, sex, ethnicity, and sleep disordered breathing on sleep architecture. *Archives of Internal Medicine, 164*, 406–418.

Seaward, B. (1994). *Managing stress: Principles and strategies for health and well being*. England: Jones and Bartlett Publishers, Inc.

Sebel, P., Stoddart, D. M., Waldhorn, R. E., Waldmann, C. S., & Whitfield, P. (1985). *Respiration: The breath of life*. New York: Torstar Books.

Segerstrom, S., & Miller, G. (2004). Psychological stress and the human immune system: A meta-analytical study of 30 years of inquiry. *Psychological Bulletin 130*(4), 601–630.

Selye, H. (1956). *The Stress of life*. New York: McGraw-Hill.

Selye, H. (1974). *Stress without distress*. New York: Harper & Row.

Silva, J. (1975). *The Silva mind control method*. New York: Simon and Schuster.

Spradlin, S. (2003). *Don't let your emotions run your life: How dialectical behavior control can put you in control*. Oakland, CA: New Harbinger Publications.

Stedman Medical Dictionary for the health professions and nursing (5th ed.). (2005). Baltimore: Lippincott Williams & Wilkins.

Thompson, D. (2002). *Hands heal: Communication, documentation and insurance billing for massage therapists* (2nd ed.). Baltimore: Lippincott Williams & Wilkins.

Travel, J., & Simons, D. (1999). *Myofascial pain and discomfort: The trigger point manual—the upper extremities*. Baltimore: Lippincott Williams & Wilkins.

U.S. Department of Health and Human Services. (2004). Weight control information network. Washington, DC: NIH Publication N. 04-5283.

U.S. Department of Health and Human Service's Office on Women's Health. Information Sheet, February 2000.

Werner, R. (1998). *A massage therapist's guide to pathology*. Baltimore: Lippincott Williams & Wilkins.

Werner, R. (2005). *A massage therapist's guide to pathology* (3rd ed.). Baltimore: Lippincott Williams & Wilkins.

World Health Organization. (1999). *The burden of occupational illness: UN agencies sound the alarm*, Press Release. Geneva: WHO.

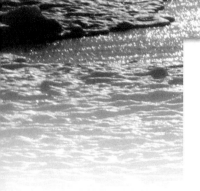

Glossary

Active assistive stretching: Clients actively move a joint through their range of motion as far as they can, and when they reach the end of their active motion the massage therapist moves them through the rest of the normal range or until an end feel is experienced.

Acute stress: The immediate physical, chemical, and mental response to a stressor or threat that a person experiences.

Aerobic endurance training: Sustained bouts of exercise to the major muscle groups that elevate the heart rate to its target range for 20–60 minutes to train cardiovascular and cardiorespiratory systems.

Agonist: The primary muscle or prime mover responsible for a specific action or movement of a joint through a range of motion.

Anorexia nervosa: An eating disorder that is essentially self-starvation brought on by the obsession with not becoming fat.

Antagonist: The muscle or group of muscles responsible for an action directly opposite to the motion produced by an agonist or prime mover.

Antigens: Any substance that invokes an immune system response.

Anxiety disorder: The chronic psychological state that occurs when a person excessively worries and irrationally anticipates that events will lead to doom and calamity. General anxiety, panic disorders, obsessive compulsive disorders, posttraumatic stress disorders, and phobias all fall under the category of anxiety disorders.

Auditory detachment: Using the repetition of sounds, mellifluous words, music, or nature sounds to help induce the relaxation response.

Autogenic training: Using the silent repetition of passive suggestions of warmth and heaviness to the arms, legs, and body to warm the distal extremities and relax the mind and body.

Autonomic nervous system: The involuntary or self-governing part of the peripheral nervous system that regulates the action of the smooth muscles in the blood vessels and the digestive tract, the cardiac muscle, and the glands. It is composed of the two directly opposed parts: the sympathetic nervous system, which prepares the organism for energy expenditure required during emergencies or stressful situations, and the parasympathetic nervous system, which counteracts the action of the sympathetic nervous system to conserve energy and reverse the effects of sympathetic nervous system arousal.

Biofeedback: Using electrical equipment that provides information on muscle tension, brain-wave activity, galvanic skin response (perspiration in the skin), and body-part temperature to help train the client to get more in tune with his or her body and learn to relax at will.

Body mass index (BMI): A common health measurement tool used to classify the potential health risks of having a body weight and waistline too great for one's height.

Bulimia nervosa: An eating disorder in which the person takes in the proper amount of food or more than they need but then vomits or purges from their system what they have ingested using laxatives, enemas, or diuretics.

Cholesterol: A type of fat produced by the body and found in meat, dairy, fish, and poultry. A certain amount is needed for normal body functions; however, too much in the bloodstream can occlude arteries and cause them to lose their flexibility and may increase a person's chance of experiencing a heart attack or stroke.

Chronic stress: A state of constant physical and or mental tension as a result of incessant sympathetic nervous system arousal that prevents the body from returning to homeostasis.

Connective tissue: Abundant tissue formed of ground substance combined with other cells that is found throughout the body and serves to bind structures together and provide support and framework. Fascia is a type of connective tissue that surrounds muscle fibers, groups of fibers, and whole muscles, and runs the length of muscles, joining to form the tendons. Tears in the connective tissue can contribute to pain.

Contract-relax-antagonist-contract (CRAC): A type of proprioceptive neuromuscular facilitation stretching that uses an isometric contraction of a target muscle, followed by 2 seconds of postisometric relaxation, followed by the contraction of the muscle group antagonistic to the muscle being stretched, using reciprocal inhibition to stretch the target muscle. CRAC is safe and effective at improving flexibility.

Contrast baths: After the acute phase of an injury the alternating application of ice and heat baths.

CPAP (continuous positive airflow pressure) therapy: Wearing a mask over the nose that is attached to a device that forces positive air pressure in to keep the air passageways open while sleeping. It is used for individuals with obstructive sleep apnea.

Crossed syndromes: Frequently seen combinations of tight and weak muscles in the cervical, thoracic, and lumbar regions that alter the body's normal balance.

Cryokinetics: Combining the application of ice with movement to help increase pain-free range of motion.

Cryotherapy: Cold therapy or the application of external sources of cold to the body to reduce pain and swelling.

Depression: A temporary or sometimes chronic mental state that is characterized by low energy, lack of initiative, and feelings of sadness, isolation, despair, guilt, dread, and low self-esteem.

Distress: Bad or negative stress that is produced by things such as unrealistic deadlines, divorce, money worries, the death of a loved one, examinations, rude and noisy neighbors, and the grind of daily commuting.

Edema: The excess accumulation of fluids in the tissues.

End feel: The texture of resistance felt when a joint reaches the end of its range.

Eustress: Good stress that comes from positive experiences or challenges that are inspiring or motivating. This stress may act as a catalyst for achievement.

Expiration: Exhaling air or moving air out of the lungs.

Fascia: A type of connective tissue that supports nerves and blood vessels and surrounds muscle fibers, groups of fibers, and whole muscles, and runs the length of muscles, joining to form the tendons. Tears in the fascia can contribute to pain.

Fight-or-flight response: A primitive mechanism, still active in modern humans, which instantly mobilizes the body's defenses to repel or avoid a threat.

Gate control theory of pain: By stimulating the area where pain originates with nonpain type of stimulation, such as the application of heat, cold, and acupressure, can create a traffic jam of sensory impulses that can interrupt pain messages by occupying the neural gate and suppressing the route that pain sensations travel.

General adaptation syndrome: The physiological changes or adaptations induced by prolonged, unchecked, chronic stress.

Golgi tendon organs: Multibranched proprioceptive nerve endings located in the tendons and at the musculotendinous junction that provide the central nervous system feedback on any active contraction or passive stretch that places tension on the tendon.

High density lipoproteins (HDLs): Referred to as good cholesterol because they capture and remove excess LDL cholesterol from the blood and bring it back to the liver for elimination.

Homeostasis: A state of balance, equilibrium, or relative consistency in the body's internal environment.

Hydrocollators: Canvas packs used to provide moist, relaxing, penetrating heat treatments.

Hyperextension: An atypical injurious motion that extends a limb or body part beyond its normal range.

Hyperlordosis: An abnormally large anterior convex curvature of the cervical or lumbar spine.

Hypertonic: Excess tension in a muscle or group of muscle fibers.

Ideal body composition: The ideal ratio of height, weight, and percent body fat.

Insomnia: The inability to experience a sound night's sleep. Some have trouble falling asleep, others wake up prematurely, and others don't feel rested after a full night's sleep.

Inspiration: Inhalation or the act of bringing air into the lungs.

Isometric: A muscle contraction occurs but the muscle length does not change.

Isotonic: The concentric and eccentric contractions of a muscle that occur when lifting a constant weight through the full range of motion.

Kinesthesia: The internal feeling or sense of how one's body and parts are aligned while standing, sitting, and moving.

Kinesthetic awareness: Also known as conscious proprioception, clients' trainable sense of their posture and how their body and its parts align. Posture realignment exercises and kinesthetic awareness training can be used to help the client improve and maintain improved body alignment.

Kyphosis: An exaggerated posterior convex curve of the thoracic spine that gives a person a humped back appearance.

Low density lipoproteins (LDL): Referred to as bad cholesterol because they carry cholesterol from the liver through the bloodstream and may adhere to the artery walls, making them sticky and more susceptible to the buildup of plaque.

Mantra: The repetition of a word or a sound to help a person abandon his or her physical senses and enter a state of deep relaxation or meditation.

Metabolic rate: Rate and efficiency in which the body converts food into energy or stores it as fat. It can be increased by lifting weights to add muscle mass and adding more activity to one's lifestyle.

Modality: A type of therapeutic agent or treatment type, such as using heat or ice, which can be applied to reduce the incidence or severity of physical problems.

Myalgic: Refers to muscular pain or points of tenderness found in a muscle.

Neti: The practice of nasal cleansing using a saline solution to help keep the sinuses clear and improve the ability to breath freely.

Neurolymphatic: A series of reflex points on the anterior and posterior of the torso along the intercostal spaces and along the spine discovered by an osteopath named Chapman in the 1930s. When pairs of these points are stimulated, they are said to increase the lymphatic drainage of the organs and glands to which they correspond.

Nociceptors: Receptors in the skin, muscles, and connective tissue that transmit information on painful stimuli to the spinal cord and then the brain, which acknowledges the sensation as pain.

Obstructive sleep apnea: A condition in which the airway is restricted or completely collapsed, which causes a person to actually stop breathing for a time while sleeping.

Paradoxical breathing: When the client breathes by expanding the chest while simultaneously contracting the abdominals and diaphragm into the chest, essentially shrinking the size of the chest cavity, producing an inefficient way to breathe.

Pathology: The science associated with the cause of disease and the structural and functional changes and abnormal conditions that they produce.

Pedometer: An inexpensive device that measures how many steps and how far a person walks in a day. Some even convert the steps taken into calories burned.

Plumb line: As a point of reference for a posture evaluation, using a weight with a line attached that is hung from the ceiling and is positioned at the client's feet and kept stationary.

Posture: Refers to the overall balance of the body and its parts or body alignment. Maintaining good posture while standing, sitting, and moving protects the body from injuries caused by the impact of gravity.

Proprioceptive neuromuscular facilitation (PNF): A variety of client-assisted stretching techniques, including the hold-relax, contract-relax, and CRAC technique. These techniques try to involve reflex neurological activity to help safely get through restrictive barriers to movement.

PRT (positional release therapy): Also known as strain–counterstrain, an indirect approach to rebalancing muscles. A muscle is placed in its position of greatest ease for at least 90 seconds or until the tissues spontaneously release. Then slowly it is returned it to its normal resting position.

Pulse: The impulses felt when touching an artery that corresponds to the heart beating. Count the number of beats in 10 seconds and multiply by 6 to determine the pulse rate.

Range of motion: The freedom of movement of a joint.

Rapid eye movement (REM): A stage of sleep in which the eyes move quickly around, the brain becomes more active, the blood pressure rises, the breathing and heart rate become irregular, and dreaming is experienced.

Reciprocal inhibition: When an agonist contracts, the antagonistic muscle is reciprocally inhibited.

Resistance training: Lifting weights on a regular basis is a great way to improve muscle tone and strength, burn more calories, prevent injuries,

and improve one's self image. As a person increases strength and endurance, he or she should progressively increase the amount of weight being lifted.

Restless legs syndrome: A central nervous system disorder characterized by an itching, tingling, jumpy, crawling, uncomfortable sensation in the legs that causes chronic sleep loss.

RICE principle: For the first 48–72 hours after an injury, treat it by using *r*est, *i*ce, *c*ompression, and *e*levation.

Scoliosis: A lateral curvature of the spine that may also include a rotational component.

Scope of practice: The legally acceptable rights, activities, techniques, services, and limits of practice of a profession.

Sleep debt: Not getting enough stage 3, 4, and REM sleep to replenish and repair our brains and bodies can lead to ill health if the deficiency is not paid back by getting extra sleep.

Stress: The body's physical, mental, and chemical reaction to circumstances that frighten, excite, confuse, challenge, surprise, anger, endanger, or irritate. The events that cause stress can be good or bad.

Stress profile: The data from the client's Personal Stress Inventory (PSI), stress log, and intake form are combined on the stress profile summary chart to conveniently list all the factors contributing to stress and to help develop the client's unique stress profile. This consolidated information aids in the design of client's personal stress reduction program and the comparison of pretreatment and posttreatment status.

Stressors: Events that trigger a stress response that may include physical dangers, political and social issues, work demands and responsibilities, environmental catastrophes, and emotional challenges.

Sympathetic nervous system: Part of the autonomic or self-governing nervous system that innervates the smooth muscles of the blood vessels and digestive tract, cardiac muscle, and the glands that is stimulated during a stress response or emergency situation and prepares the body to fight or flee from a threat by increasing energy expenditure and instituting a variety of physiological and chemical changes.

Target heart range: The range of heart beats per minute that a person should try to stay within while exercising for safety and for beneficial training effects to occur.

Tender points: Small palpable areas of hypertonic tissue located in the muscular and fascial tissues that when pressed produce localized pain.

Trendelenburg sign: A drop of the pelvis of more than 5 degrees on the unsupported side during the swing phase of gait, resulting from a weak gluteus medius muscle on the supported side.

Triceps surae: A name that refers to the combination of the two bellies of the gastrocnemius with the soleus, with the intention of considering this amalgamation the triceps muscle of the calf.

Trigger points: A painful palpable point on the body that when pressed refers pain in predictable patterns outside of the myofascial unit being pressed.

Vasodilation: The relaxation of the smooth-muscle walls in the arteries, which enlarges its diameter to allow more blood to flow to an area.

Visual Imagery: Using the natural ability to daydream and picture peaceful scenes to relax the mind and body at will.

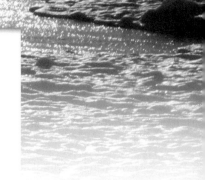

Index

A page number followed by an *i* references an illustration and a page number followed by a *t* references a table.